C000070135

1,000,000 Books

are available to read at

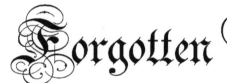

---◆---

www.ForgottenBooks.com

---◆---

Read online
Download PDF
Purchase in print

ISBN 978-0-265-81374-4
PIBN 10964980

This book is a reproduction of an important historical work. Forgotten Books uses
state-of-the-art technology to digitally reconstruct the work, preserving the original format
whilst repairing imperfections present in the aged copy. In rare cases, an imperfection in
the original, such as a blemish or missing page, may be replicated in our edition. We do,
however, repair the vast majority of imperfections successfully; any imperfections that
remain are intentionally left to preserve the state of such historical works.

Forgotten Books is a registered trademark of FB &c Ltd.
Copyright © 2018 FB &c Ltd.
FB &c Ltd, Dalton House, 60 Windsor Avenue, London, SW19 2RR.
Company number 08720141. Registered in England and Wales.

For support please visit www.forgottenbooks.com

1 MONTH OF
FREE
READING

at

www.ForgottenBooks.com

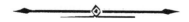

By purchasing this book you are
eligible for one month membership to
ForgottenBooks.com, giving you
unlimited access to our entire
collection of over 1,000,000 titles via
our web site and mobile apps.

To claim your free month visit:

www.forgottenbooks.com/free964980

* Offer is valid for 45 days from date of purchase. Terms and conditions apply.

English
Français
Deutsche
Italiano
Español
Português

www.forgottenbooks.com

Mythology Photography **Fiction**
Fishing Christianity **Art** Cooking
Essays Buddhism Freemasonry
Medicine **Biology** Music **Ancient
Egypt** Evolution Carpentry Physics
Dance Geology **Mathematics** Fitness
Shakespeare **Folklore** Yoga Marketing
Confidence Immortality Biographies
Poetry **Psychology** Witchcraft
Electronics Chemistry History **Law**
Accounting **Philosophy** Anthropology
Alchemy Drama Quantum Mechanics
Atheism Sexual Health **Ancient History**
Entrepreneurship Languages Sport
Paleontology Needlework Islam
Metaphysics Investment Archaeology
Parenting Statistics Criminology
Motivational

ATLAS AND EPITOME

OF

GYNECOLOGY

BY

DR. OSKAR SCHAEFFER

Privatdocent of Obstetrics and Gynecology in the University
of Heidelberg

AUTHORIZED TRANSLATION FROM THE SECOND
REVISED AND ENLARGED GERMAN EDITION

EDITED BY

RICHARD C. NORRIS, A.M., M.D.

Surgeon-in-charge, Preston Retreat, Philadelphia; Gynecologist to the Methodist
Episcopal Hospital and to the Philadelphia Hospital; Consulting Gyne-
cologist to the Southeastern Dispensary and Hospital for Women and
Children; Lecturer on Clinical and Operative Obstetrics,
Medical Department, University of Pennsylvania.

LANE MEDICAL LIBRARY
8077
SAN FRANCISCO

WITH 207 COLORED ILLUSTRATIONS ON 90 PLATES,
AND 62 ILLUSTRATIONS IN THE TEXT

PHILADELPHIA AND LONDON
W. B. SAUNDERS & COMPANY
1900

LANE LIBRARY

COPYRIGHT, 1900, BY W. B. SAUNDERS & COMPANY.

N197
S29t
1900

EDITOR'S PREFACE.

THE value of this Atlas to the medical student and to
the general practitioner will be found not only in the concise explanatory text, but especially in the illustrations.
It occupies a position midway between the quiz compend
and the more pretentious works on gynecology. The
large number of illustrations and colored plates, reproducing the appearance of fresh specimens, will give the student an accurate mental picture and a knowledge of the
pathologic changes induced by disease of the pelvic organs
that can not be obtained from mere description. Next to
the study of specimens, which for evident reasons are not
available outside of large clinics, well-chosen illustrations
must be utilized. The Atlas serves that purpose so well
that its translation and publication for the English-speak-
ing profession seemed very desirable.

The translator, Dr. W. Hersey Thomas, has carefully
followed the author's text, which, while concise, covers
the subject systematically, and with sufficient detail to give
the reader a comprehensive knowledge of gynecologic dis-
orders. The paragraphs devoted to the treatment of the
various diseases are very conservative, in some instances
perhaps too much so for the aggressive surgeon. The
author's conservatism will be appreciated, however, by
the student and the practitioner, who necessarily wish to
be informed on nonoperative gynecology.

Editorial comments have occasionally been inserted, in
order to harmonize or point out the difference between
the author's teaching and that generally approved in
America.

PREFACE TO THE SECOND EDITION.

EVERY one concerned in the production of the second edition of this volume has helped to make it represent all the advances in our technical knowledge. A statement of the latest scientific acquisitions has been incorporated into the original text. The greatest stress has been laid upon the accumulation of new illustrative material from autopsies and operations as well as from the living. The delineations of the artist, Mr. A. Schmitson, are meritorious and true to nature. The new material has been obtained partly from the Heidelberg Pathologic Institute, partly from our surgical and gynecologic clinics, and partly from my private practice. I take this opportunity to express my heartiest thanks to the Directors of the Institute, to Professors Arnold, Czerny, Kehrer, and their assistants, and especially to Professors Ernst and Jordan for the use of their instructive fresh specimens.

The publisher has spared neither trouble nor expense in the reproduction of the water-colors, which are abundant and as true to nature as possible.

O. SCHAEFFER.

PREFACE TO THE FIRST EDITION.

In spite of the existence of excellent shorter works and compends, as well as of good comprehensive atlases, the author feels that there is need of a book that will give the student and the practitioner an opportunity to elucidate and to complete his necessarily limited personal observations and examinations in the clinic and dispensary. If the entire work were carried out upon a purely diagrammatic basis, it would probably be more readily grasped by the majority of readers; not every one, however, possesses the gift of translating such pictured relations into living clinical entities. On the other hand, the strict reproduction of anatomic preparations renders difficult that clear representation which is necessary to sift the essential from the nonessential facts.

I have consequently decided, in many cases, to combine both methods of illustration—that is, to reproduce accurate anatomic specimens, and then to emphasize more sharply the changes under consideration. I have further endeavored to show every subject from as many standpoints as possible (that is, regarding their etiology, development, secondary influence, progress, and termination), and consequently have further elucidated the pictures of specimens by diagrammatic and semidiagrammatic drawings.

Thanks to my former assistantship at the Munich Frauenklinik, and in no slight degree to the indulgent permission and stimulating counsel of Professor v. Winckel, I have been able to employ, almost without exception, original anatomic and clinical material. I wish to take this opportunity to express my thanks to this

3

gentleman, and also to Professor Kehrer, who most amiably allowed me to use his clinical material.

The text has been divided into two parts. The continuous text is, without exception, written from a practical standpoint; the text of the plates, on the contrary, contains the purely theoretic, scientific, anatomic, microscopic, and chemic notes, and facts of general significance (concerning sounds, pessaries, etc.), so that in referring to the work the one text will not have a disturbing influence upon the other.

To avoid needless repetition, frequent references have been made to my " Atlas of Obstetric Diagnosis and Treatment." The necessity for this will be readily understood when we consider the identity of the anatomic data and the intimate mutual relations existing between the child-bearing process and the majority of gynecologic affections.

The material has been classified from an etiologic standpoint as far as possible; to carry this out rigidly, however, would have led to diffuseness. The chapters upon sepsis, gonorrhea, genital tuberculosis, and venereal diseases are based upon this classification. Cystitis, which comes within the domain of the gynecologist so frequently, has received special attention.

Particular effort has been directed to the clear presentation of the subject of differential diagnosis. The methods which I have chosen are the comparative and the tabular. The subject receives full attention in the chapters on Myomata, Cystomata, Carcinoma, Tumors of the Ante-uterine and Retro-uterine Spaces, and others.

At the conclusion of the work I have placed a Therapeutic Table of the ordinary remedies used in gynecology, and have indicated the appropriate methods of prescribing them—chiefly as intra-uterine pencils, vaginal and rectal suppositories, baths, and injections.

O. SCHAEFFER.

HEIDELBERG, *November, 1895.*

CONTENTS.

5

Group III.—Inflammatory and Nutritional Disturbances.

CHAPTER I.

Group IV.—Injuries and Their Consequences.

CHAPTER I.

CHAPTER IV.

LIST OF PLATES.

9

GROUP I.

ANOMALIES OF FORMATION AND ARRESTED DEVELOPMENT.

CHAPTER I.

FETAL ANOMALIES OF FORMATION.

The anomalies of formation of the female genitalia are, almost without exception, examples of arrested development. The differentiation of the Müllerian ducts is imperfect or does not occur—the customary fusion fails to take place, or the ducts unite to form a single tube of limited extent. Defects of the entire genital tract or of individual organs are thus explained, as are also the congenital atresias, fistulas, and partial or complete duplications of the genital tube (Kussmaul).

The following forms are of clinical importance :

₰ ı. APLASIA AND HYPOPLASIA OF THE FETAL RUDIMENTS.

1. Absence of the uterine appendages.
2. Absence of the uterus.
3. Absence of the entire genital tract, with or without—
4. Pseudohermaphroditism.
5. Uterus unicornis : i. e., absence of a portion of one of the Müllerian ducts (Fallopian tube attached to the uterine portion of one Müllerian duct).

6. Atresias—which may be cord-like or diaphragmatic —in the cervix (corresponding to the internal or external os), in the vagina, hymen, or vulva.

7. Congenital rectovaginal or rectovulvar fistulas (atresia ani vaginalis or hymenalis, cloaca vaginalis, or fistula rectovestibularis).

8. Feminine epispadias and hypospadias.

1 and 2. **Total absence of the uterus and its appendages** is very rare, and usually is first discovered at puberty. Solid bundles of muscle-fibers pass up from

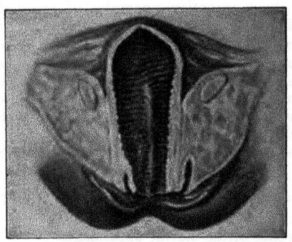

Fig. 1.—The fetal genitalia cut open in a median sagittal plane, so that the divided symphysis is thrown back on either side. Absence of the uterus (original drawing, from a preparation in the Munich Frauenklinik).

a rudimentary vagina and through the broad ligament, which can be recognized as a small transverse partition in the pelvis. The vulva is well developed, as a rule, the most striking external defects being a stunted clitoris, absence of the pubic hair, and smallness of the breasts.

The ovaries, on the contrary, are absent or but partially developed. The Fallopian tubes are patulous only in their ampullæ. In one case I found at autopsy[1] a

[1] In a fetus at the Munich Frauenklinik, "Arch. f. Gyn.," 37, 2.

total absence of the uterus and its appendages, with an elongated vagina. One portion of the fetal rudiments had formed this blind pouch, without any attempt at differentiation of a cervix. (See Fig. 1.)

Symptoms.—From the fact that the ovaries are absent it follows that the sexual instinct is usually wanting, although it may be present. The most striking symptom of all—nonappearance of the menses at puberty—may go hand in hand with the periodic appearance of the menstrual molimina.

Should such individuals indulge in sexual intercourse, new troubles arise from the forcible dilatation of the rudimentary vagina, or frequently of the urethra (incontinence of urine sometimes) (Plate 19, Fig. 2), especially since the latter often has a funnel shape, owing to a dropping back of the posterior wall.

Diagnosis.—Bimanual examination establishes the absence of the uterus. (Plate 19, Fig. 2; Plate 21, Fig. 2.) The finger is introduced into the rudimentary vagina or rectum, and counterpressure is made either through the abdominal wall or by introducing a sound or the finger into the bladder after dilatation of the urethra, or by tamponade of the vagina. The uterus and adnexa are to be sought for above the vaginal rudiment. Their recognition is by no means easy.

3 and 4. Absence of the entire genital tract renders the individual sexless, and may exist without any other malformation sufficient to endanger life. The vulva may be entirely wanting or it may be well developed. In a case that I saw the latter condition obtained, together with a hymen so yielding that it could be pushed in for several centimeters. The individual was subsequently married to her lover, who was fully cognizant of her genital peculiarities.

The clitoris may be robust; the labia majora may be fused, forming a median raphe; the nymphæ may be deformed; and the genital fissure may be closed or so shortened that the case assumes a pseudohermaphroditic character. In this event a careful examination will reveal genital glands in the labia majora; in fact, the labia majora not only resemble the scrotum, but may contain testicles.

This condition is known as **pseudohermaphroditism.** [1] If testicles and ovaries are found in the same case, we call the individual a true hermaphrodite. No such case has been established beyond a doubt. Most pseudohermaphrodites have proved themselves to be males, and some of them are capable of procreation, the latter being especially true when the genital eminence is well developed and the catheter demonstrates a culdesac in the posterior urethral wall. Female pseudohermaphroditism is always associated with vaginal atresia.

Treatment.—When the uterus does not exist, the attempt to make an artificial vagina is aimless and futile. In such a case it is the duty of the physician to explain the condition of affairs to the patient and to treat the menstrual molimina symptomatically (narcotics and external derivatives, oophorin tablets, castration). In cases of hermaphroditism the predominant sexual type should be determined as accurately as possible, since it has frequently happened that the conjugal relation has been assumed and the individual has first become conscious of his or her true sex during married life.

5. Uterus Unicornis.—It sometimes happens that one Müllerian duct remains rudimentary or imperfectly differentiated into its corresponding half of the uterus and appertinent tube. This half has a weaker muscular coat and the uterus is narrower, pointed, and possesses a horn curving toward the better-developed side. (Fig. 2.) The mildest degree of this condition is known as uterus inae-

---

[1] The germinal glands are mostly rudimentary; the other sexual attributes are those of the opposite sex. Gynandres: marked degree of male hypospadias, including scrotum; a stunted penis, testicle still in the abominal cavity or inguinal canal. Virugines: adhesion of the labia, enlarged clitoris; menstrual hemorrhages.

qualis, and arises from arrested development of one side.[1] The outcome of pregnancy and labor in such a case is portrayed in the " Atlas of Obstetric Diagnosis and Treatment" (second edition, Munich). The tube and ovary may be absent on the rudimentary side, or there

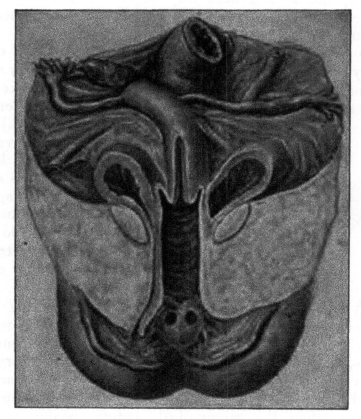

Fig. 2.—Uterus unicornis dexter; left half developed only as an elongated tube. Hymen septus (prepared as in Fig. 1).

may be a longer, undifferentiated tube, which is either solid or partly patulous. In such cases the extra-uterine

[1] In two fetal cases I found that the round ligament was not inserted into the angle between the uterus and the tube, but radiated toward the latter. The broad ligaments and tubes of the two sides were of unequal length.

transmigration of spermatic filaments or ova has been known to occur.

The early diagnosis of pregnancy is of great importance, because the rudimentary horn usually ruptures or a false diagnosis of extra-uterine pregnancy may be made.

6, 7, and 8. Atresias may be found in any portion of the genital apparatus. These may be explained in various ways :

(*a*) They represent an arrested development in early embryonic life, when the Müllerian ducts are simply solid columns of cells. Such atresias are usually cord-like and affect a considerable portion of the duct. (See obliterated vagina, Plate 19, Fig. 2.)

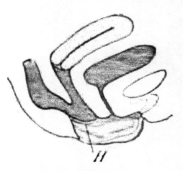

Fig. 3.—Atresia ani ; congenital rectovaginal fistula (above the hymen).

(*b*) The retarded development may occur a little later, —from the fourth to the sixth week,—and certain invaginations or openings of one hollow viscus into another do not occur, resulting in **atresia vulvæ, atresia ani,** or **atresia urethræ.**

These malformations may occur alone or in combination with other developmental errors, such as a persistent cloaca : *i. e.,* that embryonic cavity that connects the bladder with the rectum and is closed externally. (Fig. 12.) The external opening first appears when the rectovesical septum, containing the Müllerian ducts, grows down and forms the perineum. (Figs. 12 to 16.) Certain atresias combined with **congenital fistulas** may be traced back to this embryonic period—atresia ani with a rectovaginal fistula = **atresia ani vaginalis.** (Fig. 3.)

Imperfect closure of the primitive urethra toward the vagina gives rise to the rare condition known as **feminine hypospadias** (to be explained on etiologic and anatomic grounds different from those of a similar condition in the male). Imperfect closure toward the clitoris—**feminine epispadias**—is still rarer, and is usually associated with a fissured clitoris, a cleft symphysis (pelvis fissa), and inversio (ectopia) vesicæ : *i. e.*, absence of the anterior wall of the bladder, the posterior wall being plainly visible.

(c) The **fistula rectohymenalis** or **rectovestibularis** (Fig. 6) springs from a later period of the embryonic cycle, and differs from the rectovaginal fistula in that the opening is in

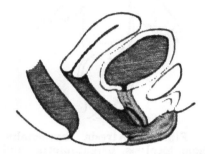

Fig. 4.—Hypospadias ; posterior wall of urethra is wanting.

the vulva, outside of the hymen. It dates from the formation of the perineum (consequently, later than the cloaca), which is formed by the union of the septum urogenito-

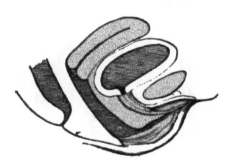

Fig. 5.—Epispadias ; anterior wall of urethra is wanting ; clitoris fissa.

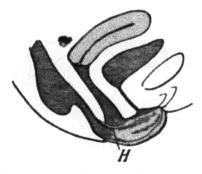

Fig. 6.—Rectovestibular or rectohymenal fistula with congenital atresia ani.

rectale with two lateral eminences, which have grown down and fused by a perineal raphe. (Figs. 14 to 16.)

(d) A fourth group of atresias originates in this fetal period, or at a much later one, in the shape of inflammatory adhesions. These are much more likely to assume a diaphragmatic character. Examples of these are seen in atresias of the vulva and of the hymen and in closure of

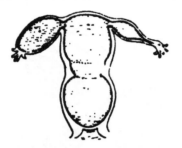

Fig. 7.—Atresia hymenalis, hematocolpos, hematometra, and hematosalpinx (both the internal and the external os may be recognized).

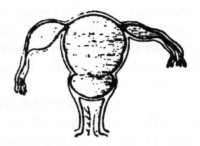

Fig. 8.—Atresia vaginalis from a transverse membrane (both the internal and the external os may be recognized). Partial hematocolpos, hematometra, partial hematosalpinx of both sides.

the vagina, of the cervix, and of the uterine orifices by transverse bridges of mucous membrane. Atresias may

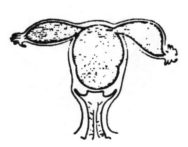

Fig. 9. — Atresia cervicalis uteri. Hematometra, hematosalpinx (internal os may be recognized; external os free).

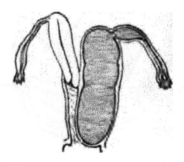

Fig. 10.—Atresia vaginalis with uterus and vagina duplex; left-sided partial hematocolpos, hematometra, hematosalpinx (both the internal and the external os may be recognized).

also be encountered in cases of uterus bicornis. (Figs. 7 to 11.)

Symptoms.—The symptoms of the genital atresias vary, and appear at different periods of life, according to their nature. Every new-born child should be carefully examined as to the permeability of the urethra and anus. This is frequently neglected, and anal atresia, or even complete closure of the urethra, is discovered only after days, either by accident or through symptoms of retention.

The hymen also deserves attention, for although atre-

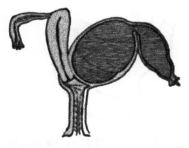

Fig. 11.—Atresia of the external orifice of a bicornuate uterus; left-sided hematometra, hematosalpinx.

sia in this situation is usually first discovered at puberty, there are recorded cases in which the menses had never appeared, owing to the presence of this anomaly, and yet the condition remained unrecognized until the patient assumed the marital relation. The cardinal symptom of all genital atresias, with the exception of those cases of uterus bicornis in which one side is patulous, is nonappearance of the menses. Increasing distention of the genital tract by mucus and by menstrual blood is the cause of the earliest disturbances. According to

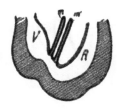

Fig. 12.—For the sake of simplicity, the two Müllerian ducts are drawn one behind the other, instead of side by side. They empty into the cloaca, which connects the bladder (allantois, *V*) and the rectum (*R*), and which has no external opening. A slight invagination indicates the position of the future anus, and a similar one, the urogenital sinus.

the location of the atresia, we have a hematocolpos, a hematometra, or a hematosalpinx.

The symptoms are as follows: Pain, at first periodic

and then continuous, with exacerbations similar to the pains of labor; vesical and rectal disturbances; indiges-

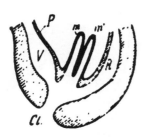

tion and vomiting, due to the pressure of the accumulated blood. Hematosalpinx occurs in uterine atresias earlier than in those of the vagina. (Plate 40, Fig. 2.) It is dangerous on account of the ease with which the tubal wall may be torn, and consequently the examination should be conducted with great gentleness. The peritoneum is

Fig. 13.—The Müllerian ducts are of larger lumen, and have descended with the rectovesical septum to empty into the open cloaca (P = peritoneum).

frequently subjected to inflammatory irritation by the escape of small quantities of blood from the tubal ostia. The same dangers exist in collections of blood in closed rudimentary cornua.

In unilateral atresia of a double genital canal (uterus septus cum vagina septa) we have less to fear, as the hematoma is more likely to rupture into the patulous side. (Figs. 10 and 11.) The bloody tumor may undergo putrefactive or suppurative changes. When only one genital canal exists, rupture commonly occurs through a thinned-out portion of the cervix. The blood may escape into the peritoneal cavity (peritonitis)

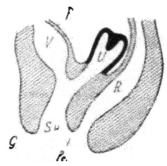

Fig. 14.—The two Müllerian ducts have fused to form the uterus (U); a septum still exists in the fundus. The sinus urogenitalis is longer (S. u.). G = genital eminence = future clitoris; Pe = perineum. The urethra opens high up, and is still more marked than the genital canal.

or beneath the peritoneum, extending down around the vagina to the floor of the pelvis—hæmatoma vulvæ or vaginæ.

In atresia ani vaginalis the feces escape through the vagina. (Fig. 3.) If the closure is sphincter-like, a periodic discharge of gas and feces occurs. When the opening is high up in the vagina, retention is impossible despite the strictest cleanliness. If the opening is small or the intestine is bent at an acute angle, inflammatory and obstructive symptoms may manifest themselves. The same is true, *mutatis mutandis*, of atresia ani vestibularis (Fig. 6) and anus perinealis. Complete absence of perineum may also be observed from failure of fusion of

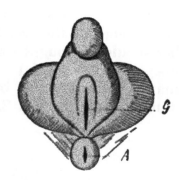

Fig. 15.—External genitalia of figures 14 and 16. Behind the relatively important genital eminence (clitoris) the opening of the sinus urogenitalis (*G*) is seen, and posterior to this, the anus (*A*).

the lateral eminences. Incontinence of urine exists with the more marked degrees of hypospadias, and especially with epispadias. (Figs. 4 and 5.)

Diagnosis.—Persistent nonappearance of the menses always demands an ocular inspection of the parts. When vaginal or hymenal atresia exists, the bluish protruding membrane is seen, while cervical atresia renders the passage of the uterine sound impossible. Should the

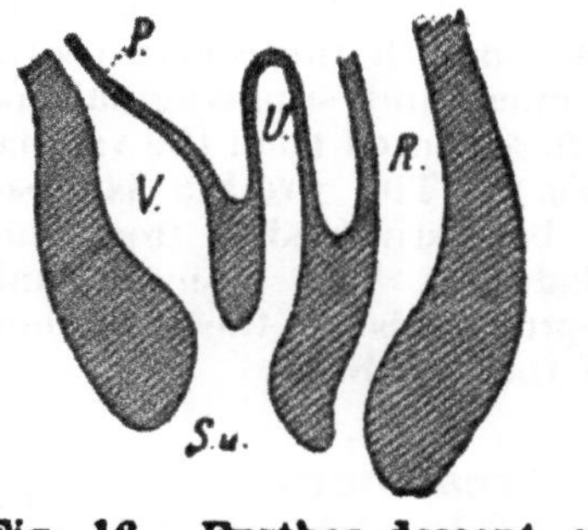

Fig. 16.—Further descent of the urogenital septum, thereby shortening the sinus urogenitalis (*S. u.*).

closure be at the internal os, the cervix alone is patulous; if at the external os, it is impervious. In unilateral atresia of duplicate genitalia one side will not permit the introduction of a sound.

Palpation completes the diagnosis. The finger is introduced into the rectum, and a firm elastic tumor is felt anteriorly, above which the uterus is recognized as a small hard body. If the distention is more marked, the uterus assumes an hour-glass shape, in consequence of the resistance of the internal os. The tubes should be sought for, exercising great care and gentleness. (Figs. 7 to 11.)

Cord-like atresia of the vagina is recognized by bimanual palpation through the rectum. (Plate 19, Fig. 2.)

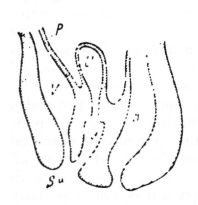

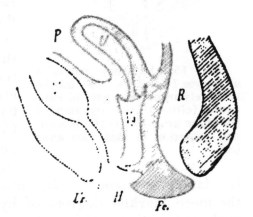

Fig. 17.—During the fifth fetal month the cervix (both vaginal and supravaginal) is differentiated from the vagina (*Vg.*). The urethra is also to be distinguished from the bladder. The vesicovaginal septum assists in the formation of the vestibule.

Fig 18.—Scheme of the completed genitalia after the formation of the hymen.

Treatment.—The gynatretic membrane should be incised without delay, and the blood should be *slowly* drained off. Collapse has followed when the latter caution has not been observed. If a tubal sac has ruptured, immediate celiotomy and removal of the blood are indicated. Abdominal section is also demanded when the hematometra is in a rudimentary accessory cornu. If uterus bilocularis or vagina bilocularis (with a septum) exists, it is better to excise the entire partition than simply to incise it.

Cases of pyocolpometra from secondary infection of the retained blood are treated in a similar manner, a drainage-tube being introduced and the cavity being washed out several times daily.

If there is a complete absence of the vagina (Plate 19, Fig. 2), its position being indicated by a fibrous cord, a new vagina must be made. Sounds are passed into the bladder and rectum, and the operator cautiously dissects up through the connective tissue. Skin-grafting should be employed to prevent a cicatricial closure of the newly formed tube. If adhesions occur in spite of this, or if, from the nature of the case, they are to be dreaded from the beginning, the ovaries should be removed by abdominal section and the uterus should be sutured into the vulvar wound, in order to prevent a subsequent hydrometra.

Congenital defects of the perineum and epispadias and hypospadias are to be repaired by plastic operations. In atresia ani vaginalis the rectum is brought down through the perineum as far as possible, and is connected with an artificial perineal anus. The fistula then closes either spontaneously or after mild cauterizations.

§ 2. HYPERPLASTIC ANOMALIES OF FORMATION.

1. Duplication of Entire Organs.—

(a) Of the whole genital tract:

    a. Uterus didelphys : *i. e.*, uterus and vagina grow as the two Müllerian ducts (Figs. 12 and 13), and remain without further differentiation as two solid cords or as two tubes ;

    β. Uterus et vagina duplex : *i. e.*, two genital tubes completely differentiated into uteri and vaginæ. These lie side by side and each possesses a tube and an ovary.

Both these malformations are seen only in those monsters incapable of independent life. At the Munich Frauenklinik I observed two examples of type *a*, with ectopia viscerum, total absence of bladder and kidneys, persistent cloaca. etc.; and one of type *β*, with eventration of all the intestines in an umbilical hernia and with atresia ani.

Duplication of the vulva is sometimes seen, but has no clinical significance. ("Arch. f. Gyn.," 37, 2.)

(b) Of the uterine appendages: ovaries, tubal ostia— arising from a division of the Müllerian ducts.

(c) Of the uterus: bicornis. (Plate 2, Figs. 2 and 19.) Those portions of the Müllerian ducts that should form

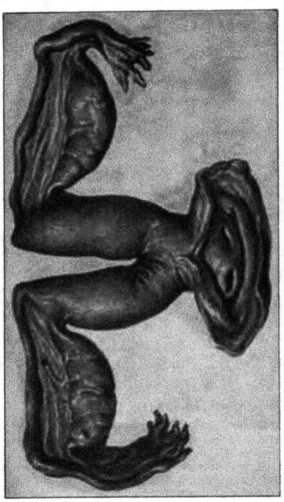

Fig. 19.—Uterus bicornis bicollis with vagina simplex (specimen from Heidelberg Frauenklinik).

the body of the uterus do not fuse, but develop separately, remaining attached to a common neck. This malformation may be associated with the one to be described presently.

In the mildest degree of duplication of the uterus the fundus simply shows a depression—uterus introrsum arcuatus.

2. Duplication by a Septum.—The Müllerian ducts fuse, but the partition dividing them does not disappear.

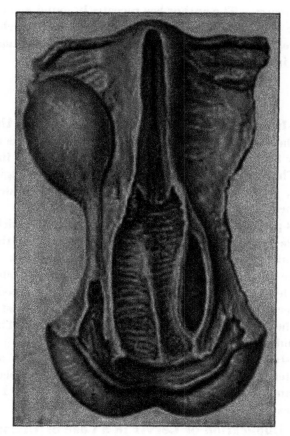

Fig. 20.—Vagina septa with atresia of one canal. Skene's glands empty into the urethral orifice (Munich Frauenklinik, "Arch. f. Gyn.," 37, 2).

(Figs. 10, 13, 14.) This disappearance usually begins in from the eighth to the twelfth week, commencing in that portion of the tube that subsequently (from the twentieth to the thirtieth week) forms the vaginal cervix. This

PLATE 1.

The Vulva of a Nonpregnant Multipara (original water-color from a case at the Heidelberg Frauenklinik). The labia majora and minora are separated. In addition to the remains of the hymen, there is to be seen a congenital blind canal, about 1 cm. in depth, at the posterior commissure. The author has repeatedly found analogous structures in the fetus (see Plate VII, Fig. 19, of the "Arch. f. Gyn.," 37, 2), as well as cysts of the hymen in the same situation. The perineum is intact.

PLATE 2.

Fig. 1.—Intravaginal Cervix of an "Infantile" Uterus. In these and the following analogous illustrations the parts are brought into view by Sims' or Simon's specula, the patient being in the dorsal position. The labia are held apart, and the furrowed vaginal wall is forced back, so that the cervix presents itself in the depth of the vaginal funnel.

The Sims position is the one best adapted for the physician without assistance, because then it is necessary to introduce the posterior speculum only, the anterior vaginal wall falling back of its own accord. The upper half of the body rests upon the left shoulder and breast; the left arm lies upon the table, parallel to the body, and can hold the speculum if necessary. The left thigh is almost completely extended; the right is strongly flexed on the abdomen. The physician stands behind the patient.

The illustration represents the pale, small cervix of a deficiently developed uterus, often combined with congenital stenosis of the cervical canal and puerile anteflexion of the uterus. (See ¿ 3, 1–4, and Fig. 22 in text.)

Fig. 2.—Duplication of Cervix in a Case of Uterus Bicornis Septus with a Single Vagina. In the embryo the Müllerian ducts do not lie quite symmetrically side by side, but the right one is nearer to the symphysis. This asymmetry may be recognized in the illustration, from the relation of the two external orifices to each other. (Figs. 10–21 in text and ¿ 2.) Where the uterus is duplicated, two cervices may present themselves in the vagina, which is usually divided by a septum. Uterus subseptus may exist with only a single external os.

Tab

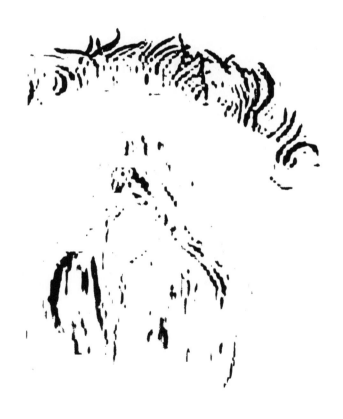

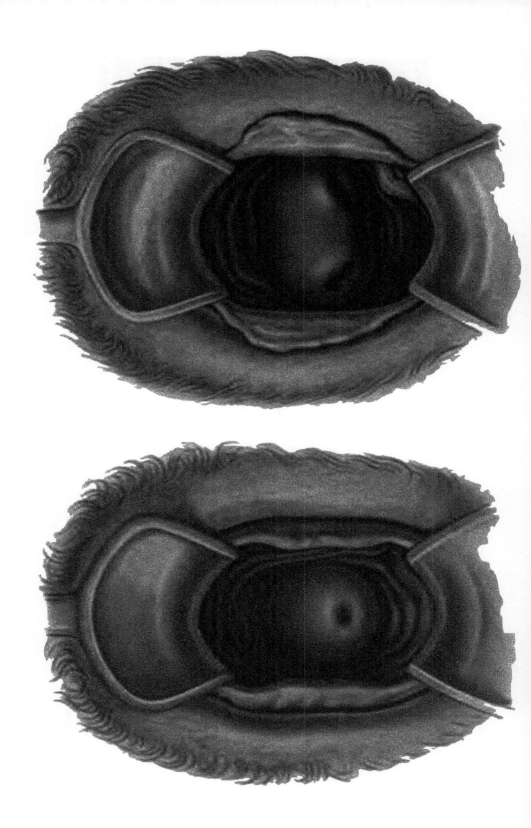

explains the association of all degrees of the bicornate uterus with septa of varying extent in the uterus or vagina. We may thus have a uterus bicornis septus or bicollis, and subseptus or unicollis, or, again, both may be combined with vagina septa or subsepta. (Plate 2, Fig. 2, and Figs. 20 and 21.) One duct may be occluded, as has been already mentioned, producing a unilateral atresia. A hymen septus or bifenestratus may be present, and, by

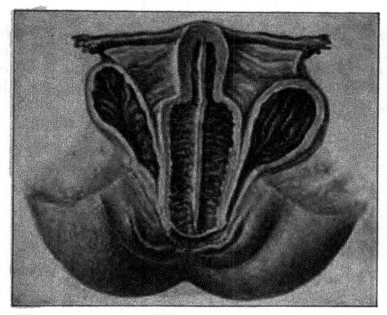

Fig. 21.—Uterus et vagina septa (Munich Frauenklinik).

reason of its resisting power, may play quite an important rôle in the pathology of the sexual life. (Fig. 2.)

Symptomatology.—The influence of these malformations upon labor has been described in my "Atlas of Obstetric Diagnosis and Treatment."

Conception frequently does not occur in consequence of the feeble development of the entire genitalia. These individuals are usually weaklings with amenorrhea, and should be advised not to marry.

3

Treatment.—Ligation or division (Paquelin) of the septa. It is to be remembered that after castration or total extirpation of the uterus for myomata the presence of a third ovary may nullify the result, or may explain a subsequent abdominal pregnancy.

CHAPTER II.

ARRESTED DEVELOPMENT AND ANOMALIES OF INFANCY AND PUBERTY.

1. Uterus fœtalis (often planifundalis).
2. Uterus infantilis and uterus membranaceus.
3. Anteflexio uteri infantilis.
4. Stenosis cervicis et orificii externi.
5. Stenosis vulvovaginalis or hymenalis.
6. Evolutio præcox.
7. Oligomenorrhea and amenorrhea.
8. Dysmenorrhea.
9. Menorrhagia.
10. Sterility.

§3. INFANTILE ANOMALIES OF FORMATION.

1 and 2.   Those formative arrests designated as **uterus fœtalis** or **infantilis** are combined with functional disturbances (symptoms)—to be described under the headings from 3 to 10—and with a generally weakened constitution,. idiocy, etc. In the fetal form the body of the uterus fails to grow, and the neck is relatively larger ; the vaginal cervix is very small, and is provided with a minute opening. The latter is also true of the infantile uterus (Plate 2, Fig. 1), but here the body has grown until its muscular coat is as well developed as is that of the neck. The body, instead of being pear-shaped and forming the largest part of the uterus, is simply a cylindric continuation of the cervix.

The **uterus membranaceus** is due to a simple primary atrophy of the organ. (Fig. 22.) All three forms are characterized by their diminutiveness.

The **diagnosis** is made by bimanual exploration (through the rectum, if necessary) and by the cautious introduction of the uterine sound.[1]

Treatment.—Treat the anemia or tuberculosis with roborants. Increase the local blood supply by massage, warm sitz-baths, stimulating vaginal douches, the stem-pessary, frequent scarifications, and mustard plasters on the thighs during the menstrual molimina. Faradization is also employed, one pole being introduced into the uterus and the other being placed upon the mons veneris.

3 and 4. Infantile anteflexion (Plate 15, Fig. 3) of a small organ is often associated with stenosis of the cervical canal or its external orifice. " Puerile anteflexion " consists in a sharp bending forward of a normal, large, flexible organ, with a shortened anterior vaginal wall, in the elongated axis of which the hypertrophic supra-vaginal cervix is found.

Symptoms.—Dysmenorrhea (8) and sterility. Both may be purely mechanical, from the narrowed lumen, or the angle of flexion, especially when the latter has become rigid from long duration and secondary inflammatory changes. The more frequent cause of both, however, is the passive hyperemia and the resulting congestive endometritis, while the sterility is still further accounted for by the frequent hypoplasia.

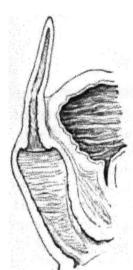

Fig. 22. — Uterus membranaceus.

Diagnosis.—After emptying the bladder the anteflexion is recognized bimanually, the form and direction of the vagina being noted. (Plate 22.) The sound demonstrates the direction of the cervix and the size of its

---

[1] The normal length of the uterus, as measured by the sound, is **six** timeters.

lumen,[1] whether it is narrowed throughout or at one of its orifices only, and whether secondary dilatation of the uterine cavity or cervical canal has taken place. (Plate 15, Fig. 3.)

Treatment.—If no other cause for the symptoms exists (an endometritis, for example), the stenosis should be removed by dilatation with metal sounds, laminaria tents, or iodoform-gauze tampons every few weeks. A more permanent result is obtained by making, immediately after the period, bilateral transverse incisions, about one centimeter deep, in the cervical commissures by means of Cooper's scissors. The mucous membrane of the cervical canal is then brought into apposition with that of the intravaginal cervix in such a manner that the two rows of stitches pass from the anterior to the posterior cervical lip and the uterine orifice gapes. The fresh surfaces are so liable to form adhesions after this operation of Sims' that it is better to make four radiating incisions (Kehrer), or to transplant a flap, with a pedicle, from the cervix to the incision. This is followed by a tamponade of ferripyrin cotton, which is nonirritating. In stenosis of the entire cervical canal faradization should be employed, with the negative pole in the cervix (fifty milliamperes for five minutes, twice a week for two months).

The anteflexion is treated by the introduction of a stem-pessary made of silver. The stem should be from 2 to 3 mm. thick, the length from 1 to 1½ cm. shorter than the uterine cavity, and the plate from 2 to 2½ cm. in diameter (v. Winckel). If the direct introduction of the stem is impossible, it may be introduced alongside of a sound. It is to be held in position for a few days by a tampon, and the patient kept quiet. If an inflammatory reaction occurs, the tampon is to be removed. This stem seems not only to remove the flexion, but also to act favorably on the dysmenorrhea and sterility (v. Winckel). It

---

[1] The normal cervical canal will accommodate a sound four millimeters in diameter.

stimulates and invigorates the organ. The vagina should be washed out daily, and the stem should be changed every few months. [The dangers involving the use of intra-uterine stem-pessaries have caused them to be abandoned by most practitioners. Forcible dilatation and overstretching of the cervical canal by means of graduated bougies or branched dilators are now usually employed. The endometritis resulting from the stenosis and aggravating the symptoms renders a thorough curetment a necessary part of the operation of dilating the cervical canal for stenosis causing dysmenorrhea and sterility.—ED.]

5. **Stenosis Vulvovaginalis or Hymenalis.**—Incision is necessary only in a marked degree of vagina infantilis, and then a flap should be transplanted. Should the hymen be too resistant and interfere with coitus, it should be incised and appropriately sutured, since forced immissio penis or the descending head has caused lateral lacerations from which considerable hemorrhage has occurred. The more insignificant stenoses are to be dilated, either quickly or slowly, with iodoform gauze. In neuropathic individuals simultaneous spasms of the constrictors often occur. (See Vaginismus.)

§ 4. ANOMALIES OF MENSTRUATION.

Physiologic menstruation commonly appears first at puberty (from the age of fourteen to sixteen years in our climate; earlier in warmer countries; in large cities earlier than in the country), and is a sign of sexual maturity. It occurs as a hemorrhage, dependent upon a regular monthly determination of blood to the genitalia, in consequence of which the uterine mucous membrane becomes more vascular, spongy, and better fitted for the reception and development of an impregnated ovum. Ovulation occurs at the same time, and is due to the escape of a mature ovum from a ruptured Graafian follicle. The entire process (ovulation and menstruation) is regulated by a nervous center, and goes hand in hand with periodic variations in the body-metabolism, which is least active at the time of the menstrual flow. The hemorrhage has its source in the mucous membrane of the uterine cavity, and recurs periodically unless pregnancy supervenes. (See "Atlas of Obstetric Diagnosis and Treatment," second edition, § 1.)

Various disturbances may precede or accompany menstruation, and are to be looked upon as expressions of fluctuations in the body-metabolism. These are : Exanthemata (herpes labialis, acne), skin irritations, chilliness, neuralgia, malaise, dizziness, borborygmus, diarrhea with suddenly appearing constipation, a preceding leukorrhea for several days, a more frequent desire to urinate, and a urine loaded with urates.

6. **Evolutio Præcox.**—In these cases menstruation may occur during childhood, and the individual may present all the appearances of sexual maturity.[1] Should she become pregnant, delivery will usually take place without special difficulty.

7. **Oligomenorrhea and Amenorrhea.—Etiology.** —In §§ 1–3 we have already found a series of causes for amenorrhea in the anomalies of development of the genitalia. These can be divided into :

(*a*) Permanent organic causes : defects of the uterus, ovaries, or Graafian follicles (either congenital or resulting from an infantile oophoritis), with otherwise completely developed genitalia.

(*b*) Functional disturbances, which persist in some cases : infantile genitalia (hypoplasia, anteflexion, stenosis, insufficient development of the uterine mucosa), anemia, especially in neuropathic individuals (lack of determination of blood to the uterus).

(*c*) Mechanical obstructions : atresias.

(*d*) Affections that cause a symptomatic amenorrhea :

---

[1] The not infrequent hemorrhages from the genitalia of the newborn should be excluded from this classification.

morphinism; obesity; severe acute diseases; excessive
disturbances of the circulation from catching cold or from
emotional excitement (fright, fear of pregnancy); diseases
of the genitalia, such as metritis (contraction of the mucous
membrane), perimetritis (ovaries and tubal ostia embedded
in exudate), and oophoritis; ovarian tumors; puerperal
hyperinvolution (atrophy of the genitalia); and pregnancy.
The latter causes a physiologic amenorrhea, but nevertheless it should be noted that ovulation and conception may
occur.

Treatment.—It should first be determined whether the
case is one of true amenorrhea or whether it is caused by
mechanical hindrances (congenital or acquired) to the exit
of blood. The treatment of the latter conditions (groups
a and c), both curative and symptomatic, has been fully
described in § 1. (See Plate 38.)

Group b (see § 3) requires a tedious yet often a fruitful
line of treatment. The careful regulation of the manner
of living is of the utmost importance. Every injurious
influence should be removed, the more pernicious being:
overexertion, especially that of a mental nature (hard study;
constant application to school-exercises, embroidery, or
sewing; frequent visits to theaters, balls, etc.); too
much or too little sleep; exhausting diarrhea or leukorrhea; masturbation; and the ingestion of improper food.
The diet should at first be bland, nutritious, and of such
a nature that constipation and tympanites are avoided;
meat diet later. The household duties are to be regularly
arranged; if possible, daily walks of one or two hours in
the country are to be recommended, taking care to avoid
fatigue; the bowels must be regulated (fruit, abdominal
massage, injections of lukewarm water with or without
soap or oil, laxatives). Certain drugs stimulate the appetite and are of value. Especially useful are blood tonics,
such as Hommel's hematogen (hemoglobinum liq.), Dah-
men's hemalbumin powder, nutrol, wine with peptonate
of iron, or Bland's pills with tincture of cinchona.

The circulation should be encouraged by warm foot-baths (95° to 100° F., with a few teaspoonfuls of salt or mustard, once or twice daily), warm sitz-baths or full baths, and the application of sinapisms to the thighs when congestion of the pelvic viscera and a mucous vaginal discharge point to a menstrual epoch. Cold baths should be forbidden. The patient should be warmly clothed. Sea air is beneficial, from its stimulating effect upon the appetite. Nervous, chlorotic girls are benefited by the rest-cure (Weir Mitchell-Playfair). For the local treatment see § 3. The importance of massage should not be forgotten.

Group d calls for treatment of the primary affection. It is in this class of cases alone that stimulating drugs are to be used : potassium permanganate, sodium salicylate, santonin, and aloes. Their use is by no means productive of uniform success. Hyperinvolution is treated by massage and electricity. (See § 3, Stenosis.)

Dependent upon the amenorrhea, the following secondary conditions are observed :

a. Marked disturbances of metabolism, which lead to dyspepsia of a severe type, tympanites, and secondary anemia.

β. Vicarious hemorrhages from other mucous membranes (renal, vesical, gastric, intestinal, nasal), and from the skin, ears, or anterior chamber of the eye. It is difficult to say whether these are results or causes of the amenorrhea, as they do not appear at strictly periodic intervals.

γ. Periodic exanthemata : erythematous, impetiginous (especially at the edge of the lip), and pustular (acne).

δ. Periodic neuroses : neuralgia, palpitation, cerebral congestion, dyspnea (asthma uterinum), cough (tussis uterina), gastric colic, digestive disturbances, etc.

Treatment.—For the vicarious hemorrhages : hot irrigations, scarification of the vaginal cervix ; for the acne : Lassar's paste,[1] sulphur ointment, pills of ichthyol (1½

[1] See "Therapeutic Table."

gr. in lozenges); for the urticaria and erythema : laxatives, salicylated alcohol, five per cent. menthol spirit, atropin, sodium salicylate (1½–2 drams daily); for the impetiginous eczema (pustules with honey-yellow crusts): diachylon ointment [1] or bismuth salve ; for the herpes : zinc oxid ointment ; for the neuralgia and asthma : caffein, antipyrin, inhalations of chloroform, infus. digitalis, and ice-bag over cardiac region. General nerve tonics and hydrotherapy are indicated.

8. **Dysmenorrhea** is characterized by violent pains (causing reflex hemicrania, nausea, vomiting, dizziness, and hysteric symptoms), which emanate from the uterine and paracervical ganglia, and are to be looked upon as symptoms from the lumbar cord. Other diseased organs (liver, heart, lung, stomach) participate in the disturbances.

From an etiologic standpoint seven forms may be differentiated :

(a) Reflex, from diseased ovaries, tubes, perimetrium, etc.

(b) In the initial stage of intramural myomata.

(c) So-called neuralgia uteri, with spasmodic flexion of the uterus (author) from fright, interrupted coitus, masturbation, thermic and mechanical insults, acute colds.

(d) Congestive, with flexions of the uterus and all conditions that occasion a hyperemia of the organ and its ligaments. The pain precedes the flow and ceases with its onset, when the blood-vessels are relieved.

(e) Inflammatory, with endometritis, metritis, parametritis, and perimetritis. The pain is most severe at the beginning of the period and gradually abates ; the uterus is very sensitive, sometimes spasmodically contracted. When the congestive (d) and inflammatory (e) dysmenorrheas have reached their height, shreds of mucous membrane, sometimes the entire mucosa, may be cast off (decidua menstrualis). This condition is designated as dysmenorrhœa membranacea with endometritis exfoliativa.

(f) Obstructive, often a result of c and d (see also §§ 3

and 4, amenorrhea), or arising from too rapid or too profuse a secretion of blood, stenosis or flexion of the cervix, or swelling of the endometrium. The pains follow the onset of the menses, and resemble those of labor. Large clots or shreds of mucous membrane are sometimes discharged.

(*g*) Exfoliatio mucosæ menstrualis or dysmenorrhœa membranacea *without* endometritis.

Diagnosis and Treatment.—Indicated under the corresponding letter.

(*a*) In every case of dysmenorrhea the constitution of the patient should be considered, and the exact condition of the entire genital apparatus should be determined by bimanual palpation and, if necessary, by exploration with the sound.

(*b*) It is impossible to diagnose small intramural myomata before they cause a projection of the uterine wall or a change in its consistence. The characteristic symptoms are violent, fixed, boring pains, without fever. These are controlled by suppositories, vaginal or rectal injections, or pills of chloral, or by use of extract of belladonna or hyoscyamin, tincture of opium, or antipyrin. Rubefacients (sinapisms, menthol, or spirits of camphor on compresses), ergotin, and salt baths are useful in the treatment of this condition. The patient should rest in bed during the attack.

(c) Potassium bromid, caffein, sodium benzoate, phenacetin, antipyrin (also as a wash), fluid extract of viburnum prunifolium, potassium permanganate (to be taken one week before the period), and the pills and rubefacients previously mentioned. Diaphoresis should be encouraged.

(*d*) Rest in bed, warm clothing, especially over the abdomen, hot sand-baths, rubefacients (see *b*). Laxatives and ipecac to prevent overfilling of the stomach, antimonials and diaphoretics for the catarrh. Local depletion of the blood-vessels by scarifications, two leeches to the cervix, copious hot vaginal injections, or glycerin and astringent tampons. Any existing cause should be appropriately treated : flexions, by pessaries, massage, etc. ; stenosis, by dilatation.

(e) Removal of the inflammation. Treatment of attack as in d; above all, blood-letting (two leeches) and laxatives, scarifications of the cervical mucosa, wedge-shaped excisions (see Metritis), atmocausis (vaporization, see Endometritis).

(f) See treatment of stenosis and amenorrhœa in §§ 3 and 4.

(g) According to v. Winckel, the application of two leeches to the cervix at repeated intervals prevents the casting off of the decidua menstrualis and allows conception and recovery to take place. Curetment and application of zinc chlorid (chlorid of iron after the operation), atmocausis, or zestocausis (see Endometritis). Symptomatic, as under b and d.

Diagnosis of Exfoliatio Mucosæ Menstrualis.—The prodromes are sensations of heat and cold, nausea, vomiting, dizziness, headache, and unconsciousness, with or without hysteric convulsions. Circumscribed pain in the lower abdomen. The discharged blood may be small in amount.

The membrane is passed with or without pain. If complete, it has a triangular shape, showing the position of the three uterine orifices (ostia tubarum, os internum). The outer surface is rough and tattered, having been torn from the uterine wall ; the inner surface is smooth, offering for inspection furrows and minute glandular orifices.

Microscopic Structure.—The connective tissue is increased, and its interstices are filled with exudate and small round cells, which push apart the utricular glands. The latter are seen in cross-section, with their cylindric epithelium and blood-vessels. Larger cells rarely appear, and then are quite isolated. The picture is practically that of interstitial endometritis. Löhlein points out that pieces of mucous membrane obtained by curetment between two periods show none of the foregoing changes.

Membranes are sometimes cast off from the vagina in *colpitis exfoliativa*, consisting of polygonal squamous epithelial cells with relatively large vesicular nuclei. Similar membranes may be exfoliated from a changed epithelial layer of the lower portion of the cervix. (See Plates 28 to 31.)

Microscopic Differential Diagnosis.—The *decidua vera graviditatis* consists of a layer of large, irregular, roundish (decidual) cells possessing large nuclei (often multiple). These completely conceal the scanty connective-tissue framework.

9. Menorrhagia.—By this term we designate those uterine hemorrhages that are so profuse in proportion to the general constitution of the individual that symptoms of anemia appear, or, if already present, become exaggerated. Its manifestations are dizziness, unconsciousness, ringing in the ears, flickering of objects before the eyes, nausea, vomiting, constipation, a striking pallor of the mucous membranes, lassitude, pain in the back, shortness of breath, palpitation, etc. The menorrhagia may be habitual or temporary.

Etiology.—(a) Diseases of the genitalia : tumors, displacements and inflammations, swellings of the endometrium ; (b) diseases of other organs that cause circulatory disturbances (heart, lungs, kidneys, spleen, liver) ; (c) associated with intestinal diseases (dysentery, constipation) ; (d) nervous hyperemia (emotion, hot drinks) ; (e) associated with constitutional diseases (Werlhof's disease, excessive development of the panniculus adiposus).

Treatment.—Symptomatic—rest in the horizontal position, a bland diet, soothing drinks (acids, effervescing powders), hot fomentations of alcohol, sinapisms.

Group a : See treatment of endometritis (especially the fungous and hemorrhagic forms), chronic metritis in the stage of engorgement, parametritis and perimetritis, fibroid and mucous polyps of the uterus, sarcoma and carcinoma, ovarian tumors, flexion and prolapse of the uterus.

If radical treatment is not adopted, the hemorrhage is to be controlled by ergotin, cornutin, secale cornutum, or hydrastis canadensis (hydrastin), stypticin, hot vaginal irrigations (113° to 125° F.) at intervals of from three to six hours, very firm tamponade of the vagina (iodoform gauze or salicylated cotton), or even tamponade of the cavity of the uterus with iodoform gauze or laminaria. The solution of ferric chlorid may be applied upon cotton, as a direct local hemostatic, or the medicated sound (aluminum or wood) may be introduced into the cervix and allowed to remain there for from two to three hours. Ferripyrin has proved itself to be of value, controlling the hemorrhage and producing no irritation. It is used as a powder or, better, as sterilized "nondraining ferripyrin-nosophen gauze."[1] Injections of gelatin solution and atmocausis (see treatment of endometritis hæmorrhagica) are to be recommended.[2]

Group b: Digitalis, expectorants, and the waters of Karlsbad, Franzensbad, Kissingen, Wildungen, Neuenahr, and Vichy have a specific action.

Group c: Laxatives (enemata of infusum sennæ, strong infusions of rhubarb, 10 : 100, oleum ricini).

Group d: Arrest hemorrhage as in group *a;* ergotin; reduction of obesity by the methods of Banting, Mendelsohn, Epstein, or Oertel ; sojourn at Marienbad ; and vegetable diet. In hemophilia and scurvy, hydrotherapy and subcutaneous injections of gelatin. Calcium hypophosphite by the mouth or rectum.

¿5. STERILITY.

The causes of sterility may be found in the physical or psychic nature of the husband or wife, or in the habitual disease of the product. They may be divided into four groups :

1. Impotentia coëundi from organic defects or from nervous or psychic influences.

HUSBAND.	WIFE.
Epispadias and hypospadias ; paresis and paralysis of the nervi erigentes from psychic influence or nervous weakness (affections of the brain and spinal cord, age, perverted habits, etc.) ; aspermatism from cicatricial stenosis ; prostatic hypertrophy.	Atresia or stenosis of the hymen or vagina ; vaginismus ; obstructing tumors or inflammations ; absence of sexual desire.

[1] Prepared under the author's direction by Evens and Pistor, of Cassel.

[2] A complete report of the indications for these new methods of hemostasis and results of their application is to be found in the author's article in the June number of "Deutschen Praxis," 1899.

2. Azoospermism or arrested formation of the genital cell.

HUSBAND.

Atrophy of the testicles (from gonorrhea, orchitis, trauma, and like causes) ; atresia of the ejaculatory duct.

WIFE.

The Graafian vesicles fail to rupture, either from congenital or inflammatory causes ; ovarian tumors.

3. The spermatic filament is deposited in the female genitalia but is unable to come in contact with the ovum.

Atresia or stenosis of the uterus or tubes (flexions of both), cervical plugs of tough mucus (endometritis) ; uterine or tubal tumors ; perioophoritic pseudomembranes.

4. The ovum fails to lodge in the uterine mucosa.

Endometritis ; uterine tumors ; weakness ; diseases of the ovum.

Examination.

HUSBAND.

Since gonorrhea is a frequent cause of azoospermism and cicatricial stenosis, the previous history is to be carefully considered and the number of well-formed spermatic filaments in the semen is to be determined.

WIFE. (See ¶ 1 to 4.)

Character of the menses ; presence of fluor albus (gonococci) ; uterus, by speculum and sound ; uterus and adnexa, bimanual.

The treatment depends upon the cause demonstrated. If no reason can be found, advise the patient to hold the semen in the vagina as long as possible (with the knees together), as Marion Sims proved that the posterior vaginal vault acts as a seminal receptacle, the intravaginal cervix (in the normal position of the uterus) being here bathed in the spermatic fluid. In some cases coitus must be practised with the pelvis of the female elevated, or *a posterioribus.*

GROUP II.

CHANGES OF SHAPE AND POSITION.

CHAPTER I.

HERNIA.

The abdominal organs may be invaginated into natural, preformed canals,—being covered by the enveloping soft parts,—and may present themselves in the abdominal wall, in the gluteal region, in the course of the femoral vessels, in the vagina, or in the labia. For vaginal hernia see also Inversion of the Vagina, § 7.

§ 6. HERNIA AND OTHER CHANGES OF SHAPE OF THE VULVA.

The hernial contents may consist of the uterus—especially one horn of a uterus bicornis—and its adnexa (ovary, see § 1, Pseudohermaphroditism), with or without the intestine and its appendages, or of the intestine alone.

The more frequent path is through the inguinal canal (Fig. 23); less often in front of the broad ligament and along the levator ani. In the first case we speak of a hernia inguinalis labialis (anterior); in the latter, of a hernia vaginalis labialis (posterior). The hernia may attain the size of a melon.

Diagnosis.—Varying changes of size of the tumor, reduction of contained intestine (usually filled with gas and fluids) with a "gurgle," the characteristic form and

48

sensitiveness of the ovary, impulse on coughing, etc., all establish the nature of the swelling.

Treatment.—Just as in other hernias—taxis and retention by a truss (Scarpa) or by a large, hollow, vaginal ring (hard-rubber). If reduction is impossible, open the sac and replace, or an abdominal section may be performed, the hernia reduced, held by fixation sutures, and the orifice closed.

Other changes of shape are seen in the duplication and enlargement of individual parts—the nymphæ and clitoris—which may give rise to irritation, excoriation, edema, etc.

Treatment.—Frequent washings, using astringents if necessary, and applications of oak-bark decoctions or lead water, constitute the preventive treatment. Boric ointment or bryolin, sitz-baths with bran, dermatol, bismuth-talc, nosophen-starch, or applications of solutions of cocain are to be used for their curative action.

CHAPTER II.

INVERSION AND PROLAPSUS.

These conditions hold a certain mutual relation, inasmuch as the former is a weighty predisposing cause of the latter. The inverted vagina easily drags the uterus to the vulva, while in other cases the inversio vaginæ and the prolapsus may be traced to a common cause. On the other hand, the uterine prolapse, or apparent prolapse, due to hypertrophy of the cervix, may lead to protrusions of the vaginal mucous membrane.

₹ 7. THE INVERSIONS OF THE VAGINA AND UTERUS.

Inversions of the lower half of the vagina mostly lead to the formation of hernias ; the most frequent are those of the posterior wall of the bladder (Cystocele, Plate 5, Fig. 1) and of the anterior wall of the rectum (Rectocele, Plate 5, Fig. 2). The upper half of the vagina is far less often the seat of inversion, the other organs carrying the rectovesical or vesico-uterine folds of peritoneum ahead of them. In the "Atlas of Obstetric Diagnosis and Treatment" (Figs. 102 to 105) cases of incarcerated retroflexed gravid uteri and of extra-uterine pregnancy are illustrated in which the gestation sac causes a protuberance of the vaginal wall.

Among the rarer cases brought to our notice are ovariocolpocele, enterocolpocele (Plate 19, Fig. 1), hydrocolpocele, pyocolpocele (Plate 58, Fig. 1, and Plate 59, Fig. 3), and those bulgings of the vaginal wall that are brought about by tumors of Douglas' pouch (Plates 58 and 59), or of the rectovaginal or vaginovesical septa. (Plate 58, Fig. 3; Plate 88, Figs. 5 and 6.)

If the ovary, intestine, or omentum becomes fixed in the pouch of Douglas, it may cause the vaginal wall to bulge, so that in extreme cases it presents itself at the vul-

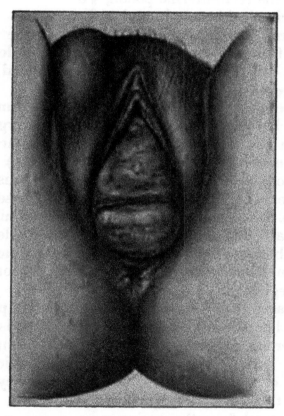

Fig. 23.—Inversion of both vaginal walls and inguinal hernia of the right labium in a case of lacerated perineum (photograph of an original water-color). The two conditions are not infrequently associated, as they have a common cause—relaxation of the supporting tissues.

var opening. This is particularly true in cases of retroflexion or prolapse of the uterus. The simultaneous inversion of the anterior and posterior vaginal walls is rare, because it could be caused only by an influence exerted at

the same time on both recto-uterine and vesico-uterine cul-
desacs. It is rarely caused by ascites (with a retroflexed
or vertical uterus), more frequently by pus or an encapsulated peritoneal exudate (pyocolpocele).

Diagnosis.—See scheme and differential diagnosis of
tumors of the recto-uterine pouch, § 35.

In ovariocele bimanual exploration reveals a characteristic form, sensitiveness, and relation to the tube and
uterus. If the ovary is enlarged or embedded in exudate, other differential points must be considered (exploration per rectum).

Enterocele is recognized by the signs common to all
intestinal hernias, palpable and audible gurgling and
changes in the tension of the tumor, with variations of
intra-abdominal pressure (impulse on coughing).

Hydrocolpocele and pyocolpocele are to be suspected if
the symptoms of ascites and peritonitis are present. (See
Peritonitis.) Carefully examine the previous history.

Prognosis and Treatment.—An enterocele can become troublesome only during delivery. Reduction from
the rectum if necessary; colporrhaphy, in some cases
during pregnancy.

A displaced ovary should be reposited, the patient being in the lateral or knee-chest posture (narcosis if necessary, finger in rectum). The difficulties encountered are
dependent entirely upon the number of adhesions. The
reposition of ovarian tumors during pregnancy or labor
may lead to serious consequences. If it fails, the tumor
must be tapped from the vagina.

The prognosis and treatment of hydrocolpocele and
pyocolpocele are the same as those of the causative disease.
Puncture from the vagina if condition is analogous to
cases just mentioned.

Inversion of the posterior vaginal wall may lead to
rectocele. As the two organs are connected only by loose
connective tissue, this displacement does not always

occur ; indeed, the rectum generally induces it.   As usual causes may be mentioned relaxed vaginal walls, gaping of the vulvar cleft, with or without perineal laceration, and prolapse of the uterus.   It presents itself to the examining finger as a pocket, which causes constipation and tenesmus.   (Plate 4, Fig. 1 ; Plate 5, Fig. 1 ; Fig. 27.)

The **treatment** consists in the repair of the perineum and pelvic floor and in the shortening and narrowing of the vagina.   (See operations described under Prolapse of the Uterus.)   When the muscular coat of the vagina is relaxed from colpitis : astringents, either as injections (solutions of aluminum acetate, 10 to 20%) or upon tampons (glycerite of tannin).   A pessary should be looked upon as a temporary makeshift.

Inversion of the anterior vaginal wall is more frequently by far associated with cystocele, because the two organs are firmly connected, and the intra-abdominal tension causes the bladder to follow the vaginal wall.   The bladder is divided into two pouches, one lying behind the pubic symphysis, the other in the cystocele.   The latter draws the urethra down with it, causing it to assume an S-shape.   The greater concavity looks downward and leads into the cystocele.   (Plate 4, Figs. 2 and 3 ; Plate 3, Fig. 5 ; Plate 5, Figs. 2 and 4 ; Plates 8 and 9, Catheterization ; Plate 12 ; Plate 13, Condition in Artificial Prolapse.)   The disturbances of the circulation in the inverted parts sometimes cause dysuria, and, together with the inability completely to empty the bladder, may lead to cystitis and to the formation of vesical calculi.

Treatment.—Plastic operations to narrow the anterior vaginal wall and to retain the bladder and the vaginal wall in their proper places.

INVERSION OF THE UTERUS.

This is an affection, severe in its nature, arising under quite similar circumstances.   The chief etiologic factor is

PLATE 3.

FIG. 1.—**Impressio fundi uteri** as an initial stage of inversion of the uterus arises when the organ is relaxed, and Credé's method is too forcibly exercised, or traction is made upon the cord.

FIG. 2.—**Partial Inversion of the Uterus.** A portion of the cervix has not yet become invaginated. The inverted uterus already forms a considerable peritoneal pocket; this "funnel" is filled by the tube and ovary.

FIG. 3.—The uterus has become invaginated as far as the external os; the latter, however, has not descended.

FIG. 4.—The completely inverted uterus protrudes from the vulva; the upper portion of the vagina has also become invaginated as far as the constrictor cunni and levator ani.

FIG. 5.—**Complete Prolapse of the Retroflexed Uterus and of the Vagina with Laceration of the Perineum; Cystocele.** (See Fig. 28 and Plates 8-10.) The apex of the bladder approaches the fundus; the vesical diverticulum reaches to the internal os; the pouch of Douglas lies in the prolapse, containing, however, no intestinal loops (enterocele), as sometimes occurs in rare cases; the intestines are held back by the retroflexed corpus uteri. The external os is everted; the cervix is swollen.

This illustration represents one of the extreme possibilities of prolapse, and at the same time the most frequent manner of its development.

---

a relaxation and dilatation of both the uterine and cervical walls. The direct cause is most frequently an acute one, occurring in the puerperium (precipitate birth, forced Credé's method, traction on the cord); or one chronic in its nature, such as traction upon the fundus uteri from the expulsion of a fibroid polyp. If the tumor is submucous, the mucous membrane alone is drawn down; if it is intramural, the muscular coat, or even the serous covering, may be invaginated, so that a peritoneal "funnel" is formed in which the adnexa or intestinal coils (only in puerperal inversions) may lie (Kehrer). The latter may contract

Tab. 3.

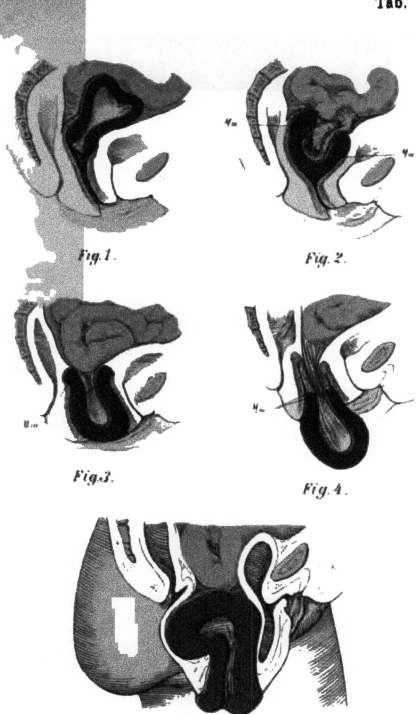

Fig.1.

Fig. 2.

Fig.3.

Fig. 4.

Fig.5.

Lith. Anst. F. Reichhold. München

inflammatory adhesions in cases of long standing. (Plate 3, Fig. 2 ; Fig. 24.)

Different degrees of inversion may be differentiated : complete, including the entire cervix ; complete, with inversion of the vagina (inversio uteri cum prolapsu); incomplete, as far as the internal os. The slightest degree is the *impressio fundi uteri*. (Plate 3.) The acute puerperal inversion may become chronic.

Symptoms.—The mucosa swells and proliferates from the constriction. It bleeds easily, and ulcers arise from friction. The ulcerated surfaces may grow fast to the vaginal mucosa, or gangrene may appear. The acute puerperal form occurs with violent symptoms resembling shock.

The chief symptoms are pain and hemorrhage, dependent upon the nature of the tumor. They render the patient anemic and force her to stay in bed.

Diagnosis.—An exact portrayal of the existing conditions is demanded, as an inverted uterus has been repeatedly confounded with a polyp, and cut off.

In complete inversion with prolapse we find a red, solid-elastic tumor, which bleeds easily and is sensitive to pressure. The uterine orifices of the Fallopian tubes may probably be recognized.

In incomplete inversion the sound may be passed into the cervix, beside the tumor (corpus uteri), for quite a distance—further in front than behind (from 3 to 4 cm.). Bimanual palpation is of importance ; it demonstrates the absence of the uterus from its usual position and the presence of the peritoneal "funnel."

Treatment.—If due to a tumor, enucleation of the same, whereupon the uterus usually reinverts itself spontaneously. If irreducible from proliferative thickening of the uterine wall, amputation of the organ close to the external os, carefully closing the peritoneal funnel with sutures. In acute puerperal inversion, manual reposition (as in phimosis), trying to push back the portion in contact with the external os first, and making counterpressure from the abdomen to prevent elongation and possible laceration of the vagina.

The earlier the attempt is made, the more likely is it to be crowned with success. If manual reposition fails, the parts are to be carefully disinfected and pushed back by

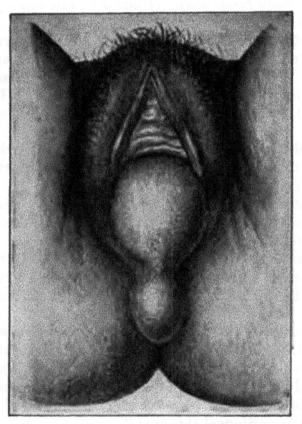

Fig. 24.—Complete inversion of the uterus from a myoma of the fundus. (See Plate 3.) (Original diagrammatic drawing.)

the colpeurynter (always to be filled *after* introduction) or by means of astringent tampons. These are held in position until the tumor is partly reduced, when the reinversion is completed by cold-water injections. Massage of the uterus assists the action of the colpeurynter, and ergot effects the contraction of the organ. Elevations of temperature give warning of the onset of pelvic peritonitis, when all attempts at reduction must be discontinued.

Celiotomy is indicated only in extreme cases. A better method is that of Küstner, who makes an incision in the posterior vaginal vault, which enables him to incise the posterior uterine wall throughout its entire length, and to reinvert the organ. Kehrer attacks the uterus through the anterior vaginal vault.

¿8. PROLAPSE OF THE VAGINA AND UTERUS.

When the external os sinks below the interspinous plane, we speak of descensus uteri. If in addition to the descent of the uterus the lower portion of the vagina protrudes at the vulva, the case is one of incomplete or partial prolapse of the vagina ; if the vaginal vault also protrudes, complete prolapse.

In incomplete prolapse of the uterus the cervix alone protrudes at the vulva ; in complete prolapse the entire organ—with the completely inverted vagina, and cystocele or rectocele, or both—lies outside of the introitus.

The Normal Situation and Position of the Uterus.

The normally situated uterus lies in the true pelvis in a position of anteversion. The anterior surface is obliquely placed, facing the bladder ; the posterior surface is strongly convex, and is parallel to the upper sacral curvature. The longitudinal axis of the organ passes from above downward, and from before backward. If fixed points are desired, the fundus marks the center of the conjugate vera, and the external is in the interspinous plane, being somewhat nearer to the sacrum than to the symphysis. (Plates 14 and 22.)

This position is not a constant one, however ; the uterus is in a condition of unstable equilibrium, the fundus descending with every inspiration. In the upright position the fundus is still lower, while the cervix becomes more elevated. It is balanced upon an axis of fixation corresponding to the internal os, this portion of the neck being suspended from the pelvis and sacrum by the supravaginal connective tissue and the involuntary muscle-fibers of the uterosacral ligaments. In the dorsal position the fundus goes backward and the cervix approaches the symphysis. The position is also dependent upon

PLATE 4.

Fig. 1.—**Incomplete Prolapse of a Retroverted Uterus; Marked Rectocele; Vaginal Inversion.**

Fig. 2.—**Incomplete Prolapse of the Uterus, Due to Hypertrophy of the Intermediate Portion of the Neck; Inversion of the Vagina with Cystocele.** (See Plate 12.) The fundus of the uterus is nearly at its normal height. The sound shows the uterine canal to be longer than normal (longer than 5 or 6 cm.). The distance from the internal to the external os demonstrates the elongation to be in the intermediate portion of the cervix. The portion of the neck that is elongated is further shown by the relation of the anterior and posterior vaginal fornices to the external os and to the internal os.

The illustration shows the posterior vaginal vault at its usual height in the pelvis; the anterior, however, is lower, and yet holds its usual relation to the external os; consequently, it is not the intravaginal cervix that is hypertrophied, but the middle portion of the neck, situated between the anterior and posterior vaginal fornices and lying higher up.

Fig. 3.—**Total Prolapse of Anteflexed Uterus and of the Anterior Vaginal Wall, with Cystocele; Characteristic Flexion of the Urethra.** (See also Plates 8 and 9, Introduction of Catheter.)

Fig. 4.—**Complete Prolapse of Retroflexed Uterus (First Degree) and of Vagina.** Small rectal and vesical diverticula.

PLATE 5.

Fig. 1.—**Prolapse of Posterior Vaginal Wall; Rectocele; Descent of Retroflexed Uterus (Second Degree).** The posterior vaginal wall seldom becomes inverted first; a rectal diverticulum may form in the pouch, demonstrable to the introduced finger.

Fig. 2.—**Prolapse of the Anterior Vaginal Wall; Extreme Grade of Cystocele; Anteflexion of the Uterus (First Degree); Descent of the Uterus.** Evidence of the existence of a cystocele is obtained by the catheter. (See Plates 8 and 9.)

Fig. 3.—**Reposition of Prolapsed Uterus by a Martin Stempessary.** (Original diagrammatic drawing, modified according to Schröder.) This pessary is applicable when the genitalia are roomy or relaxed. The stem rests upon the levator ani, receiving lateral sup-

Tab. 4.

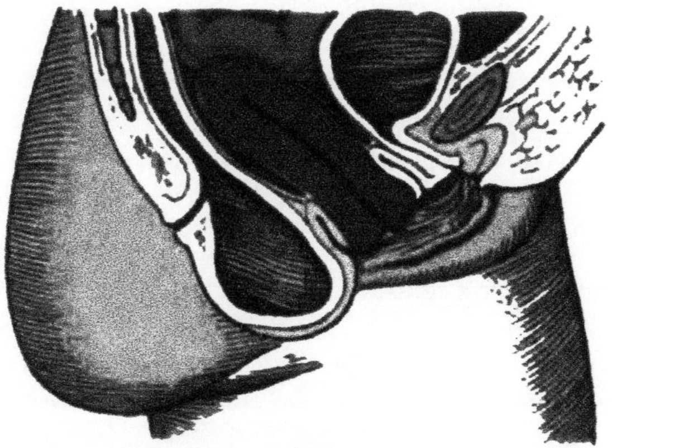

Fig.1.

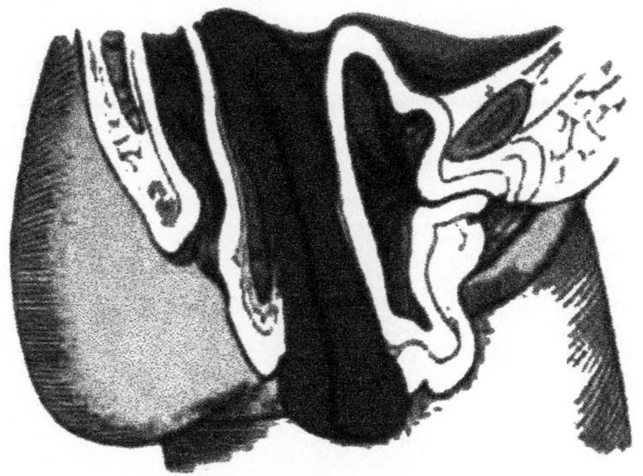

Fig.2.

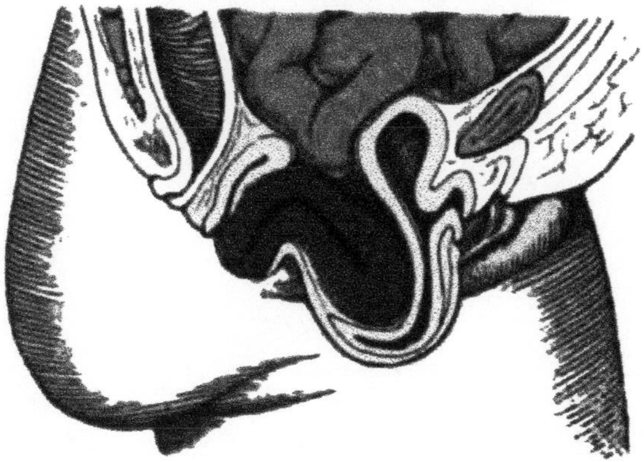

Fig.3.

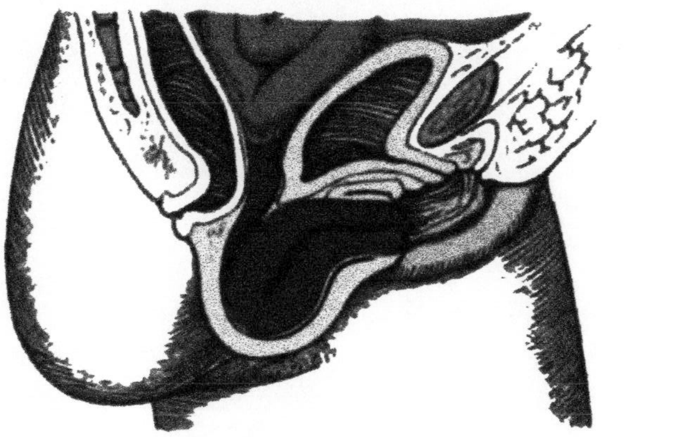

Fig.4.

Lith. Anst P. Reichhold, München.

Tab. 5.

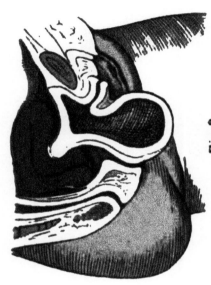

Fig. 2.

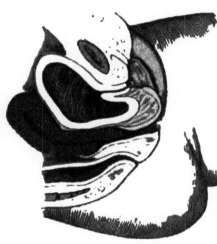

Fig. 4.

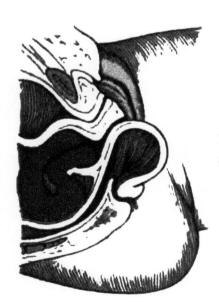

Fig. 1.

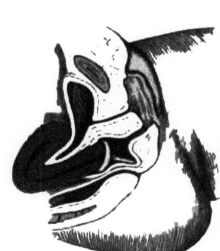

Fig. 3.

Lith. Anst. F. Reichhold, München.

port if it slips to one side. This case is one of pseudoprolapse, because the reposition unduly elevates the fundus, anteflexes the body, and draws up a diverticulum from the bladder. The condition is really elongation of the neck, and amputation is indicated.

FIG. 4.—Hypertrophy of the Anterior Lip of the Uterus, Producing Inversion of the Anterior Vaginal Wall and Cystocele. (Original diagrammatic drawing modified according to Schröder.)

---

the degree of distention of the bladder and rectum. (See §§ 10 and 11, Plate 17, Fig. 2 ; Plate 14, Figs. 1 and 4)

The uterus is not really "suspended," but the ligaments limit the excursions of the organ beyond a certain point. It really rests indirectly upon the floor of the pelvis, the external os pressing against the posterior vaginal wall, and the cervix being grasped by the connective tissue surrounding the vaginal vault. The latter is partly held up by ligaments, but more particularly by the vaginal walls themselves, these in turn deriving their support from the pelvic floor (constrictores cunni, levatores ani) and perineum. The integrity of the perineum is consequently a most important factor in preventing the descent of the internal genitalia, the ligaments being a secondary consideration. It is not to be forgotten that the uterine supports may be insufficient to withstand an increased pressure from above (tumors) or traction from below. These structures are assisted by atmospheric pressure when the patient is in the knee-elbow position, and Sims' speculum is introduced. The round ligaments resemble a bridle, having no supportive action.

The size of the uterus also influences the existing conditions.

The recto-uterine fold of peritoneum is normally 7 cm. above the anus ; the vesico-uterine, 7½ cm. above the urethral orifice. Note the following measurements :

Length of the uterus (external measurement) :

    In virgins . . . . . . 6– 8 cm. ; weight, . . 40 gm.
    In married women . . 8–10 "   "   . . 100 "

Width :

    Of the fundus { in virgins . . . . 4 –5 cm.
                   { in married women . . . . 5½–6½ "
    Of the neck . . . . 2 –2½ "
    Thickness { in virgins . . . . 2 –3 "
               { in married women . . . . 3 –3½ "

Length of uterine cavity :

	Entire.	Body.	Neck.
In the immature uterus	2.6	0.8	1.8
In the mature virginal uterus	5.4	3.2	2.2
In the uterus that has been gravid	5.9	3.3	2.6

The corporeal secretion of the uterus is thick and oily ; the cervical, albuminoid or mucoid. Both are alkaline and contain mucin (coagulated by acetic acid).

The prolapsed mucous membrane of the vagina and vaginal cervix becomes either excoriated (Plates 8 and 10) or covered with a thickened layer of epithelium, the superficial strata of which are horny in character. (Plate 28, Fig. 2.) The lips of the cervix are everted. (Plates 10 and 12, Figs. 28 and 29.) The introitus vaginæ (about 1 or 2 cm. of the vagina) maintains its normal position, even in extreme cases, forming a swollen ring about the prolapsed tumor. The latter consists of the vagina and uterus, and contains diverticula from the bladder and rectum. (Plates 10 and 13.) The urine (or fecal matter) stagnates in these pouches, inducing catarrh and the formation of calculi; especially as the urethra is usually sharply bent upon itself. If the lower and posterior half of the bladder forms the diverticulum, the ureters are likewise bent at an acute angle and may give rise to hydronephrosis. (Plate 4, Fig. 3; Plate 5, Fig. 2; Plate 12.) Retroversion of the uterus acts as a predisposing cause for this condition of affairs (and for prolapse generally), especially when it is combined with laceration of the perineum (loss of support for vaginal wall) or descensus uteri. (Plate 4, Fig. 1; Plate 5, Fig. 1; Plate 13; Plate 19, Fig. 1.) Even the apex of the bladder and the vesico-uterine fold of peritoneum may be in the tumor. As the pouch of Douglas is in close contact with the posterior vaginal vault, it is likewise well down in the prolapse, and may accommodate a loop of intestine. (Plate 4, Fig. 4; Plate 13.)

The **development of the prolapse** is as follows: The anterior vaginal wall loses its normal support, either from perineal laceration (Plate 54) or from weakness of the pelvic floor. (Plates 6, 7, 25, 27.) The tuberculum vaginæ sinks down first, and remains between the nymphæ. Then the upper portion of the vagina begins not only to descend, but also to invaginate itself, as may be demonstrated every time the patient bears down. The cervix of the still normally anteverted uterus is drawn downward and forward. (Plate 54, Figs. 2 and 3.) By this time the posterior vaginal wall commences to prolapse, making traction upon the posterior vaginal vault and, through it, upon the uterus. (Plate 54, 4.) This organ assumes first a vertical position, and then one of retroversion, its long axis running parallel with that of the vagina, which is now more vertical. At this time the slightest sudden pressure from above, a fall, or a series of similar factors acting in a like manner is sufficient to effect prolapse of the uterus. (Fig. 26.) The same pressure from above, together with the usually existing relaxed uterine wall, causes a bending of the body toward the cervix—retroflexio uteri. The relations of the bladder and peritoneal folds are shown in plates 4 and 5, and in figures 27 and 28.

If the prolapse is complete, the pressure acts still further, everting the cervical mucosa (in extreme cases as far as the internal os), which swells and becomes eroded. (Plates 8, 10 ; Fig. 28.) A lividity of the cervix results from the circulatory disturbances. (Plate 10.) In chronic cases this congestion leads to inflammation and proliferation ; giving rise not only to polyps of the mucous membrane, but also to secondary enlargements and elongations of the uterine neck—elongatio colli. (Plates 4, 5, and 12 ; Fig. 25.)

The body of the uterus takes little part in the process. The superficial epithelial layer becomes horny. (Plate 28, 2.) The muscular coat of the vagina becomes thickened, and the adipose tissue disappears.

Symptoms.—When the patient stands or walks, she feels as though the descending organ would fall out ; if the prolapse is complete, it impedes her movements ; it becomes ulcerated and painful from rubbing—the same is true of the thigh. The vaginal and cervical mucosæ become inflamed, not only secreting mucopus, but causing profuse and painful menses. The prolapsed parts are much enlarged—at first from stasis, later from prolifera-

PLATE 6.

Inversion of the Posterior Vaginal Wall. Leukorrhea; intact perineum. (Original water-color.)

tion of the connective tissue. (Chronic Metritis, Plates 28 and 32.) The dragging upon the adnexa calls forth nervous and dyspeptic symptoms. Defecation and urination are interfered with from secondary retention. Aside from its subjective discomfort, secondary inflammation of the peritoneum, by encapsulating the tubes and ovaries in exudate, leads to sterility. Structural changes in the uterine mucosa and the difficulties attendant upon cohabitation and upon retention of the semen are productive of the same result. The organs become fixed in their abnormal position.

Etiology.—Congenital prolapse of the uterus is one of the greatest rarities. I found such a case in a child with hydromeningocele at the Munich Frauenklinik (Fig. 25); I saw a second in the Heidelberg Frauenklinik in 1894.[1] It is also a rare condition in the virgin, being here caused by heavy lifting. The most frequent causes are found in puerperal injuries and too early attempts at straining, since at this time the uterus already has a tendency to assume or maintain a retrodeviation. Severe labors (forceps) lead to perineal lacerations and to stretching and relaxation of the genital walls and suspensory apparatus. (See explanations of Plates 13, 17, and 54; also p. 57.)

Retroversion of the uterus is easily produced by puerperal subinvolution with a relaxed vagina, chronic inflammatory conditions, frequent labors in delicate women, and tumors that force the uterus downward. Immediately after every normal labor the anterior lip of the cervix may be palpated, just within the introitus vaginæ.

---

[1] Described in "Arch. f. Gyn." by Dr. Heil. At that time I knew of only a third similar case (Qviesling, "C. f. Gyn.," 1890); since then several have been published.

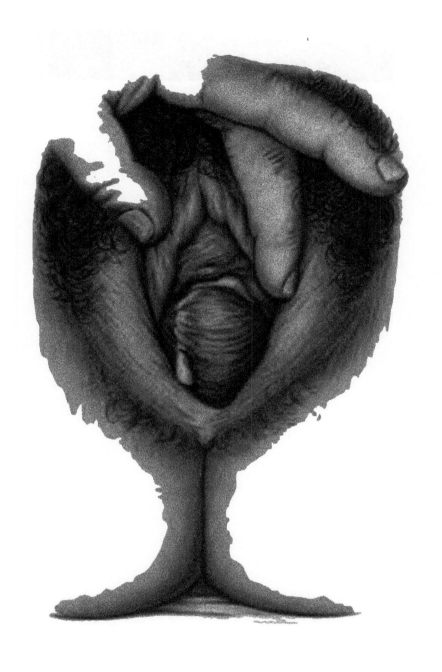

Lith. Anst. K. Reichhold, München

Prognosis.—The danger of acute gangrene from constriction is a remote one. The condition is weakening from all the preceding manifestations. The excoriations predispose to epithelioma (v. Winckel).

Diagnosis.—In many patients the prolapse recedes when they lie down or remain quiet; but any increase of the intra-abdominal tension (coughing, lifting, straining at stool) causes it to descend, or to protrude from the vulva.

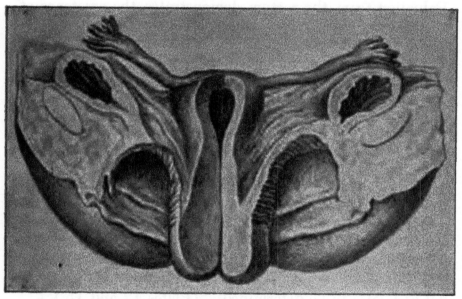

Fig. 25.—Congenital incomplete prolapse of the uterus from a mature fetus with hydromeningocele (Munich Frauenklinik, 1889; "Arch. f. Gyn.," 37, 2). Hypertrophy of the middle portion of the neck; inversion of the vaginal vault; marked development of the ovarian arteries, with iliac arteries of small lumen. The os is notched, and a slight ectropion is present.

The exact contents of the prolapse must be determined. Does it contain the uterus? How much of the vagina? Are vesical or rectal diverticula present? A number of conclusions may be drawn from inspection. (Figs. 26 to 29; Plates 8 to 10.) The external os, the cervical canal, and the length of the uninverted portion of the vagina are recognized by exploration with the finger and sound.

PLATE 7.

FIG. 1.—**Inversion of the vagina from a perineal tear of the third degree** (into the rectum); the tuberculum vaginæ has descended. (Original water-color.)

FIG. 2.—**View of the Cervix in a Case of Elevation of the Uterus.** The cervix does not present itself as a free projection into the vagina, but forms the apex of the vaginal funnel. The oval external os gapes slightly.

Palpation from the rectum demonstrates the existence of a proctocele and, in doubtful cases, the absence of the uterus from its usual position. The direction taken by the vesical diverticulum is shown by the catheter.

If the uterus is completely prolapsed, it may be grasped outside of the vulva, and a retroflexed (common), anteflexed, or vertical position may be recognized. (Figs. 26 to 29.)

In an incomplete prolapse the differential diagnosis from **cervical hypertrophy** must be made. The distance from the external to the internal os is to be measured with the graduated sound (the normal uterus has a cervical canal 6 cm. long). The internal os is recognized by the resistance that it offers to the passage of the knobbed tip of the sound. The distance that the anterior and posterior vaginal vaults extend above the external os is also to be determined. (Plates 12 and 15.)

Finally, it must be ascertained whether the uterus is freely movable in its hernial sac, or adherent to its adnexa and to the descended coils of intestine.

Treatment.—Prophylactic.—Perineal lacerations are to be repaired at once. If the puerperal uterus is inclined to retrodeviation, keep the patient on her side as much as possible. She should never get up before from the tenth to the fourteenth day, and if the foregoing predisposing causes of prolapse exist, she should be kept in bed for two or three weeks, and then forbidden to lift or to do hard

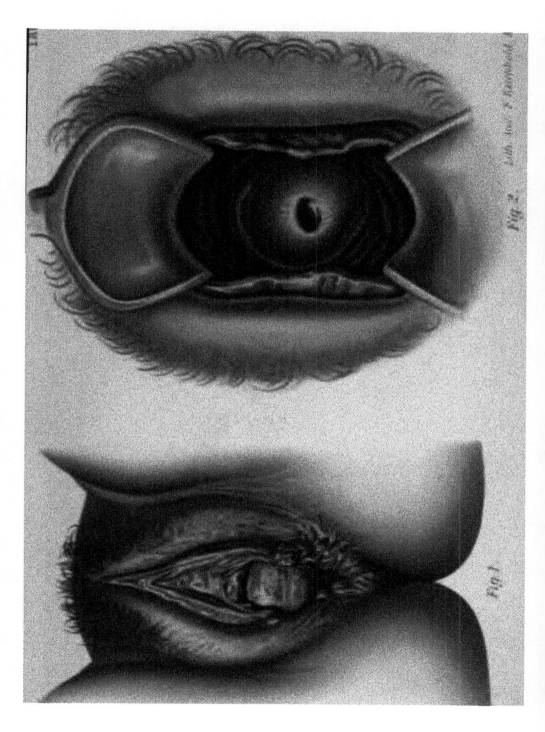

Fig. 1.

Fig. 2.

work for some time. When the genitalia are relaxed and the vagina threatens to invert, support the perineum with a T-bandage; on the eighth day of the puerperium a pessary may be introduced. Catarrh, constipation, and tumors are to be appropriately treated.

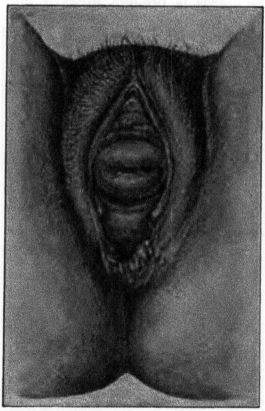

Fig. 26.—Incomplete prolapse of the uterus; inversion of the vagina from perineal tear of the third degree (into the rectum). The os is notched (photograph from original water-color).

If the prolapse is beyond the preventive stage, an apparently rational therapy—from our knowledge of the supports of the internal genitalia (based upon the author's experiments and those of Kimmel [1])—would be the

[1] Kimmel, Inaug. Dis., 1894, Heidelberg.

strengthening of the muscles of the pelvic floor by massage. This has, nevertheless, been followed by but few permanent results. At the present time it is better to treat these cases with the pessary or by operation.

The **operative treatment** is radical and sure. In retro-deviations the uterus is brought forward into its normal

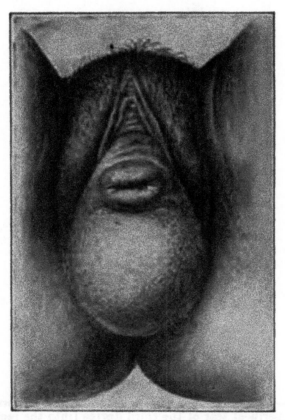

Fig. 27.—Complete prolapse of a retroflexed uterus, with rectocele. The os is notched (photograph from original water-color).

position by retrofixatio colli uteri, with or without opening of the recto-uterine pouch; by shortening the round ligaments, either in the inguinal canal or after an anterior colpotomy. By the latter route the broad ligaments may *be shortened* or a thickened uterus may be anteflexed by

excision of a wedge-shaped piece from its anterior wall.
After the menopause the uterus may be separated from the
bladder and stitched to the vagina or bladder (*vaginofixation* or *vesicofixation* of Dührssen, Mackenrodt). If the
organ is held by strong adhesions, or if the ligaments and

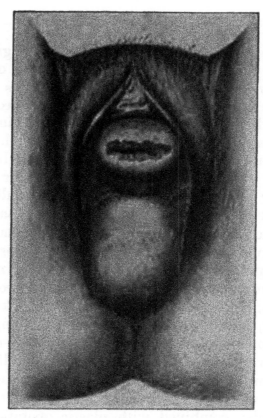

Fig. 28.—Complete prolapse of a retroflexed uterus; simple erosion,
without rectocele. (See Fig. 27.) (Photograph from original water-
color.)

vaginal walls are greatly relaxed, *ventrofixation* should be
performed; the best method is that of Czerny-Leopold,
which consists in stitching the uterine serosa (Sänger
stitches the round or broad ligament) directly to the
parietal peritoneum of the abdominal wall.

PLATE 8.

Complete Prolapse of an Anteflexed Uterus; Cystocele.
Ascertained by the introduction of the sound into the diverticulum
(note direction of sound ; latter held like a pen).   Excoriation of the
inverted mucous membrane.   (Original water-color.)

Retention is secured by narrowing the vagina and repairing the perineum ; *anterior colporrhaphy* of Sims, in
cystocele, by excising a portion of the mucous membrane
(shaped like a myrtle leaf) and bringing the edges of the
wound together ; [An oval denudation (Martin), reaching
from the meatus urinarius to the cervix, and closed by tier
sutures of catgut, to narrow the vagina and to leave a firm
support for the bladder, is the most popular method in
America for repairing the anterior vaginal wall.   Except
where great elongation of the anterior vaginal wall has
occurred, the purse-string operation of Stoltz has been dis-
carded, because it necessarily shortens the anterior vaginal
wall by approximating the meatus and cervix, and thus
tends to retrovert the uterus.—Ed.] *posterior colporrhaphy*
of G. Simon, Hegar, Bischoff, Martin, v. Winckel, Fritsch,
Neugebauer, Kehrer, either by excising a triangular piece
of mucous membrane, the base corresponding to the perineum, or by excising pieces of irregular outline and removing so much of the lateral wall that the posterior wall
is narrowed and the perineum raised.   Posterior colporrhaphy is also combined with plastic operations on the
perineum—*colpoperineauxesis* (Hegar, Kaltenbach) or *col-
poperineoplasty* (Bischoff).   [The anatomic and physiologic principles embraced by Emmet's colpoperineorrhaphy
have been so thoroughly appreciated by American surgeons that Emmet's operation is usually chosen to the
exclusion of all others.—Ed.]   These operations should be
most carefully planned and carried out.   The portions to
be excised are first outlined, then removed, the edges of the

Tab. 8.

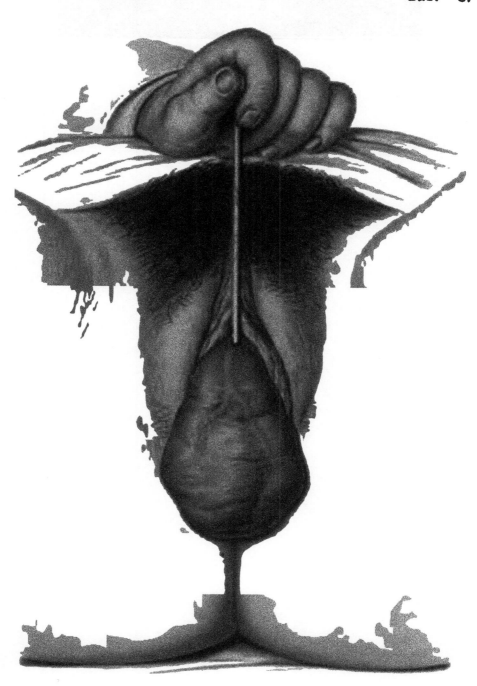

wound freely loosened up, and the sutures accurately placed.

Considerable experience is necessary to enable the operator to remove neither too much nor too little tissue. When the operation is completed, the vulva should not gape, and the vaginal walls should be well supported by

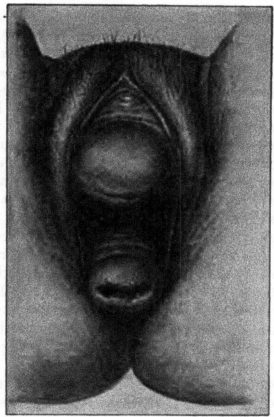

Fig. 29.—Complete prolapse of an anteflexed uterus; simple erosion. (See Plate 28.) (Photograph from original water-color.)

the new perineum. Buried catgut or fine silk may be used as suture material in the vagina; in the perineum, silkworm gut or silver wire is to be employed.

If an ectropion or an ulceration exists, the incision may be made to include this portion of the cervix. Not only

PLATE 9.

Extreme Inversion of the Vagina, with Cystocele and Incomplete Prolapse of the Retroverted Uterus. (Original water-color.) Density of the mucous membrane. Thickening of the vessels.

superficial parts of the mucous membrane, but also extensive wedges of muscular tissue (see Metritis), or conic pieces of the hypertrophied cervix, may be excised, and deep sutures of silk or silkworm gut may then be inserted.

The preparation of the patient and the after-treatment must receive as much care as the operation. Before the operation, laxatives, vagina well scrubbed out with antiseptics (three times, including the cervical mucosa), and the prolapse returned, are measures to be employed because the parts are then less vascular. After the operation, three weeks in bed; in the first days, liquid diet and a few drops of laudanum; removal of the perineal stitches at the end of the first week; if nonabsorbable sutures have been used in the vagina, they are taken out later. Vaginal irrigation, if discharge is fetid; laxatives, to avoid tension on the sutures.

If the uterus is so strongly adherent to the hernial sac that its reposition is impossible or can not be borne (in spite of massage and stretching and tearing the pseudo-ligaments), and the subjective disturbances are great, nothing remains but total extirpation (Kehrer).

If the operation is refused, **pessaries** and **rings** may be used for retentive purposes. Among these may be mentioned :

1. The round ring of Mayer (Plate 20, Fig. 3), when the lower part of the vagina is still narrow. It is harm-

PLATE 10.

Incomplete Prolapse of the Uterus; Simple Erosion; "Circular" Thickening of Cervix; Rectocele. (Original water-color *from a* case at the Heidelberg Frauenklinik.)

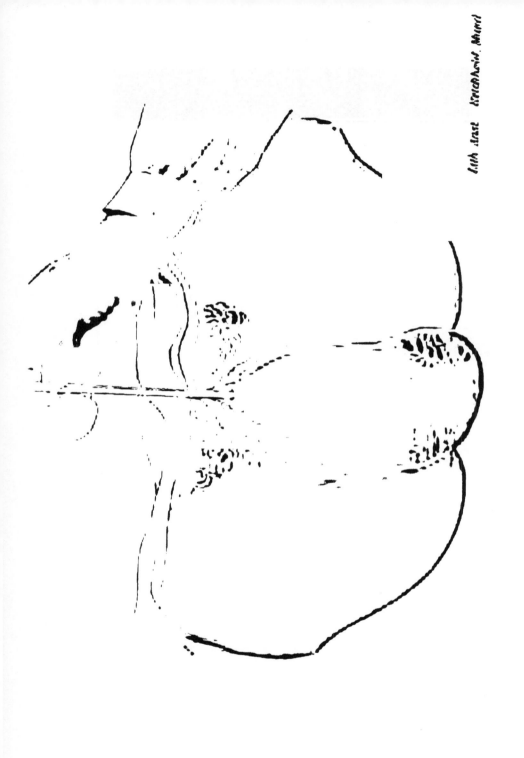

lith state Erichson. Munri

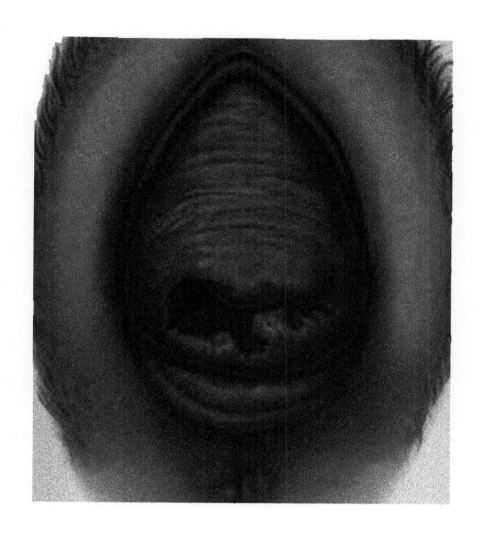

ful, inasmuch as it dilates the vagina. Those made of celluloid or hard rubber are better than the soft-rubber variety.

2. The B. S. Schultze sledge pessary (Figs. 32 and 33) corrects the retrodeviation of the uterus and allows a natural range of motion when the vagina is very large and relaxed. It is better for prolapsus than—

3. Schultze's 8-shaped pessary, which is so constructed that it is supported by the perineum. (Fig. 31.) It is of greatest utility when the introitus vaginæ is intact.

4. Hodge's lever pessary, especially applicable in inversion of the anterior vaginal wall (Plate 20, Fig. 4 ; Fig. 30), because it does not dilate the middle portion of the vagina, but puts it on the stretch.

5. The Zängerle-Martin stem-pessary (Plate 5, Fig. 3) rests upon the levator ani and is applicable in obstinately recurring prolapse, and roomy, relaxed genitalia. The old stemmed hysterophore is worthless, and is at best to be looked upon as a last resort, when the lower vagina is dilated.

The following two pessaries, on the contrary, are not sufficiently appreciated in practice :

6. Hewitt's cradle or clamp pessary (VI-shaped, a ring bent upon itself), and—

7. Breisky's egg-shaped pessary of hard rubber (especially Nos. 2 and 3), which are especially adapted to inoperable cases beyond the menopause. It is held in position by a T-bandage, and must be removed with forceps.

See Directions for the Application of Pessaries, §11.

The **reposition** of the prolapsed organ is accomplished with the patient in the dorsal position. The pressure upon the cervix acts in the direction of the vaginal axis, upward and backward, pushing back first the posterior vaginal wall, then the uterus, and lastly the anterior vaginal wall. Tampons (saturated in glycerin, renewed twice daily) retain the prolapse temporarily, the dorsal position being maintained. Breisky gave his patients a tampon-

PLATE 11.

Anteflexion of the Uterus in a Child. View of Douglas' pouch. (Original water-color, from cadaver.)

---

carrier, enabling them to introduce the tampons themselves.

As a supplement to the foregoing, **elevatio uteri** will now be considered. The uterus plays an entirely passive rôle in this change of position, as tumors of the organ itself, or of adjacent organs, or peritoneal residues, and pseudoligaments lift it wholly or partly above the pelvic inlet. (Plate 16, Fig. 1.)

The **diagnosis** and the **treatment** are the same as those of the causal affection. The former is often difficult, and as the condition is usually associated with structural changes, the organ becoming thinner and softer, the sound is to be used with caution. The uterus may be *pushed* up from below, or *drawn* up from above. The cervix often projects into the vagina as a mere cone. (Plate 7, Fig. 2.)

Tab. 11.

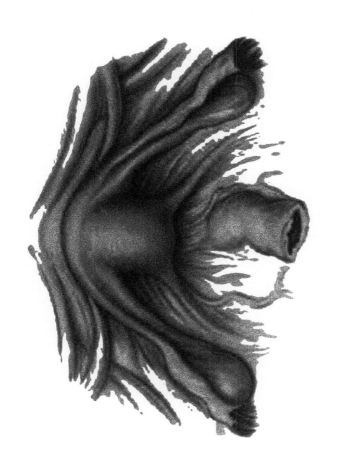

Lith. Anst. F. Reichhold. München.

CHAPTER III.

THE PATHOLOGIC POSITIONS, VERSIONS, AND FLEXIONS OF THE UTERUS.

Pathologic positions are displacements of the uterus *in toto*, the individual portions of the same holding their normal mutual relations. They may be forward, backward, or to one side. Versions are turnings of the uterus, as a whole, about an imaginary axis passing through the internal os. This axis may have a transverse or a sagittal direction. In the condition known as a flexion, on the contrary, the body of the uterus forms an angle with the cervix. These three forms may be observed in combination with one another or with a "high position." (Compare with Elevatio Uteri on p. 72.) Three degrees are differentiated, dependent upon whether the fundus is above, at the same level with, or below the external os.

§9. THE PATHOLOGIC POSITIONS OF THE UTERUS AND ITS ADNEXA.

The uterus as a whole may be displaced forward, backward, or to one side : antepositio, retropositio, and lateropositio (dextropositio and sinistropositio).

The displacement of the organ is a passive one, the most frequent cause being perimetritic or parametritic exudates. These may be either recent, tumor-like masses forcing the uterus away from them, or contracting bands of scar-like adhesions pulling the organ toward them. (Plates 44 and 45.) It can thus be seen that the uterus may be forced consecutively in two opposed directions at

73

PLATE 12.

Incomplete Prolapse of the Uterus; Elongation of the Intermediate Portion of the Neck with " Circular " Hypertrophy of the Vaginal Portion; Inversion of the Anterior Vaginal Wall; Cystocele. The posterior vaginal vault is almost at its normal height. (See Plate 4, Fig. 2.) (Original water-color from a specimen in the Munich Frauenklinik.)

---

different stages of the disease. (Plate 16, Figs. 1 and 2 ; Plate 17, Fig. 1 ; Plate 58, Fig. 2.)

Tumors act in the same manner. There may be tumors of the uterus itself (antepositio from a myoma of the posterior wall, Plate 58, 4), tumors of neighboring organs (Plate 59, 2 and 4, Ovarian Cystomata), or tumors of Douglas' pouch, especially those of the rectum and sacrum. Finally, excessive distention of adjacent organs may produce the same result. The bladder (Plate 17, 2, and Plate 14, 4), the rectum in cases of chronic constipation, and a pyosalpinx (Plate 59, 3) furnish examples.

A special variety of lateroposition is of a congenital and physiologic nature, brought about by unequal growth of the Müllerian ducts and their adnexa (tubes, ligamentum latum).[1] (See Fig. 2 in text.)

PLATE 13.

Artificial Prolapse for Operative Purposes, with the Arising Inversion of the Vagina and with Cystocele. The uterus first assumes a position of retroversion. Further traction directs the organ downward in the direction of the vaginal axis (see the dotted lines, which show the normal position of the uterus at the beginning and its subsequent stages of transition). The pathologic process proceeds in the same way. (Original diagrammatic sketch making partial use of a drawing of Beigel's.)

[1] In 130 postmortem specimens of adult female genitalia, I found the adnexa of the right side longer in 31.5% ; of the left side, in 27%.

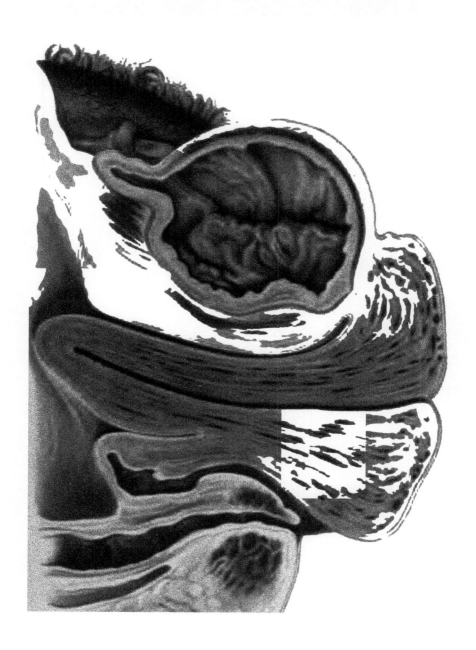

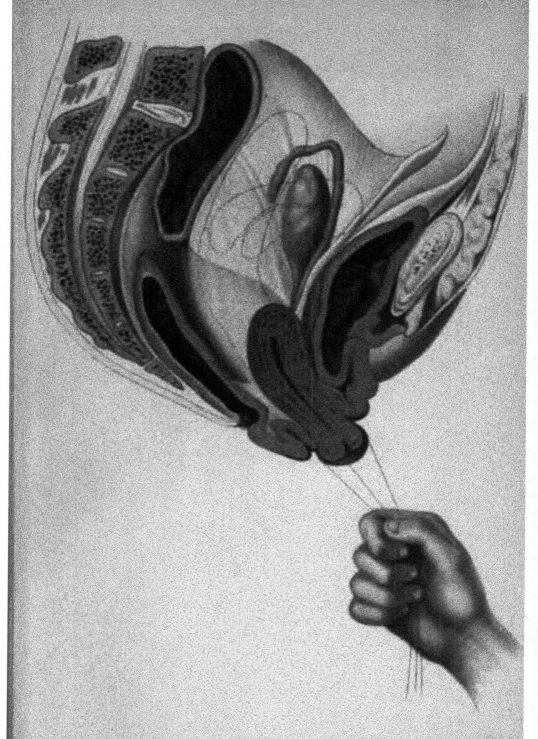

Tab. 13

Lith. Anst. F. Reichhold, Münch.

Diagnosis.—The presence or absence of a flexion is first determined bimanually, and then the cause of the displacement is ascertained. The changed position of the uterus is quite frequently combined with retroversion (Plate 17, 2), elevation (Plate 14, 4), or both (Plate 16, 1). Extra-uterine pregnancy must be excluded if tumors of the adnexa or of Douglas' pouch are present. The sound is to be employed only after the position of the body of the uterus has been accurately determined. It is clear from the foregoing that an exact differential diagnosis, especially of the tumors of Douglas' pouch (see p. 74), must be made. In uncomplicated changes of position both vaginal vaults retain their normal form and relations; the position of the vagina, on the contrary, is changed, its curve being lessened and its walls being placed under greater tension (anteriorly in antepositio).

The **treatment** consists in the removal of tumors and the extension of cicatricial bands by massage.

The **tubes and ovaries** are frequently displaced by inflammatory processes or through relaxation and congestion of their ligaments. The inflammatory virus (mostly gonococci, staphylococci, and streptococci) escapes from the abdominal ostium of the tube, and causes perimetritic, perisalpingitic, and perioophoritic exudations. Its contraction dislocates the movable adnexa, and agglutinates them with the intestine and with the serosa of Douglas' pouch. (Plates 44 and 45.) The process may cause the tubes to be bent at an acute angle. Ovariocolpocele and pyocolpocele have already been mentioned; they can, with or without the uterus, form the contents of almost any variety of abdominal hernia. (See § 6; § 7, Inversio Uteri Prolapsi; Plate 3, Fig. 2.)

The ovaries usually change their position with the uterus, and consequently displacements (one side or both) in all directions are encountered. Descent of the ovary, combined with retroversion of the uterus, is the most frequent one (Plate 19, Fig 1); the ovary may be palpated beneath the uterus. They may also be displaced by tumors that proceed from the ovary itself (with or without adhesion to adjacent viscera) or from neighboring organs. The normal position of the internal genitalia is described on page 57.

The **symptoms, diagnosis,** and **treatment** will be found in the chapter upon inflammation of these parts.

§ 10. THE ANTEVERSIONS AND ANTEFLEXIONS OF THE UTERUS.

Every anteversion or anteflexion is not pathologic. By pathologic anteflexions are meant only those that are permanent, and that are commonly associated with a lessened mobility of the corpus uteri. This lessened mobility may refer to its position in the pelvis or to the relation that it holds to the cervix. The latter is designated as a " rigid " angle of flexion if it has arisen from an inflammatory proliferation of connective tissue in an abnormally flexible organ. This variety of anteflexion was described in § 3 (3 and 4) as that of infantile and puerile uteri.

Etiology.—With the exception of the abnormally flexible infantile form, there is always some cause for the displacement outside of the uterus.

1. Cord-like residues of parametritic or perimetritic exudates are most common causes. The latter may either bind the corpus uteri down to the bladder or to the anterior pelvic wall (Plate 14, Fig. 4), or may fix the neck posteriorly (this being more frequent). Anteflexion results if traction is made upon a still flexible uterus by an adhesion of the posterior wall corresponding in position to that of the internal os. (Plate 15, Fig. 1.) It also follows fixation of the neck anteriorly, as shown in plate 15, figure 2 ; this is a rare occurrence, however.

2. Tumors likewise produce anteversions and anteflex*ions in different* ways : either by the pressing downward

and forward of tumors of other organs (ovarian cystomata), or by a myoma of the anterior uterine wall, which
can simulate a flexion (determine course of uterine canal
with sound, see Plate 14, Fig. 3), or by submucous
polyps, as shown in plate 15, figure 4. Anterior myomata cause anteversion or anteflexion, according to their
situation in the cervix or the corpus uteri.

3. The body of the uterus may likewise tip forward and
sink down, from an increase of its own weight (metritis,
hyperemia of menstruation, first weeks of pregnancy).

4. Küstner found marked congenital anteflexion of the
uterus in strong, vigorous children ; my experience confirms
this, and I have frequently been able to demonstrate, in
addition, a profuse secretion of glairy mucus in the cervical
canal and follicular cysts in the ovary.

Diagnosis.—Certain symptoms and objective signs,
mentioned in § 3 (3 and 4), are to be emphasized : Dysmenorrhea, sterility, constipation, and vesical disturbances
are not so frequently the result of mechanically changed
conditions (flexion at the internal os with stenosis, pressure
of the corpus uteri upon the bladder ; Plate 14, Fig. 2 ;
Plate 15, Fig. 3) as of endometritic and parametritic hyperemia and proliferation. Constipation, associated with
violent pain and digestive disturbances, and due to the
cicatricial contraction of pararectal exudates, is one of the
most constant concomitant phenomena. Catarrh of the
bladder is also quite frequent. Disturbances of innervation play a frequent and important rôle.

The pathologic character of the anteversion or anteflexion must be established : the lessened mobility of the
body of the uterus ; the neck, usually higher and bound
down posteriorly ; the cause of the fixation, commonly
parametritic masses of exudation about the cervix (Plate
59 ; Plate 61, Fig. 2), and its pararectal extensions. The
sound determines the direction of the cervical canal, and
the relation that the fundus holds to the long axis of the
neck is revealed by bimanual palpation.

PLATE 14.

Fig. 1.—**Anteversion of the Uterus.** Normal position, when the bladder is empty and the uterus is not bound down. The vagina passes in a normal manner from behind forward and from above downward.

Fig. 2.—**Anteversion of the Uterus** (pathologic, as the fundus is lower than the cervix). The os looks backward and upward. Cervix elevated. Bladder pressed upon.

Fig. 3.—**Myoma of the Anterior Uterine Wall Simulating an Anteflexion of the Second or Third Degree.** Differential diagnosis by the sound. Pressure on the bladder.

Fig. 4.—**Anteversion (or Anteflexion) of a Fixed Uterus (at the Same Time Retroposition from a Full Bladder).** The corpus uteri, bound down to the bladder, is elevated by the filling of the same ; when the angle of flexion is not rigid, extension of the uterine axis occurs.

Treatment.—The cause must be removed as far as possible. See sections on parametritis, perimetritis, metritis, myomata, and § 3 (3 and 4). The symptomatic treatment is that of the uterine catarrh (see endometritis), the pain (see parametritis and § 4, 8), the vesical disturbance (see cystitis), and the constipation. The latter must be dealt with energetically : tepid injections of water ($\frac{1}{4}$—$\frac{1}{2}$ of a liter), oil, or occasionally infusion of senna ; abdominal massage ; vegetable diet ; and medication by the mouth, commencing with the milder drugs. (See therapeutic table.) The intestinal tenesmus is treated with the same narcotics as those used for the parametritic pains and dysmenorrhea ; these are given in the form of suppositories or intestinal injections. Hydrotherapy is of value. During the inflammatory exacerbations and attacks of pain the patient must be kept in bed.

Contracting scars in the vaginal vault must be excised. (Plate 55, Fig. 1.) The treatment with the intra-uterine stem-pessary has been portrayed in § 3 (3 and 4). It is furthered by the introduction of the round ring of Mayer.

Tab. 14.

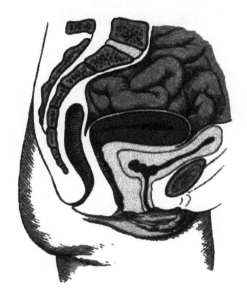

Fig. 1.

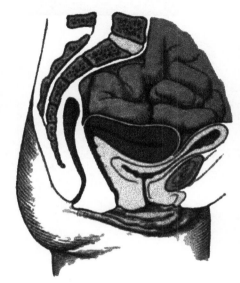

Fig. 2.

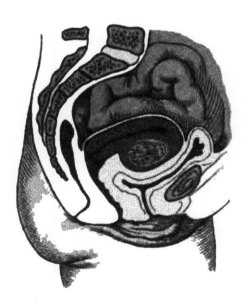

Fig. 3.

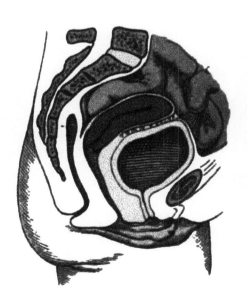

Fig. 4.

Lith. Anst. F. Reichhold. München.

Cicatricial bands situated high up are to be stretched or torn by massage.   (Plate 23.)

§ II. THE RETROVERSIONS AND RETROFLEXIONS OF THE UTERUS.

When the fundus uteri is placed vertically above the neck, or passes backward from it, and the condition is a permanent one, we speak of retroversion.   We consider that its different degrees, as well as those of retroflexion, are independent of the absolute height of the fundus.

Etiology.—Congenital retroversion, or a vertical position of the corpus uteri, is found in feebly developed organs.   Congenital retroflexions are likewise described (Saxtorph, C. Ruge, v. Winckel), and puerile retroflexions are more frequent than the later pathologic ones.   Von Winckel and Küstner explain that some of the latter arise from the former by the action of pernicious influences, as a habitually full bladder and premature excessive straining. The puerperium may have a similar effect, from the dorsal position and the relaxed uterine walls.

The puerperal process, however, operates in another manner, furnishing one of the most frequent causes : namely, inflammation in combination with injuries of the vaginal vault, and stretching, tearing, and relaxation of the genitalia.   (Fig. 3 of Plates 16 and 17.)

Weakened conditions, either general or local (chronic diseases, dyscrasias, postpartum subinvolution, neuropathies, masturbation), are also predisposing causes of relaxation.   In this group belong those cases of simple retroversion in which spasmodic flexion has been observed by the author.

The neck may be drawn anteriorly by contracting scars (Plate 15, Fig. 2 ; Plate 17, Fig. 4), pushed forward beneath the corpus uteri by tumors (chronic distention of the rectum, etc.), or the organ may be bound down to the rectum or posterior pelvic wall by perimetritic adhesions. (Plate 16, Figs. 1 and 2 ; Plate 38.)

PLATE 15.

Fig. 1.—**Anteflexion of the uterus of the second degree** (fundus uteri at same height as vaginal cervix) from posterior peri-metritic adhesions or contracting parametritic exudates of Douglas' folds at the level of the internal os. Gaping of external os. Pressure on the bladder. The pararectal adhesions produce pain and constipation.

Fig. 2.—**Anteflexion of the uterus of the first degree with the neck lying horizontally** (rare condition); the body drawn toward the bladder by parametritic adhesions; a vesical diverticulum is drawn toward the internal os. The corpus uteri is vertical. The os looks forward and a trifle upward. The vaginal vault is drawn anteriorly, so that the vaginal axis is vertical.

Fig. 3.—**Anteflexion of the Infantile Uterus with Stenosis of the Cervix and Internal Os ; Dysmenorrhea** (more frequent condition, see § 3, 3 and 4).

Fig. 4.—**Anteflexion of the uterus of the third degree** (fundus lower than the vaginal cervix), caused by a submucous uterine polyp (fibromyoma).

PLATE 16.

Fig. 1.—**Retroversion of a Fixed Uterus.** The uterus is verti-cal and is fixed by sacro-uterine and recto-uterine adhesions—the contracted and shortened uterine ligaments. Vagina put on the stretch by the elevation of the uterus.

In retroversions the chief causes for the deviation are changes in the ligaments ; in retroflexion, changes in the uterine parenchyma, together with changes in the ligaments. Retroversion easily passes into retroflexion. If the adnexa are not bound down in Douglas' pouch, they usually lie above the uterus and laterally.

Fig. 2.—**Retroflexion of a fixed uterus** (first degree, fundus higher than the cervix) ; uterus bound down throughout its entire length to serosa of Douglas' pouch by perimetritic adhesions. Cervix forced anteriorly, anterior lip thinned, the anterior cervical wall like-wise ; posterior lip thickened. Vagina thrown into folds by the descensus. Pressure of the intestines upon the uterus.

Fig. 3.—**Slight retroflexion and descent of the puerperal uterus from relaxation of the genitalia** (dorsal position, pressure

Tab. 15.

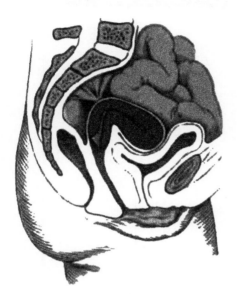

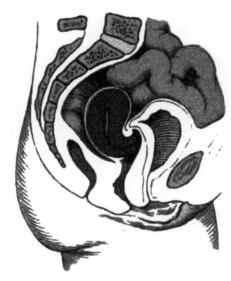

Fig. 1.

Fig. 2.

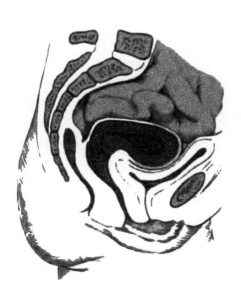

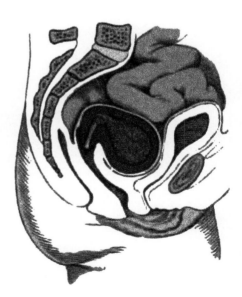

Fig. 3.

Fig. 4.

Tab. 16.

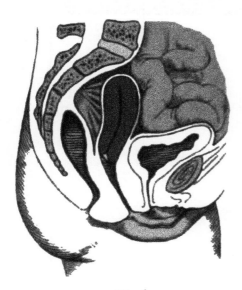

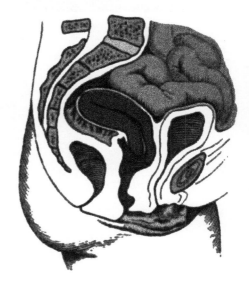

Fig.1.

Fig.2.

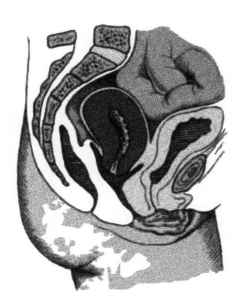

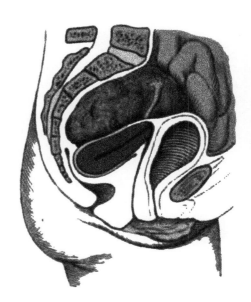

Fig.3.

Fig.4.

of the abdominal organs ; later, hard work, etc.). Puerperal metritis is very often the cause of subinvolution.

FIG. 4.—**Retroversion of the Uterus (Third Degree, Fundus Lower than the Cervix) from Pressure of an Ovarian Cyst.** The os is directed forward and upward. The vagina is vertical and extended. Pressure upon the rectum.

Uterine myomata (Plate 18, Figs. 1 and 2) or tumors of the vesico-uterine space pressing down from above may effect retroversion and retroflexion. (Plate 16, Fig. 4.) The dorsal position, a heavy, relaxed, puerperal uterus, and the weight of the intestines, usually combined with descensus uteri (Plate 16, Fig. 3), may bring about prolapse of a retroflexed uterus. (Plate 4 ; Figs. 27 and 28.)

Apart from primary inflammatory processes, secondary adhesions of the posterior serosa of an already retroverted uterus may also occur.

Symptoms.—Menorrhagia from hyperemia of inflammation or relaxation, and secondary proliferation of the mucosa as a result of the latter ; dysmenorrhea, partly as a result of the proliferative changes, partly from the mechanical obstruction of the flexion, and spasmodic uterine contraction ; catarrhal secretion ; sterility, less common than in anteflexion.

The pressure of the vaginal cervix produces urinary disturbances from angulations of the urethra and the ureters (Plate 19, Fig. 1), and the displacement also interferes with defecation (flattened, ribbon-like stools).

Reflex nervous disturbances appear,—not only those of digestion (vomiting with migraine, dyspepsia), but also those of the respiratory and circulatory organs (tachycardia, uterine cough, uterine asthma, neuralgia, etc.),—as well as a host of hysteric symptoms : convulsions, unconsciousness, hystero-epilepsy, cardialgia, paraplegia, aphonia, spasmodic cough, globus and clavus hystericus, and hypersensitiveness. Motor and sensory disturbances of the lower extremities (weakness, formication, cramps of

6

PLATE 17.

Fig. 1.—**Encapsulated Peritoneal Exudate in Douglas' Pouch. Descent and Anterior Position of a Fixed Uterus (Furrowed, Curved Vagina).** A circumscribed peritonitis, or a gravitating peritonitis from other abdominal organs, causes an accumulation of exudate in the recto-uterine space ; the overlying intestines roof in the culdesac, and by an adhesion of the serous surfaces an encapsulation of the pseudotumor is brought about. The uterus is adherent to the bladder as far as the fundus.

Fig. 2.—**Retroposition of the Uterus by a Full Bladder.** From its normal attachment to the bladder the uterus is at the same time elevated and the vagina extended. The uterine body is directly over the vagina, and their longitudinal axes correspond. This position predisposes to prolapsus uteri ; consequently, the frequent habit of the young of imperfectly emptying the bladder may help to bring about a descent of the uterus.

Fig. 3.—**Descent and Retroflexion of the Uterus of the First Degree, Brought About by Relaxation of the Folds of Douglas.** To be recognized by the low position of the vertically situated vaginal cervix and by the curvature of the vagina. These symptoms make up the picture of relaxation of the genitalia and their supporting apparatus (ligaments and pelvic floor), which predisposes to prolapse of the genitalia. The external os gapes—ectropion of relaxation.

Fig. 4.—**Retroflexion of the uterus of the first degree,** with a normally directed neck, caused by the contraction of parametritic adhesions that bind the latter to the bladder (see ₹ 11, Etiology). The weight of the intestines, combined with relaxation of the uterine wall, and the dorsal position (as in puerperium) force the body of the uterus backward.

---

gastrocnemius) are also observed. They are due to reflex action, pressure, or inflammation.

Diagnosis.—By bimanual examination, after vaginal palpation and inspection have shown the anterior cervical lip to be thinned and shortened, the posterior lip thickened, and the os directed toward the symphysis. The body of the uterus is palpated either by allowing the abdominal hand to sink into the pouch of Douglas or from

Tab. 17.

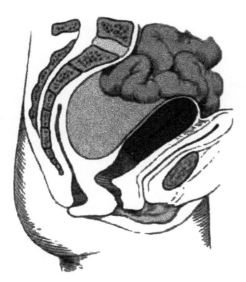

Fig. 1.

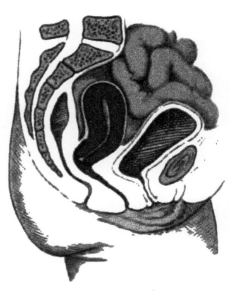

Fig. 2.

Fig. 3.

Fig. 4.

Lith. Anst F. Reichhold. Mü

the rectum. The presence or absence of adhesions must be determined.

Treatment.—The manual treatment of the retrodeviations is fully demonstrated in plates 21 and 22. By this method a freely movable uterus may be replaced : *i. e.*, its body laid upon the anterior vaginal vault. Massage may be instituted if the organ is bound down by adhesions (Thure Brandt, Plate 23), the latter being forcibly torn if necessary ; or the contractile elements of the uterus, of its ligaments, and of its vessels, may be stimulated.

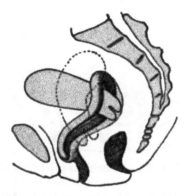 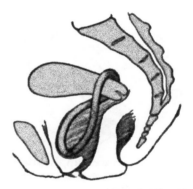

Fig. 30.—Hodge's lever pessary in retroflexion of the uterus, first degree. It effects a normal position chiefly by causing tension of the posterior vaginal vault.

Fig. 31.—Schultze's 8-shaped pessary fixes the cervix in normal position ; it is supported by the vaginal wall and the pelvic floor.

If the free uterus can not be replaced by this method, the bullet forceps of Küstner is used, or the sound is cautiously employed. (See explanation to Figs. 1 and 2, Plate 20.)

When the uterus is brought back into its normal position, a lever-pessary is introduced as a retentive measure. (See Figs. 30–33.) Cold douches to the cervix and sacrum, alternate hot and cold vaginal douches, ergotin subcutaneously, and tamponade to strengthen the uterine walls and their ligaments are useful adjuvants.

The **lever-pessaries** are tried in the following order:

1. The S-shaped Hodge pessary (rather sharply curved), when the sacro-uterine ligaments are not sensitive.

2. The 8-shaped Schultze pessary, when the pelvic floor is normal and the vagina is not too relaxed. Sometimes the instrument must be quite long.

3. The sledge-shaped pessary of Schultze, when the vagina is relaxed or the pelvic floor is defective.

4. Hewitt's clamp pessary. (See p. 71.)

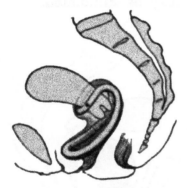

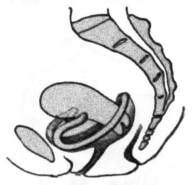

Fig. 32.—Rarer application of Schultze's sledge-pessary with firm pelvic floor.

Fig. 33.—Usual application of Schultze's sledge-pessary. It is supported by the vaginal wall and the symphysis. The cervix is fixed between the anterior and the posterior bar. Employed in retroflexed descended uterus.

Directions for the Application of Pessaries.—The appropriate pessary is to be introduced with the patient in the dorsal or knee-elbow position, and the vagina should be held open by a duck-bill speculum, allowing the uterus and adnexa to fall forward.

1. The round, flexible caoutchouc ring of Mayer is compressed with the fingers or the Fritsch forceps (Plate 20, Fig. 2), introduced beyond the constrictor vaginæ, and placed so that the cervix rests within its opening, which should not be too small. The ring should slightly dilate the vagina.

2. The S-shaped pessary of Hodge and the more curved one of Thomas with a bulbous enlargement of the upper bar (made of hard rubber or celluloid, rendered flexible by hot water, or of copper wire covered with caoutchouc) are introduced into the vagina in the sagittal plane. (Plate 20, Fig. 4.) When the pessary is above the constrictor vaginæ, it is rotated 90 degrees, so that the upper and broader bar comes to lie in the posterior vaginal vault, as shown in figure 30.

It acts as follows: The broad posterior bar lifts the uterus and pries it anteriorly; the cervix is drawn posteriorly by the longitudinal and transverse traction upon the vagina, and especially upon the uterosacral ligaments. From the new position of the cervix and from the pressure of the intestines upon the posterior uterine surface the uterus rests firmly upon the posterior vaginal wall; the descent of the organ and the accompanying disturbances consequently cease, even if the retrodeviation is not wholly removed. The tension upon the sacro-uterine ligaments resulting from the descent is relieved by the transverse tension and elevation of the vaginal vault. In married women the simple curved pessary, allowing of cohabitation, is the more applicable, the lower bar resting upon the pubic symphysis. Should this render the emptying of the bladder difficult, it may be provided with a curve (concave anteriorly). If the upper bar makes the vaginal vault too tense, it should be bent backward.

3. The 8-shaped Schultze pessary is inserted with its smaller half about the cervix. (See Fig. 31.) It is made of hard rubber or of copper wire covered with caoutchouc, and rests upon the pelvic floor.

4. The sledge-shaped pessary of Schultze is so introduced that the longer bar lies above and behind the cervix, the shorter bar being in front. (Fig. 33.) The shorter curvature rests against the pubic symphysis. This pessary is used instead of the 8-shaped one when the pelvic floor is relaxed. If the vagina is too roomy, the longer bar is

PLATE 18.

Fig. 1.—**Retroversion of the Uterus from Two Intramural Myomata.** By palpation, the condition simulates a retroflexion of the second degree. The sound demonstrates the course of the uterine canal, and consequently the true condition. External os directed anteriorly. Rectum pressed upon; constipation; Douglas' pouch filled up. Urinary disturbances also ensue.

Fig. 2.—**Transition from Retroversion to Retroflexion of the Uterus from an Intramural Myoma of the Anterior Wall.**

Fig. 3.—**Retroflexion of the Uterus of the Third Degree (Fundus at the Height of the Cervix).** Descent of the uterus recognized by the folding of the vaginal wall (the os is below the interspinous plane also). Pressure upon the rectum. The os looks anteriorly. The uterine body fills the pouch of Douglas. Thickening of the posterior uterine wall and lip; thinning of the anterior one.

Fig. 4.—**Retroflexion of the Uterus of the Third Degree (Fundus Lower than the Cervix).** Inveterate case; os looks anteriorly, gapes widely (ectropion); anterior wall of the neck and lip of the os thinned. High position of the cervix; extended, vertical vagina. Douglas' pouch filled by the uterine body.

PLATE 19.

Fig. 1.—**Retroversion of the Uterus; Vaginal Ovariocele.** Angulation and dilatation of the ureters. Vertical position of the vagina. (See §§ 7 and 11.)

Fig. 2.—**Bimanual Examination from the Rectum of a Case of Cord-like Total Atresia of the Vagina with a Rudimentary Solid Uterus.** During cohabitation the immissio penis has taken place into the urethra—probably congenitally funnel-shaped—and dilated it as far as the internal sphincter. The palpating finger can be pushed into the bladder without difficulty, and its withdrawal is followed by a quantity of urine. A slight incontinence exists. (Original diagrammatic drawing from a case.)

Tab. 18.

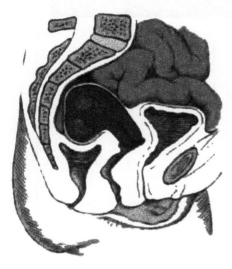

Fig. 1.

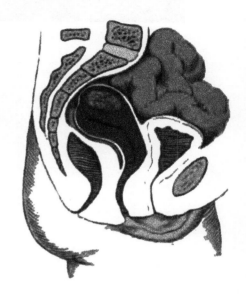

Fig. 2.

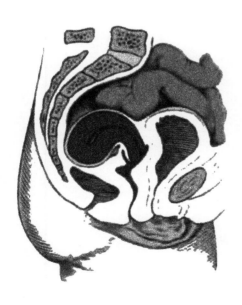

Fig. 3.

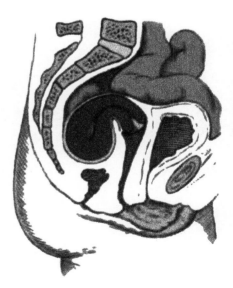

Fig. 4.

Lith. Anst. F. Reichhold. Mü

Tab. 19.

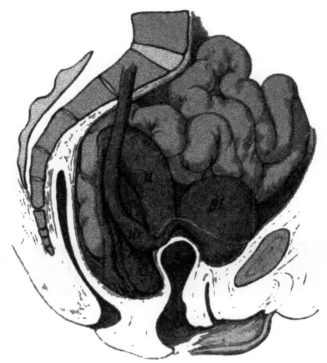

Fig. 1.

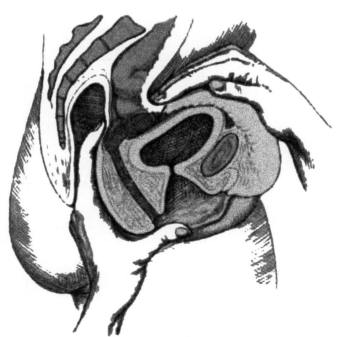

Fig. 2.

Lith. Anst F. Reichhold, Munche

brought forward and used as a support, while the smaller
one holds the cervix in its concavity. Material same as
preceding : the 8-shaped pessary is made of rings from 8½
to 19 cm., the sledge-shaped of rings from 10½ to 14 cm.,
in diameter (from 7 to 10 mm. thick).

A ring is in good position if its lower end is not visible
at the vulva ; if it does not threaten to fall out ; if it does
not overdilate the vagina, but may be easily rotated on its
longitudinal axis ; if the upper half of the vagina is rendered moderately tense ; finally, if the fundus uteri is anterior and the cervix posterior, since otherwise the folds
of Douglas are not relaxed.

If the foregoing conditions are complied with, the disturbances soon disappear. In only one-fifth of the cases
is a really permanent cure obtained, so that the uterus
remains anteriorly without support.

Disadvantages.—If the ring is improperly constructed
(uneven, too large, too thin, or made of wool, hair, leather),
or remains in position too long, it excites hypersecretion,
ulcerations, and abscesses. Fistulous tracts communicat-
ing with neighboring organs may result. Even with a pessary made of good material, I have seen this occur after
the menopause. If the ulcers cicatrize, embedding the
ring, or if the latter becomes incrusted with phosphates
from the secretions or with dried masses of mucus and
blood, it is difficult to remove the instrument. After removal of the wall of granulations the ring is to be seized
with dressing forceps and extracted by rotatory movements. It is sometimes necessary first to break it *in situ*.

To obviate these difficulties the ring should be removed
and cleaned after each period, although a pessary may
remain in the healthy genitalia for two or three months
without harmful results. Repeated vaginal irrigations of
nonirritating fluids must be made : daily, if leukorrhea
exists.

The ring is to be immediately removed upon the appearance of pain.

PLATE 20.

FIG. 1.—Reposition of a Retroverted Uterus by Means of Küstner's Bullet Forceps. The uterus is first brought into the vertical position by traction ; the cervix is then pushed backward, and the fundus uteri, if freely movable, comes forward.

FIG. 2.—Reposition of a Retroverted Uterus by Means of the Sound. The latter is introduced with its concavity directed anteriorly, and is pushed in until its knobbed end has passed the internal os. The concavity is now turned posteriorly, corresponding to the pathologic course of the uterine axis. If 5 or 6 cm. of the sound have passed into the uterus, its knobbed end lies in the fundus. The curvature of the sound is now cautiously (!) rotated anteriorly, the handle of the sound being depressed at the same time.

FIG. 3.—Introduction of the Elastic Ring of Mayer by Means of Fritsch's Forceps. The ring should lie about the cervix.

FIG. 4.—Introduction of Hodge's Pessary. This is bent into the shape of an S, as shown in the adjacent figure (Thomas' pessary is still more sharply bent at the upper bar). (See Fig. 30.)

It is very important to determine whether the displacement or its complications cause the existing trouble, or whether hysteria alone exists.

The inflammations of the bladder, endometrium, and perimetrium are to be treated in the usual manner. If adhesions render the reposition impossible, the condition is made bearable by firm tamponade of the posterior vaginal vault with glycerin tampons.

If pregnancy occurs, the pessary is allowed to remain until the fifth month ; the retroflexed gravid uterus is to be similarly controlled in order to prevent incarceration beneath the sacral promontory.

Operative measures are adopted, partly to dispose of very resistant adhesions, which usually elevate the uterus considerably, partly to fix the organ anteriorly, either by celiotomy or per vaginam.

If the uterus is freely movable [Alexander's operation.—

Tab. 20.

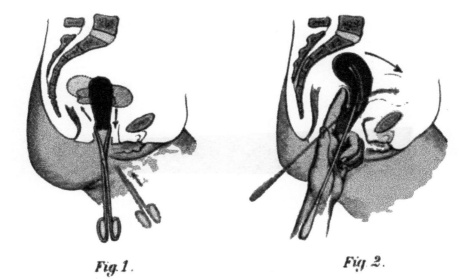

Fig. 1.

Fig. 2.

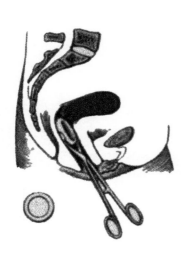
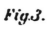
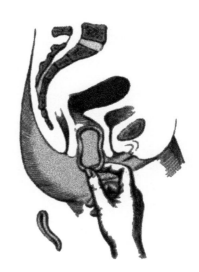

Fig. 3.

Fig 4.

ED.], retrofixatio colli or vaginofixation is indicated; if it is markedly adherent, ventrofixation (suspensio uteri) is to be performed. (See p. 67.)

The Applicability of Pessaries with Respect to Certain Complications of Retroversion.

1. Retro-uterine Adhesions.—These are to be slowly stretched by massage three or four times for at least twelve sittings. First elevate in retroposition, to stretch or tear the adhesions, then anteflex the uterus, introduce a ring, and keep the patient in bed with an ice-bag upon the hypogastrium (remember the possible production of a hematocele l). The tamponude of the posterior vaginal vault is a palliative measure.

2. Chronic perimetritis furnishes a *noli me tangere;* it must be cured first (absorption cure).

3. Parametritic bands and scars from lacerations (Plate 55, Fig. 1) are excised, the longer diameter of the denudation being transverse, and the edges are so brought together that the row of sutures is in the longitudinal axis of the vagina, producing an elongation of the same (Martin).

4. Chronic Metritis.—This is to be treated first by wedge-shaped excisions, and then a pessary is to be applied; if the pessary is not well borne, glycerin tampons. In acute metritis antiphlogistic treatment until the pain has disappeared.

5. Endometritis.—This will require astringent and antiseptic vaginal douches twice daily; the pessary should be frequently removed; treat the uterus by cauterization, intra-uterine irrigation and medication, atmocausis, etc. Erosions of the os are to be cauterized or excised.

6. A stenosis of the cervix is to be dilated or incised.

7. If the cervix is too short, it exerts insufficient leverage upon the body, which becomes flexed, or the cervix slips away from the ring and displacement occurs; reversed introduction of the Hodge pessary with the upper bar posterior is recommended.

PLATES 21 AND 22.

Manual Reposition of a Retroflexed Uterus (First and Second Degrees). First step: The body of the uterus is palpated from the posterior vaginal vault by the index and middle fingers. Second step : While these two fingers push the organ upward, the other hand covers in the pelvic inlet, passes behind the uterus, and presses down along its posterior surface until (third step) it touches the fingers in the vagina. In this manner the uterus is held from above, and is hindered from slipping backward. Fourth step : The fingers in the vagina may now leave the posterior vaginal vault and push the cervix upward, while the external hand presses the fundus toward the apex of the bladder, thus forcing the uterus into its normal position. The position of the adnexa may be determined by analogous steps. The abdominal walls should be relaxed (full bath if necessary), and the limbs should be flexed at an angle of 60 degrees. The tubes are felt as round cords ; the ovaries (which can not be fixed) as bodies of the size of an almond. The ovaries lie 2 or 3 cm. laterally and behind the uterus, on the inner margins of the psoas muscles. The healthy ovaries exhibit a characteristic sensitiveness to pressure.

---

8. The anterior vaginal wall being too short, it may be lengthened by the operation mentioned under 3 (Skutsch).

9. The abnormally roomy, relaxed vagina is to be narrowed by colporrhaphy ; if not permitted reversed application of the sledge-pessary, as in figure 32.

10. The puerperium is an appropriate time for the treatment of the organs and ligaments, which at this period are capable of being modeled and stretched. Replace by the method of Schultze—pushing back the cervix, elevating

---

PLATE 23.

Massage (Thure Brandt). By steps similar to those shown in plates 21 and 22 the finger-tips meet behind the retroverted uterus and rub and stretch the adhesions between the latter and the rectum. At first the blood supply of the adhesions is increased ; they become softer and more easily stretched. The uterus is finally "lifted " (Fig. 2) in order to lengthen the parametritic bands.

Tab. 2

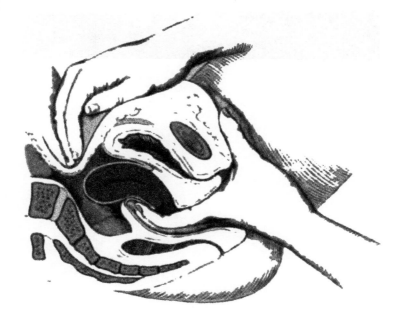

Fig. 2

Fig. 1

Lith. Anst F. Reichhold.

Tab. 22.

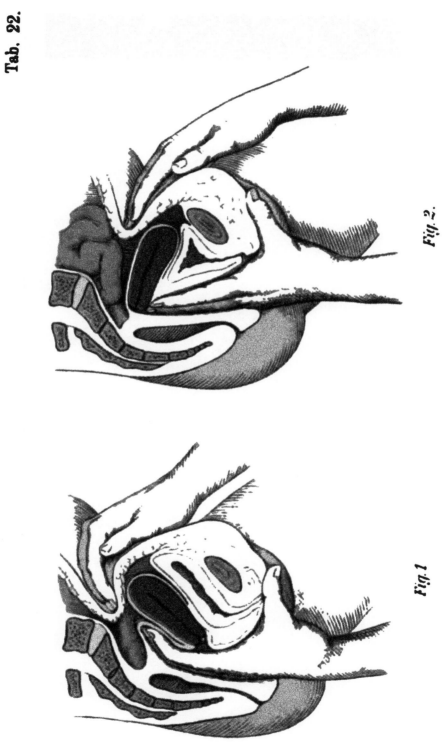

Fig. 2.

Fig. 1

Lith. Anst. v. Reichhold, München.

Tab. 23.

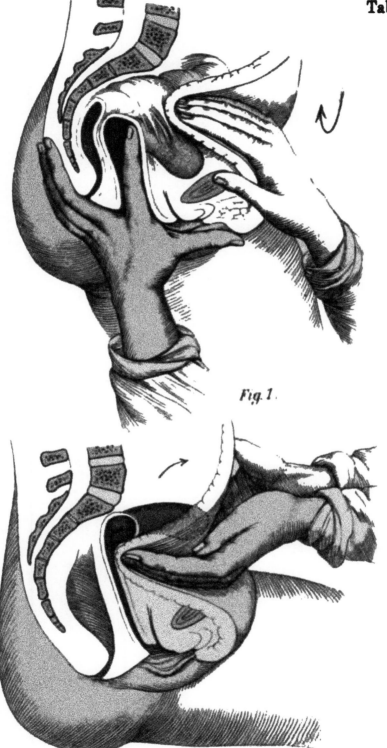

Fig. 1.

Fig. 2.

Lith. Anst. v. Reichhold. München

Tab. 28.

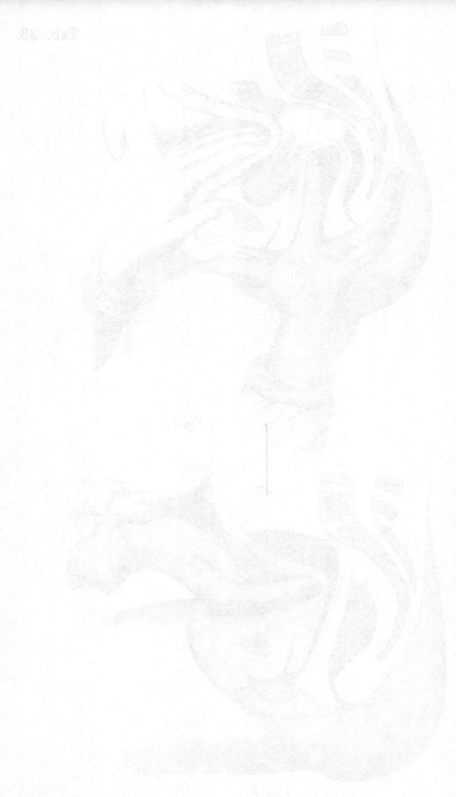

the fundus, and thus causing the body to spring forward. Retention is maintained by two glycerin tampons placed transversely in the anterior, or, at other times, the posterior, vaginal vault. Enforced lateral position.

During pregnancy it is necessary for the ring to remain only until the fifth month, because the uterus then holds itself in proper position from its increased size.

11. In *narrowing of the introitus vaginæ* (stenosis of the hymen, vaginismus) operative measures are to be adopted and a ring is to be introduced.

12. The combination of perineal defect with vaginal inversions and prolapsed uterus is to be treated by operation; otherwise, the sledge-pessary.

13. *Tumors* and *senility* are contraindications.

14. If the ring is in good position and the patient still complains, it is to be removed and another cause for the disturbances (hysteria) sought.

Torsion of the uterus is a pathologic turning of the uterus about its longitudinal axis, caused by tumors or abnormal distention of neighboring organs, or by parametritic or perimetritic fixations. (Plates 44 and 45.) It is usually combined with other displacements. The vaginal cervix shows the effect of the torsion. (Plate 55.)

There is a **physiologic torsion** (cause of the first vertex position), since the anterior surface of the uterus, usually in dextropositio, is turned toward the right, and the left margin approaches the symphysis (the child consequently has more room for its back on the left side than on the right, which is narrowed by the spinal column).

PLATE 24.

FIG. 1.—**Gonorrhea.** Papilloma of the hyperemic cervix; purulent discharge (from Mraçek).

FIG. 2.—**Gonorrheal Cervicitis.** Bloody discharge. Erosio simplex. (Original water-color.)

FIG. 3.—**Gonococci and Pus-corpuscles.**

(Plate 24, 3.) The vulva and the vestibule are covered with thick, yellow, creamy pus, which wells out of the vagina upon separation of the labia. As the disease progresses the discharge becomes more fluid, but remains yellow. (Plates 24 and 27.) The parts are swollen, strikingly red, and sensitive. If the finger is introduced into the vagina and stroking movements are made against the pubic symphysis, pus can be stripped from the urethra. (Plate 25.) Urination causes marked ardor urinæ followed by vesical tenesmus; every quarter or half hour the desire to urinate returns; the emptying of the bladder never seems complete. The symptoms of vesical catarrh present themselves; the urine becomes cloudy and has a pungent ammoniacal odor (neutral or even alkaline reaction).

Bartholin's glands do not become inflamed until a later period (Plates 25 and 26), and in comparatively rare cases proliferation of the papillæ of the skin occurs (condylomata acuminata). (Plate 24, Fig. 1.)

The vaginal mucosa is likewise inflamed, sensitive, and dotted with red points, corresponding to the hyperemic papillæ. The greater portion of the purulent secretion does not come from the vagina (which has no glands), but from the cervix, which becomes infected at the same time. (Plate 24, 2.) The swollen cervical mucosa is deep red and protrudes at the external os; a cervical endometritis consequently exists. At first the process stops at the internal os.

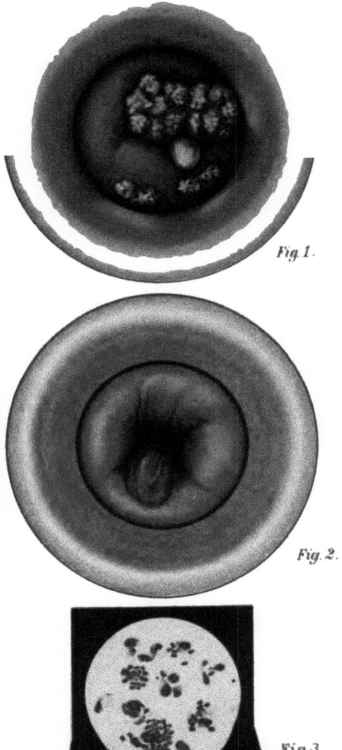

Fig. 1.

Fig. 2.

Fig. 3.

Lith. Anst. K. Kreichbold. München

Gonorrheal vaginitis, properly speaking, is a more chronic process and occurs only in children.

A different course is taken by infection from a **latent gonorrhea** (gleet of the male, *goutte militaire,* consisting of a very short stricture of the pars membranacea with a painless, scanty secretion, especially noticeable as the "morning drop"; rarely, sensitiveness of the urethra and epididymis; during sexual excitement darting pains at the root of the penis). A creeping inflammation arises, the first symptoms of which (ardor urinæ and discharge) are usually overlooked. The disturbance becomes more marked as the process invades the mucous membrane of the body of the uterus.

In this situation both forms of the disease pursue a similar course.

Endometritis of the body of the uterus causes irregularities of menstruation, the various pathologic varieties alternating (see §4); at the same time, as a result of the inflammatory hyperemia of the uterus, a sensation of a heavy body—of a fullness in the pelvis—presents itself; later, there is actual uterine pain. These pains, however, may also proceed from inflammations of the tubes, as the cocci quickly invade the latter from the uterine cavity.

Here the process halts for a second time, and the latent gonorrhea may remain stationary, just as the acute form does at the internal os. The gonococci may, however, penetrate into the myometrium, or may gain access to the blood and set up new areas of infection, especially in the joints. The gonorrhea becomes a lurking chronic inflammation with a dubious prognosis. The discharge is increased and purulent.

Frequently the inflammation does not extend to the peritoneum from the tube because the isthmus or the fimbriated extremity of the latter becomes agglutinated. In this way a closed sac is formed, which becomes filled with pus—a **pyosalpinx.**

PLATE 25.

Bartholinitis Dextra Gonorrhœica. Perforation of the abscess on the inner surface of the nymphæ; urethritis; relaxation of the vaginal walls. (Original water-color.)

If the peritoneum is affected, it occurs in one of two ways: either through the tissues of the tubal wall by means of its lymphatic paths, or by continuity of structure, creeping out upon the peritoneum and ovary. The latter may likewise be infected by means of the lymphatics or from the peritoneum.

Painful, chronic, circumscribed inflammations of the serosa of Douglas' pouch arise—**perimetrosalpingitis** and **perimetro-oophoritis.** Interstitial inflammation of the ovary may terminate in abscess. These changes are accompanied by attacks of fever and considerable pain, and lead to serofibrinous exudates in the recto-uterine space, which subsequently form adhesions between the serous surfaces of the pelvic organs. These are responsible for the manifold displacements and anomalies of position of the uterus, its adnexa, the intestinal coils, and the rectum.

The disease of the tubes (it is usually bilateral) is the cause of a new symptom—sterility (one-child marriages).

It is worthy of note that the gonococci prepare the way for the pus cocci, so that in the later stages we have to do with a mixed infection.

Symptoms.—Ardor urinæ (finally vesical catarrh and bartholinitis, the former being recognized by the cloudy, alkaline urine containing crystals of triple phosphate and acid urate of ammonium, numerous micrococci, and mucus-, pus-, and blood-corpuscles; the latter, by the increased

---

PLATE 26.

Bartholinitis Sinistra Gonorrhœica. Abscess formation (from Mraçek).

Tab. 25.

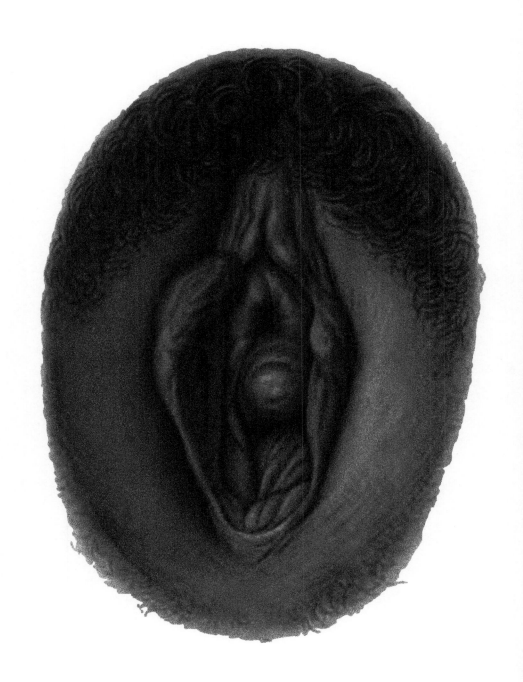

Schmidt

Lith. Anst. v. Reichhold München

tenderness, redness, swelling, and finally fluctuation at the lower third of the labia majora, see Plates 25 and 26); purulent discharge from the vagina, irregularities of menstruation, pain, and sterility.

Diagnosis.—Demonstration of the gonococci (by staining for half a minute in an effective alcoholic solution of methylene-blue—see Plate 24, Fig. 3; it is the only coccus decolorized by Gram's method; above all, it is found *within* the pus-cells); a general or punctiform reddening of the vagina; the pus is seen to come from the cervix; pain is localized in the uterus, adnexa, or peritoneum of Douglas' pouch.

Treatment.—In fresh cases with colpitis alone: Vaginal irrigations with a 5% solution of protargol (five times daily for two weeks, then twice daily with potassium permanganate); keep the parts clean, especially the vulva (cervicitis is usually present, however). Dilatation of the cervical canal by means of metal dilators, after having carefully disinfected it and the vagina by means of antiseptic solutions; intra-uterine irrigation with two liters of a 0.5% to 2.5% (even 5%) solution of protargol (increase the strength gradually for two or three weeks). Following this, the introduction of 5% to 10% protargol salve or bougies, wiping out the vagina with a 10% protargol solution and gauze tamponade with protargol salve or protargol glycerin. In the third week of this treatment the application of astringents to remove the remaining swelling of the mucous membrane mentioned on page 93: Aluminum acetate solution (2 to 5%), bismuth subnitrate (2 to 3%). This treatment is to be carried out with caution, the patient being kept at absolute rest in bed for the greater part of its duration, to prevent the disease from spreading to the adnexa. It is based upon Neisser's recommendation of the silver albuminates (especially protargol) as specifics.

If for any reason this treatment can not be properly carried out, we must return to the earlier method of treat-

7

PLATE 27.

Gonorrheal Vulvitis and Vaginitis. Old perineal tear of first degree ; external hemorrhoids ; intertrigo. (Original water-color.)

PLATE 28.

FIG. 1.—**The Microscopic Structure of the Parts of the Vulva.** (1) Stratified squamous epithelium with the excretory ducts (2) of the numerous sebaceous glands of the labium majus, whose connective tissue (3) is sparingly supplied with blood-vessels. (4) Stratified squamous epithelium of the nymphæ (still without sebaceous glands in the fetus), covering numerous connective-tissue papillæ ; the cavernous tissue is traversed by numerous capillaries, which form a mass of erectile tissue at (6). This is surrounded by dense bundles of fibers receiving their blood supply from (10) and passing to the outer lamella (8) of the hymen, the squamous epithelium (9) of which is likewise stratified. The inner lamella of the hymen is composed of bundles of fibers and vessels, which come from the vagina (12). (Original drawing from a specimen obtained from a newly born girl.)

FIG. 2.—**Longitudinal Section Through the Cervix in a Case of Old Prolapse of the Uterus.** The stratified squamous epithelium of the cervix shows a superficial horny degeneration. The transition from the squamous epithelium of the outer wall of the cervix to the cylindric epithelium of the cervical canal is seen at (3). Its displacement inward is due to the slight ectropion of the lips of the os. The stasis of the blood and lymph in prolapsed uteri is apparent from the dilated vessels (4). (Original drawing.) (See Plates 10 and 12.)

FIG. 3.—**Simple, Papillary, and Follicular Erosion of the Cervix.** (Original drawing combined from different specimens.) At the left are seen the intact stratified squamous epithelium of the vaginal cervix ; this is continuous with cylindric epithelium, which is formed by the cuboid cells of the matrix after desquamation of the squamous epithelium has occurred (erosio simplex). Further to the right are seen papillary elevations with cylindric epithelium (erosio papilloides). Glandular follicles showing cystic dilatation from retained mucus, or filled with exudation, are seen in the inflamed connective tissue, which is traversed by dilated vessels with round cells (erosio follicularis). Some muscle-fibers are above and to the left. (See Plate 29, Fig. 4 ; Plates 33, 35, and 37 ; Plate 60, Fig. 2 ; and Plate 90, Fig. 1.)

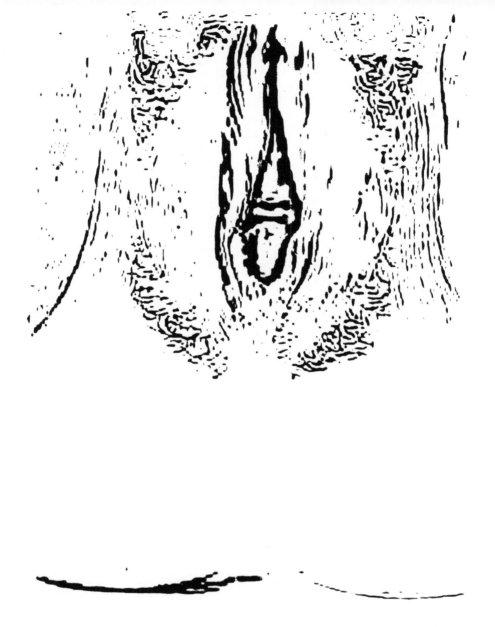

K. Retchfield.

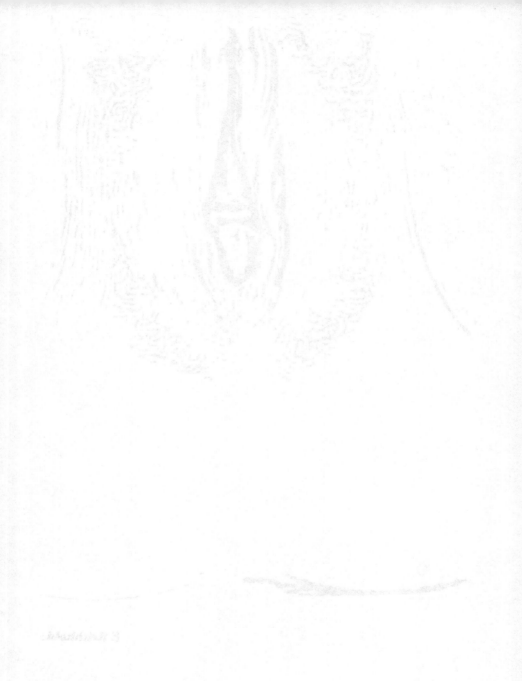

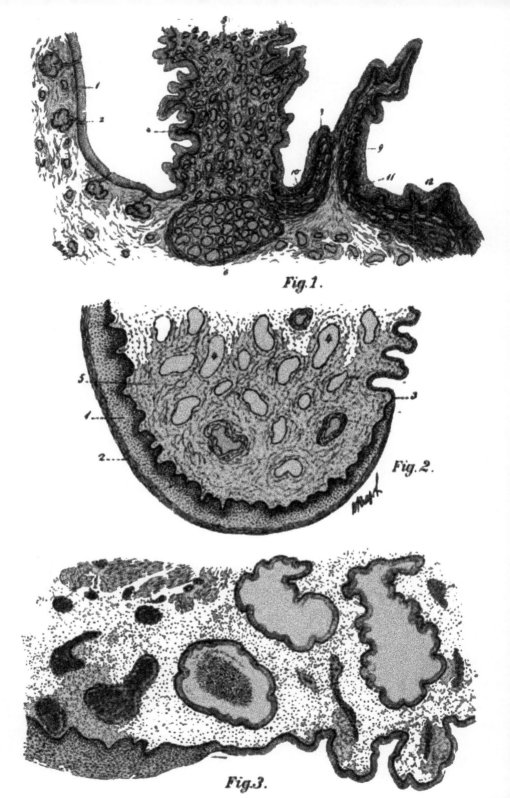

Fig. 1.

Fig. 2.

Fig. 3.

Lith. Anst. F. Reichhold, München

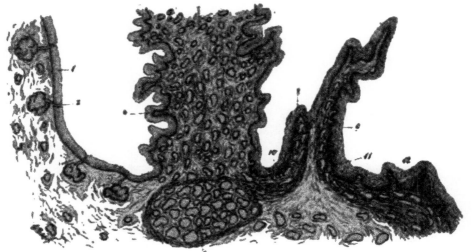

Fig. 1.

Fig. 2.

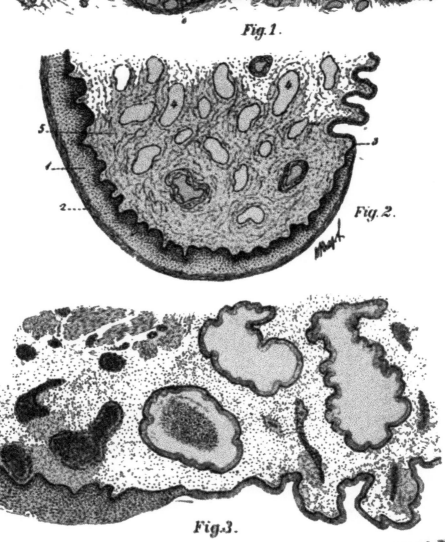

Fig. 3.

Lith. Anst. F. Reichhold.

ment : let the cervix alone, wash away the secretions several times daily with 2 or 3 liters of solutions of silver nitrate, potassium permanganate (bright red), bichlorid of mercury (1 : 2000 to 1 : 4000), the patient being in the recumbent posture ; wipe out the vagina several times a week and pack with protargol gauze (10 %) ; finally, the patient is allowed to introduce tampons of protargol glycerin.

The husband must have his urethra appropriately treated.

Argonin—also an albumin-silver combination—contains less silver than protargol. Argentamin, on account of its greater penetration and its ability to excite inflammation, is adapted only to neglected cases, in which it is of considerable service. Nitrate of silver is of value in the after-treatment because of its astringent qualities. Largin contains 11.1 % silver in combination with nucleo-albumin, and excels all others in its power of killing the gonococci ; it is, however, inferior to them in rendering the soil unfit for the organism.

For the urethritis (female) : wipe out the urethra with a 5 % protargol solution, sublimate 1 : 5000, or a 2 % solution of silver nitrate, and introduce a 5 % protargol bougie every day for a week ; the bladder may eventually be washed out with a 1 % to 2½ % protargol solution.

If the bartholinitis goes on to abscess formation, incise when fluctuation occurs and pack with iodoform gauze ; if it recurs, excise it entire and bring the edges of the wound together.

Condylomata are removed with scissors or cauterized with 25 % chromic acid, concentrated carbolic acid, or nitric acid.

Cystitis : Wash out the bladder as previously directed ; later, with a 1 % or 2 % silver nitrate solution and a 2½ % solution of cocain (¼ to ½ liter, lukewarm, using catheter and Hegar's funnel, or Küstner's urethral funnel).

Internally, diuretic drinks (milk, tea, juniper berries, etc.) and urotropin—0.5—three times daily.

In the second group of cases—the older ones—only

PLATE 29.

Fig. 1.—**Elephantiasis Vulvæ.** (Original drawing.) (1) Stratified squamous epithelium covering the connective-tissue papillæ. Numerous lymph capillaries (3) are seen in the connective-tissue stroma (2). Some round-cell deposits are present, due to the proliferation. (See Plate 51, Fig. 1.)

Fig. 2.—**Condyloma Acuminatum.** (Original drawing.) (See Plate 24, Fig. 1.) Fine dendritic proliferation of the connective-tissue papillæ (2), which are covered with a very thick layer of stratified squamous epithelium (1).

Fig. 3.—**Vaginal Secretion.** (1) Polygonal squamous epithelium (seen from the side at 6); (2) red blood-corpuscles; (3) leukocytes; (4) oidium albicans; (5) staphylococci; (7) bacilli; (8) trichomonas vaginalis.

Fig. 4.—**Cross-section of an Ovule of Naboth Situated in the Wall of the External Os.** (Original drawing from a specimen.) (1) Simple cylindric epithelium of the cervical mucosa; (2) partly desquamated cylindric epithelium from dilated cervical glands (ovula Nabothi); (3) cervical glands; (4) stratified squamous epithelium of the vaginal cervix. (See Plate 37, Fig. 2; Plate 60, Fig. 2; Plate 90, Figs. 1 and 3.)

---

after the vagina has been washed out for weeks do we proceed to treat the uterus on the principles laid down under endometritis and metritis. (See §13.) If affections of the adnexa are not rigidly excluded by careful bimanual examination, every intra-uterine therapeutic measure will be replied to by these organs with an exacerbation of the trouble. The salpingitis, etc., must be first treated. (See § 16.)

In commencing joint affections the temporary constriction of the extremity is to be carried out according to the method of Bier.

§ 13. CHRONIC ENDOMETRITIS. EROSION AND ECTROPION OF THE EXTERNAL OS.

Endometritis is an affection of the uterine mucous membrane alone; it may appear as a disease *sui generis* without

Tab. 29.

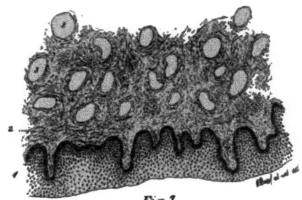

Fig.1.

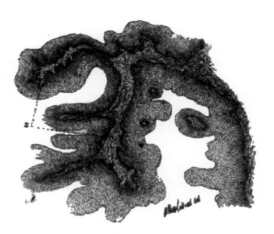

Fig.2.

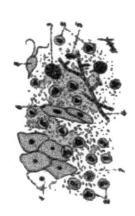

Fig.3.

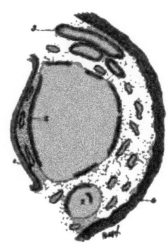

Fig.4.

Lith. Anst. F. Reichhold, Mün

Tab. 56.

affecting other organs, and causes little general disturbance.

Although gonorrhea plays the most important rôle in the etiology of the infectious uterine inflammations, there are, nevertheless, an important class of cases in which we must seek another cause. This is especially true when they occur in the virgin. Pyogenic organisms, not infrequently owing their introduction to the practice of masturbation, are partly responsible for them.

Another group of cases frequently leading to a general disease may be traced to a septic infection, whether it occur in the puerperium, or as the result of operative measures or of trauma.

Clinically, we are able to differentiate :

1. Catarrh (*a*) of the cervical mucosa ; (*b*) of the corporeal mucosa, usually of a nonbacterial nature.

2. Purulent inflammation (*a*) of the cervical mucosa ; (*b*) of the corporeal mucosa, almost without exception of a bacterial nature.

From an anatomic standpoint the first form is synonymous with the pure glandular inflammation ; the second, with the interstitial inflammation accompanied by some glandular change. (See explanation to Plates 30 and 31 and p. 107.)

The affections of the cervix are the more frequent ; those of the mucous membrane of the uterus, the more severe.

(a) Catarrh of the Cervix and Chronic Cervicitis and Their Consequences : Erosion and Ectropion.

The acute inflammation of the mucous membrane and wall of the cervix is, without exception, of an infectious nature, and is due to the invasion of gonococci or streptococci following puerperal lacerations, trauma, or operations upon the cervix. In the latter case either the ulceration of the vaginal cervix or the inflammation of the entire uterus and its surrounding connective tissue may be the more prominent manifestation.

PLATE 30.

Fig. 1.—Normal Uterine Mucosa. (Original diagrammatic drawing.) The mucous membrane of the entire uterus is covered with a single layer of ciliated cylindric epithelium. In the cervix these cells are club-shaped and considerably higher than in the corpus uteri. Both forms produce mucus, which ascends from the more easily stained protoplasm about the nucleus to the upper portion of the cell, from which it is emptied. As this process goes on, the nucleus of the utricular cell ascends and descends, while the more actively secreting cervical cell possesses two constituent parts: a lower rounded portion, always containing the nucleus, and devoted to secretion; an upper portion, connected with the former by a narrow isthmus, and devoted to the storage of the secretion. This upper portion consequently does not take the nuclear stains. The nuclei of the cervical cells are necessarily all at the same level, while in the utricular cells this is not the case. The cervical cells are fixed by means of processes that extend underneath the contiguous epithelium. In the intact healthy uterus the cylindric epithelium extends to the external os, where the squamous epithelium of the vagina commences.

The uterus may be anatomically divided into two parts—the body and the neck. Corresponding to the utricular and cervical cells, we also have two specific forms of glands: large, acinous glands in the cervix (cervical glands); long, narrow, tubular glands, chiefly in the body (utricular glands). These glands are distributed as follows:

In the body of the uterus, only tubular utricular glands with low epithelium, the nuclei being centrally situated. In the cervix above the plicæ palmatæ, both cervical and utricular glands, the former having unusually high epithelium. In the plicated region, simply folds and recesses, no real glands; the plicæ are studded with slender, thread-like papillæ, which are covered by a low, almost cuboid, cylindric epithelium

In the lowest portion of the cervix both acinous and tubular glands are found; there is also another variety of papillæ—low, fungiform, and covered with large club-shaped cervical cells.

The secretion of the healthy uterus is scanty. The vagina contains no glands, or only a few (*glandula aberrantes*) at its junctions with the uterus and with the vulva.

The mucous and submucous connective-tissue stroma is richly supplied with round cells and vessels, which allow of considerable varia-

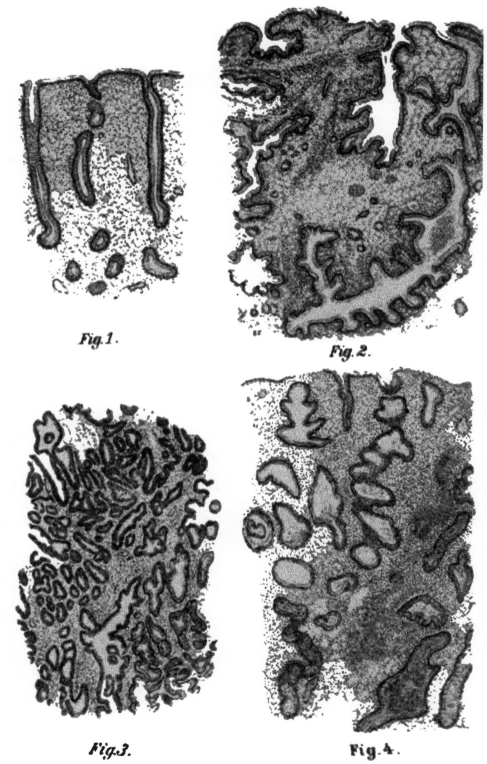

Tab. 30

Fig.1.

Fig.2.

Fig.3.

Fig.4.

Lith Anst F. Reichhold

tion in the degree of swelling of the mucous membrane, whether it be momentary or corresponding to the periodic congestions. This also explains its rapid regeneration. The muscularis is situated beneath the submucosa.

FIG. 2.—**Hyperplastic Glandular Endometritis.** (Original drawing from a specimen.) The individual glands are more numerous and are increased in extent by lateral pouchings (Ruge); the walls are enveloped in a connective-tissue capsule, which is richly infiltrated with leukocytes and round cells; the remaining stroma shows practically no inflammatory or proliferative process. If the stroma gave evidences of the latter, the condition would be known as endometritis fungosa (Olshausen), the mucous membrane being considerably thickened. If the proliferation of glandular and interstitial tissue is circumscribed, the condition is known as endometritis polyposa.

FIG. 3.—**Malignant adenoma (glandular cancer)** (original drawing from a specimen) differentiates itself from hyperplastic endometritis by the fact that the glandular (epithelial) proliferation exceeds that of the connective-tissue stroma; the relative proportion between the two differs from the normal. The glandular tissue eats up the stroma, so to speak, destroys the muscularis, and finally invades other organs or gives rise to metastases along the lymphatic channels. The stroma always shows marked round-cell infiltration; the glandular spaces are lined with stratified squamous epithelium—an evidence of the active proliferation. There is a striking irregularity in the form of the glands and in the picture as a whole.

FIG. 4.—**Hypertrophic Glandular and Interstitial Endometritis.** (Original drawing from a specimen.) The glandular hypertrophic form rarely occurs alone, and consists of an enlargement (no increase or marked pouching) of the glands (Ruge); they become coiled like a corkscrew, showing, at most, a serrated pouching. In this specimen the interglandular tissue shows proliferative round-cell infiltration; hemorrhages have occurred in both glandular and connective tissues. The superficial epithelium has undergone partial desquamation.

Chronic cervicitis arises as a sequel to such an inflammation, especially if the external os has been lacerated and gapes.

The noninfectious inflammations of the cervix present

PLATE 31.

Fig. 1.—**Acute interstitial Endometritis.** The interglandular connective tissue is in active proliferation, and consists of densely packed round cells. The glands are partly pressed aside and partly converted into retention cysts (ovula Nabothi) by distortion of their excretory ducts. Hemorrhage into the stroma. Epithelial desquamation. (Original drawing from a specimen.)

Fig. 2—**Chronic interstitial endometritis** is the continuation of the former, the round cells becoming changed into rigid connective tissue. The glands atrophy. The vessels become thick-walled. The superficial epithelium is absent or almost squamous (the squamous epithelium of the external os can be seen at the left of the illustration).

Fig. 3.—**Postabortive Endometritis.** An island of decidual cells may be seen under the partly regenerated superficial epithelium. Few glands, many round cells, strongly dilated capillary blood-vessels.

---

the same clinical picture. A condition of relaxation is the primary cause; it may lead to ectropion even though no laceration exists. If the inflammation is limited to the mucous membrane, we speak of catarrh of the cervix.

Symptoms.—The discharge is the first and most constant symptom. In uncomplicated catarrh it is mucoid; in purulent cases (mixed infection) it is mucopurulent as a result of the admixture of pus-corpuscles. This discharge in time weakens the individual and hinders conception by the formation of a cervical plug of tough mucus. The blood-vessels are overfilled and are easily torn on account of the inflammatory proliferation of the mucous membrane. (Plate 30.) Reflex menorrhagia and dysmenorrhea occur, as well as slight hemorrhages from contact. Pain is present, however, in the intervals between the periods, if the swollen mucous membrane protrudes from the external os—ectropion. (Plate 28, Fig. 3 ; Plates 35 and 56.)

Ectropion usually occurs when the commissures of the os uteri have been lacerated. I have repeatedly seen it

Tab. 31.

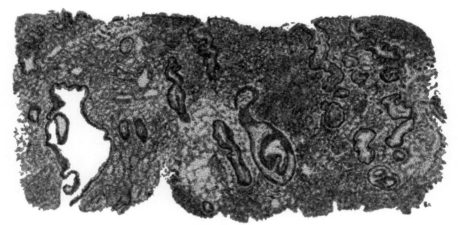

Fig.1.

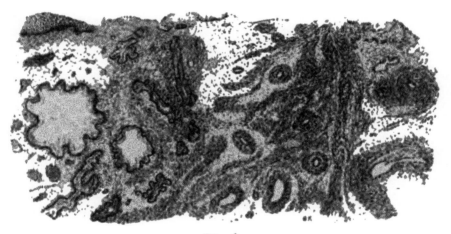

Fig.2.

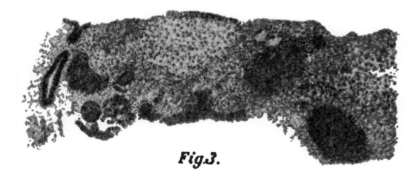

Fig.3.

Lith. Anst F. Reichhold. München.

Tab. 31.

Fig. 1.

Fig. 2.

Fig. 3.

Lith. Anst. F. Reichhold, München.

arise in the intact uterus if pessaries were introduced when
the organ was relaxed and in a lower position than usual.

Diagnosis.—Palpation discloses the thickening of the
cervix, and the examining finger is covered with mucus or
pus. Changes of structure can be felt only in the older
ectropions, and such a condition should always lead one
to suspect a beginning cancer.

Inspection (Speculum).—In a multipara with ectropion the examination of the mucous membrane is easy;
in the closed orifice of the nullipara we discover, at most,
retention cysts of the cervical glands—ovula Nabothi.
(Plate 29, Fig. 4; Plate 56, Fig. 1; Plate 69, Figs. 1
and 3.) In these cases we must draw the os well down
by means of forceps, evert the lips with tenacula, or dilate
the external os.

The cervical cavity is distended by the profuse, tena-
cious secretion; this may be demonstrated by the sound.
(Plates 47 and 67.)

The secretion also causes a desquamation of the superficial layers of the squamous epithelium about the os uteri,
and erosio simplex is produced. (Plate 28, Fig. 3; Plate
33, Fig. 1.) If the cells of the matrix become cylindric
and arrange themselves in glandular formations, we have
to do with an erosio papilloides. (Plate 90, Fig. 1.) If
either one is combined with the formation of ovula Nabothi,
we speak of erosio follicularis. (Plate 37, Fig. 2.)

Differential Diagnosis.—Between erosion and ectropion: In the former the external os is centrally situated
within the erosion; in the latter it is outside of, and
pressed away by, the ectropion. (Plates 33, 37, and 56.)

Differentiation between erosio papilloides and epitheliomatous papilloma is best made by the microscope. (Plate
28, Fig. 3; Plate 79, Figs. 1 to 3.) The follicular form
may produce polypoid excrescences by a circumscribed
elevation of portions of the mucous membrane. (Plate
90, Fig 3.)

Between ectropion (Plates 34, 35, and 56) and incipient

PLATE 32.

Fig. 1.—**Marked Congestion and Beginning Simple Erosion of the Posterior Lip of the Os, as a Sign of Uterine Inflammation: Endometritis and Metritis.** The simple erosion (see Plate 33 also) consists of a casting-off of all the epithelial cells above the cuboid layer, allowing the cutaneous capillaries to shine through more distinctly. The constant irritation of the uterine secretion is the cause of the desquamation.

Fig. 2.—**Slight Congestion of the Cervix of a Multipara with a Characteristic, Broad, Fissured External Orifice.**

---

cancer : Touch is not to be depended upon, since both conditions offer the sensation of hard, solitary nodules. (Plates 81, 83, 84, and 90.) Inspection shows ovula Nabothi in ectropion ; nodules with destructive ulceration in carcinoma. If ulceration does not exist, all that remains is the microscopic examination of an excised piece.

Prognosis.—It is of importance to remember that catarrh of the cervix is cured with difficulty, and that the inveterate forms have a tendency to malignant degeneration.

Treatment.—The local treatment of the cervical mucosa is exactly the same as that of the uterine mucous membrane. (See p. 109.) The swelling of the vaginal cervix and of the ovules of Naboth is greatly lessened by multiple punctures and scarifications. If the external os is narrow, lateral incisions are to be made—*to* the vaginal vault, if necessary.

Erosions are to be treated by cauterization : Acetic acid, to which 4 % carbolic acid has been added, is poured into the

---

PLATE 33. ˙

Fig. 1.—**Congenital Simple Erosion of the Cervix of a Virgin.** (Original water-color from a case.)

Fig. 2.—**Leukorrhea and Simple Erosion.** (Original water-color from a case.)

Tab. 32.

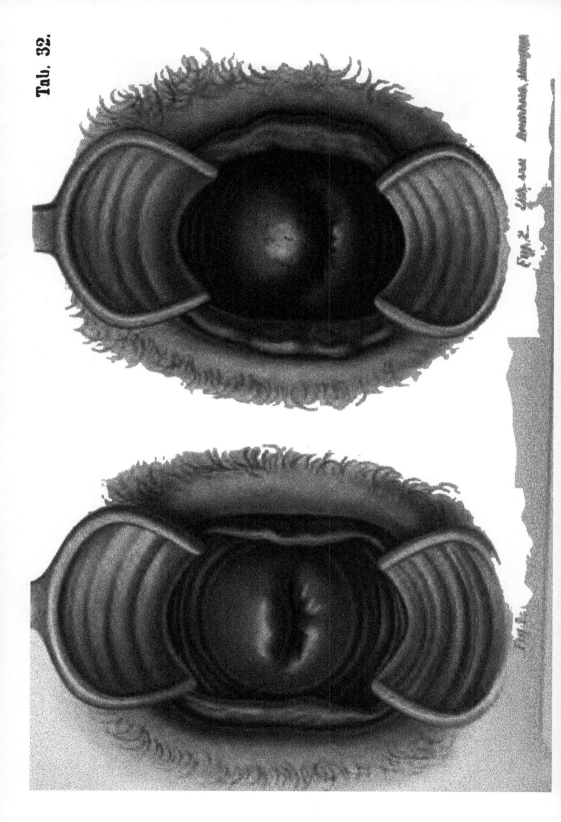

Fig. 2. *Lithorea americana*

Tab. 23.

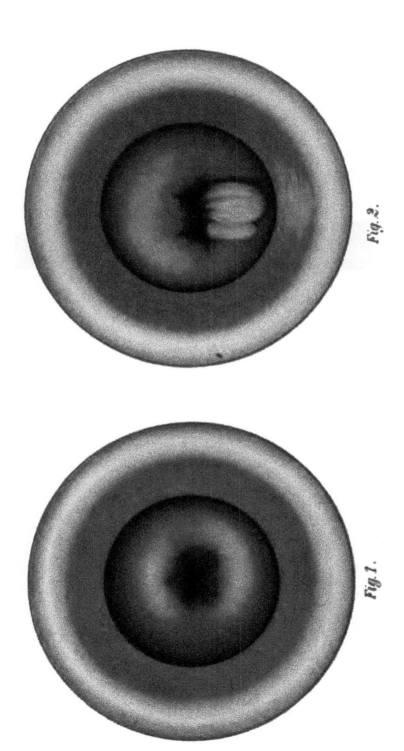

Fig. 1.

Fig. 2.

Lith. Anst. Reichhold. München

speculum and allowed to act for several minutes (daily, for a few weeks). The reddened ulcerated patches gradually disappear as the pathologic cylindric epithelium is replaced by epidermoid cells. Weak solutions of cupric sulphate or zinc chlorid act more quickly. If the epithelial covering is cast off in deeper ulcerations, cauterize with one drop of fuming nitric acid, afterward washing out with warm water; otherwise, excise. Above all, remove the cause—the discharge.

Ectropion and follicular hypertrophy of the mucous membrane, if present in but a slight degree, vanish when the catarrh is treated with caustics. The severe forms are treated by operative measures : by removal of the swollen mucous membrane by means of a wedge-shaped excision from the entire thickness of the cervical wall (see Metritis under § 14) ; by excision of the connective-tissue commissures of the gaping os uteri followed by suture. In other cases the pessary should be removed and an operation for prolapse should be performed.

(b) Endometritis Corporis Uteri.

Any endometritis, whether it be cervical or corporeal, may appear as an acute or a chronic process, or in milder or severer forms.

The latter division denotes not only difference of grade, but also qualitative change :

The milder forms produce no structural change ; the secretion is more profuse and is mucoid and glairy ; hemorrhages occur.

The severer forms lead to proliferation and to a purulent discharge.

There are certain histologic peculiarities that explain these differences (see Plates 30 and 31) ; these are as follows (Ruge, Veit) :

I. *Endometritis glandularis:* (1) Hypertrophic—*i. e.*, the glands proliferate in length only, becoming rolled up between the surface of the mucosa and the muscularis. Their longitudinal section resembles

PLATE 34.

Ectropion with Extreme Relaxation of the Cervical Wall and Intact Commissures of the External Os. Anemic cervix following climacteric menorrhagias from myomata. (Original wat color from actual case.)

a corkscrew. (2) Hyperplastic—the glands proliferate in length and breadth, forming lateral pockets.

II. *Endometritis interstitialis:* (1) Acute round-cell proliferation leads to purulent secretion; (2) chronic or cirrhotic connective-tissue formation, contraction, leading at last to atrophic endometritis.

The glandular forms occur as mixed forms, especially with acute interstitial endometritis ; if the hyperplasia and proliferation are pronounced, we have:

III. *Endometritis fungosa* (mixed form), if the proliferation is diffuse ; or—

IV. *Endometritis polyposa* (mixed form) and *endometritis follicularis* (Plate 90, 3), if it is circumscribed.

From groups II and III the following varieties may be separated, their most striking symptom being either hemorrhage or a casting-off of the mucosa :

V. *Endometritis exfoliativa* (dysmenorrhœa membranacea, see § 3).

VI. *Endometritis dissecans* with phlegmon.

VII. *Endometritis hæmorrhagica:* scanty secretion : fungous mucosa ; after abortion in acute infectious diseases.

If the endometritis is the result of an abortion, we designate it as :

VIII. *Endometritis post abortum*, to be recognized by the large decidual cells.

The ovules of Naboth arise (Plate 29, Fig. 4 ; 56, Fig. 1 ; 69, Figs. 1 and 3):

1. From excessive proliferation and secretion in I (2).
2. From a too narrow excretory duct in I (1).
3. From occlusion of duct by angulation in I (1).
4. From compression of duct by inflamed connective tissue in II (1).
5. From cicatricial closure in II (2).

The **symptoms** of chronic endometritis corporis uteri are the same in infectious and noninfectious cases :

1. Pain, at the time of the menses (dysmenorrhea),

PLATE 35.

Mucous Polyp and Ectropion of the Anterior Lip of the Uterus. The cervical walls are relaxed and anemic ; the commissure of the os uteri is intact. (Original water-color from actual case.)

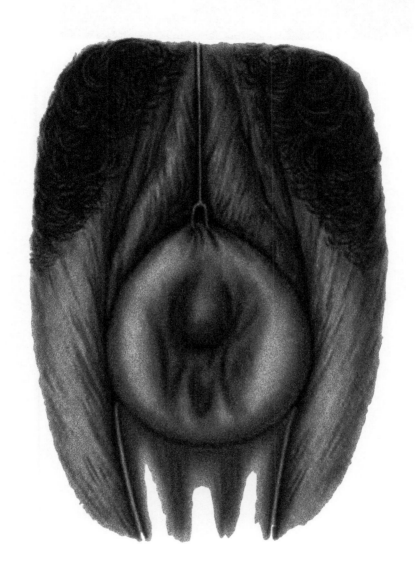

F. Reinhold Müller

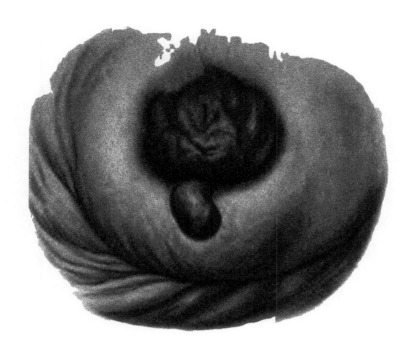

Lich. Anst. F. Reichhold, München.

with or without casting-off a decidua menstrualis; or, rarely, in the interval (intermenstrual pain); or permanent, ceasing with the beginning of the flow, so that the menstrual period is the only time at which there is no pain; or permanent, with exacerbations at the menstrual epoch. (See § 17.)

2. Discharge, mostly bloody, serous, mucoid (Küstner, Schröder) and purulent (B. S. Schultze). Determined by means of tampons.

3. Changed character of menstruation; menorrhagia and dysmenorrhea.

4. Sterility.

5. Reflex nervous disturbances : pains in the umbilical region, dyspepsia, all varieties of hysteric troubles.

As the myometrium is usually involved, the symptoms of myometritis may complicate the clinical picture.

Diagnosis.—1. The sound causes characteristic pain as it passes the internal os; the entire uterine mucosa is hypersensitive. The sound also reveals the size of the uterine cavity and any roughenings or fungosities that may be present.

2. Abrasio mucosæ (curetment, raclage, excochleation) —the tissue is removed and its structure examined with the microscope.

3. In doubtful cases the cervical canal is dilated (metal dilator of Fritsch, Küstner's adjustable dilator, laminaria—well sterilized) and the entire uterine cavity is palpated.

Prognosis.—Serious results follow from the hemorrhage and from the discharge, as well as from the occurrence of malignant degeneration.

Treatment.—Above all, provide for a regular and sufficient discharge of the secretions. The external os, and especially the internal os (normally 4 mm. in diameter), are usually constricted from the inflammatory swelling of the mucosa, and may require mechanical dilatation. To aid in removing the secretions, vaginal irrigations

PLATE 36.

FIGS. 1 *a*, 1 *b*, 1 *c*. —**Different Molds of the Uterocervical Canal as Shown by Swollen Laminaria.** The end to which the silk thread is attached lay in the external os. (Original water-color from actual cases.)

FIG. 2.—**Curetment in Fungous Endometritis.** Relaxed, anemic cervix; sharp, although irregular limitation of the squamous epithelium at the external os. (Original water-color from actual case.)

with astringents (alum, tannin, bismuth subnitrate, zinc sulphate) or antiseptics (potassium permanganate, solution of aluminum acetate,[1] formalin, 1 : 4000 to 1 : 2000 corrosive sublimate), exciting the uterus to contraction and washing the cervical mucosa.

The character of the diseased mucous membrane must be changed by using astringents or caustics. The stronger caustics (10% zinc chlorid, for example) should not be used, as they may produce strictures, stenoses, and pathologic adhesions. These substances are best applied in liquid form (sesquichlorid of iron in 50% solution or pure, 2% solution of silver nitrate, 5% solution of zinc chlorid, fuming nitric acid) by means of cotton and the aluminum sound.

At the same time the infectious virus must be removed, either by the foregoing caustics or by antiseptics. In addition to intra-uterine irrigation (Fritsch's two-way catheter), pencils of itrol or iodoform may be introduced.

The cervix may be dilated and the uterine cavity may be disinfected at the same time by packing the uterus with itrol or iodoform gauze (following Abel, to be removed daily). Landau introduces yeast cultures.

The changed and infected mucous membrane may be removed by radical methods—abrasion, curetment (raclage, excochleation).

[1] See Therapeutic Table.

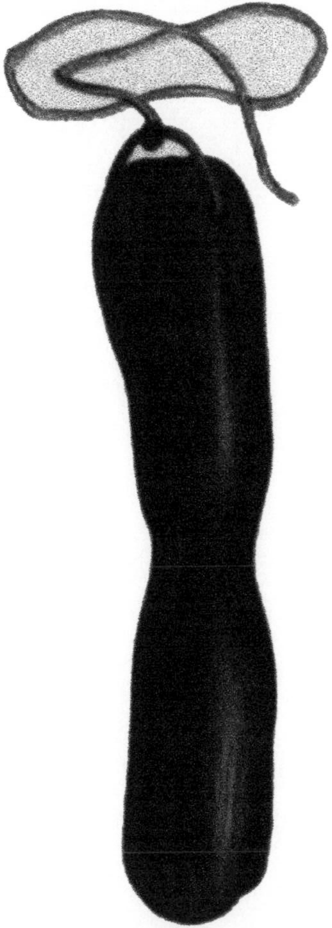

Fig. 1

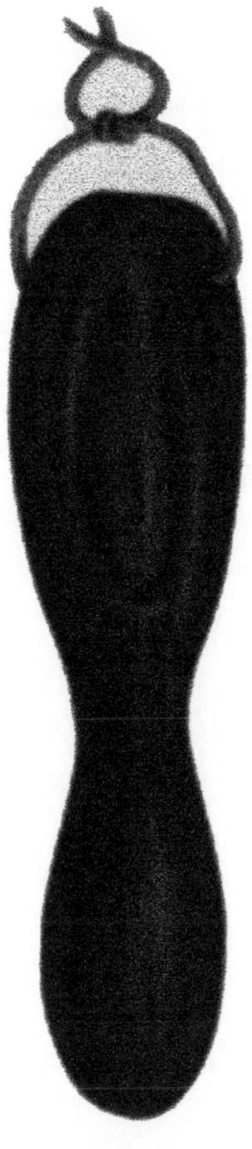

Fig. 1

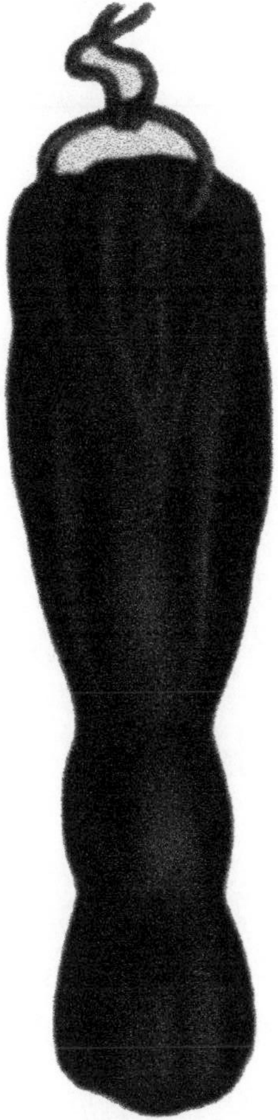

Fig. 1c

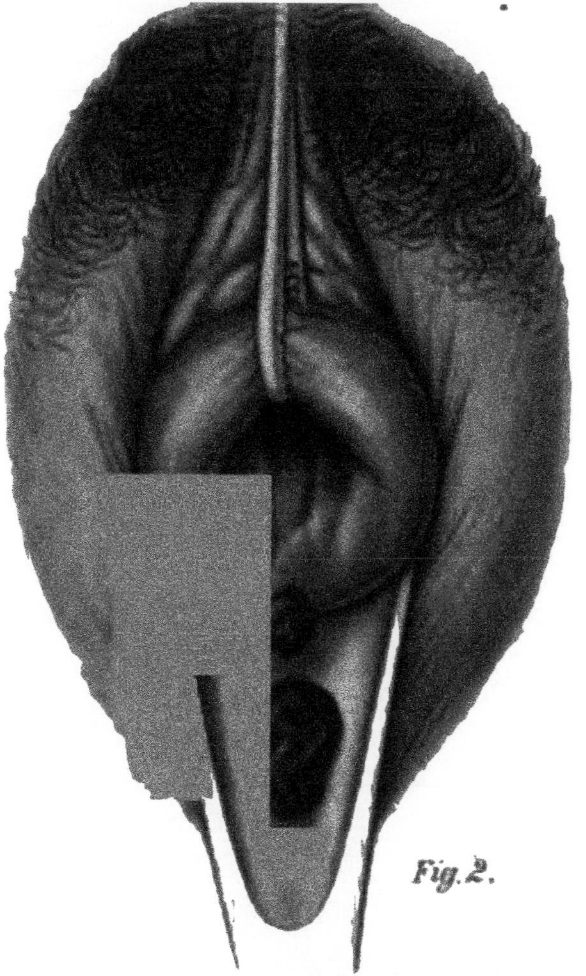

Fig. 2.

Lith.-Anst. F. Reichhold, München

TREATMENT. **111**

After careful disinfection and dilatation the cervix is fixed with bullet-forceps and the uterine walls are carefully and evenly scraped. Simon's sharp spoon or the dull wire curet may be used. [The dull wire curet is practically useless.—Ed.] The various portions of the cavity should be cureted in some definite order. The cureting is to be immediately followed by packing with antiseptic gauze (itrol, iodoform) or with gauze saturated with some caustic (solution of ferric chlorid, formalin). This controls the hemorrhage, acts as a disinfectant, and brings the medicament in contact with the remaining diseased mucous membrane. It is still better to follow up the curetment with atmocausis or zestocausis. (See Treatment of Chronic Metritis.)

Narcosis is necessary in the majority of cases. The intra-uterine irrigations may sometimes cause colic.

For three or four days after the curetment daily intra-uterine douches of 2% carbolic acid act favorably ; in the marked cases of proliferative fungous endometritis the process is kept within bounds by washing out the uterine cavity twice daily, and then applying astringents (solution of sesquichlorid of iron, tincture of iodin) by means of the sound.

According to my experience, atmocausis and zestocausis (vaporization, vapocauterization) are productive of better and more permanent results than these scraping and cauterizing methods.

§ 14. CHRONIC METRITIS.

The clinical picture of chronic metritis consists of inflammatory hyperemia and swelling and sensitiveness of the entire organ. It leads to a connective-tissue hyperplasia rather than to a proliferation of the muscle-cells. The inflammation progresses slowly, with acute and subacute exacerbations, and in some cases ends in cirrhosis. The endometrium is nearly always diseased, and consequently

PLATE 37.

FIG. 1.—**Chronic Metritis with Ovula Nabothi.** Metritis is an inflammation of the uterine muscularis. If the process is of long duration, the muscle-cells are partly replaced by scar-tissue (see Plate 31, Fig. 2), which in our illustration retracts the cervical mucosa and causes a visible wrinkling. The ovula Nabothi are retention cysts, resulting from distortion of the ducts by contracting connective tissue. (Plate 29, Fig. 4.)

FIG. 2.—**Gonorrheal Endometritis with Simple Erosion and Ovules of Naboth; Inflammatory Hyperemia.** (Plates 29, 30, and 31.) Thick, yellow, creamy pus flows from the os and fills the vagina. The ovula Nabothi are also filled with pus. The erosion is the result of the endometritis. The simple infection with gonococci soon gives place to a mixed infection with staphylococci and streptococci, the former organisms having prepared the soil for the latter. The process creeps up the tubes and then progresses to the nearest peritoneal surface (metritis, oophoritis, perisalpingitis), at first producing exudations, then adhesions and cicatricial bands. (Plates 44 and 45, Fig. 36.) The gonococci, as a rule, invade only the superficial layers of those membranes covered with cylindric epithelium.

The adhesions of the tubes and ovaries lead to the formation of abscesses (Pyosalpinx, Plate 42) and sterility. The perimetritic process causes displacements of the uterus and its adnexa.

---

the symptoms of myometritis and endometritis are inseparably associated.

There are two stages: (a) The stage of hyperemia and round-cell infiltration: the uterus is soft and easily torn, as a result of the edema and fatty degeneration of the muscularis. (b) The stage of cirrhotic induration: the uterus is tough, anemic, or livid from venous stasis

---

PLATE 38.

Retroversion of the Fixed Uterus (First Degree) and Agglutination of the Cervix (Acquired). A peritoneal pseudoligament holds the uterine fundus in retroversion. Caustics or senile processes cause adhesions and, later, atresia of the cervix. Changed direction of the vagina in retroversion of the uterus. (Original water-color from a specimen in the Munich Frauenklinik.)

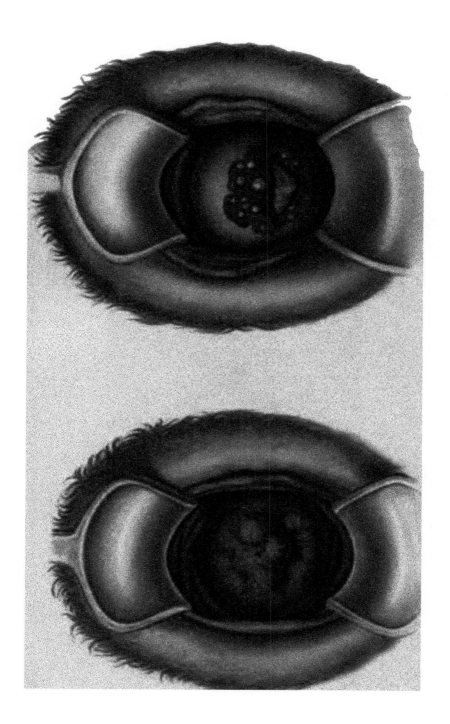

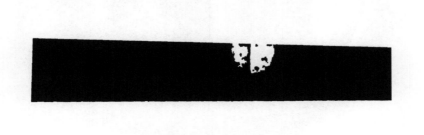

München

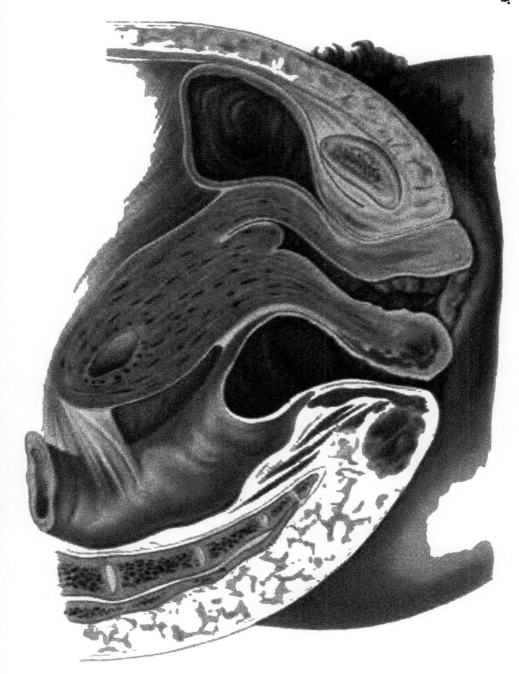

(arterial walls thickened, their lumen narrowed, muscularis partly replaced by connective tissue).

Etiology. — (1) From puerperal subinvolution ; (2) from the irritation of a chronic endometritis ; (3) from the penetration of infectious germs (especially gonococci) ; (4) from other hyperemic irritations, such as masturbation ; (5) from venous stasis in flexions, prolapse, or other displacements accompanied by engorgements (habitually full bladder, chronic constipation, or secondary stasis from circulatory disturbances in other organs) ; (6) rarely, from an acute metritis.

Prognosis.—Although the disease does not cease at the menopause, but usually several years later, this time is the best for effective treatment. The prognosis is more favorable if the second stage appears early, as the disturbances then disappear.

Symptoms.—A sensation of fullness (as if a heavy body were in the abdomen), pains in the side and sacral region, discharge, menorrhagia, dysmenorrhea, dysuria, and constipation. The symptoms are more pronounced at the menstrual epoch or when obstinate constipation exists. They are favorably influenced by rest in the dorsal position.

Diagnosis.—The cervix is soft, thickened, and hyperemic, with swollen lips, from the accompanying endometritis—ectropion, erosion, ovula Nabothi. (Plates 32 and 56.) In the second stage the cervix is livid, hard, and wrinkled. (Plate 37, Fig. 1.)

Hypersensitiveness is not always present, but a peculiar softening and enlargement of the organ occur, causing it to resemble a gravid uterus at the second and third months. The sound reveals the elongation of the uterine cavity and a thickening of its wall.

Any variety of inflammation of the surrounding tissues and organs may occur. Conception takes place with difficulty, and leads to abortion or to premature delivery.

Differential Diagnosis.—In the first months it is dif-

8

PLATE 39.

Acute Purulent Pelvic Peritonitis (Peritonitis of Perforation). View of pouch of Douglas and the posterior wall of the uterus and left broad ligament with its tube and ovary. The pus has been wiped off of the uterus but allowed to remain on the serosa of Douglas' pouch. (Original water-color from a specimen at the Heidelberg Pathologic Institute.)

---

ficult to differentiate a gravid uterus from an inflamed organ; the former is softer, especially at the cervix and internal os (bimanual from the rectum), and rests upon the cervix like a round, thickened body; the latter is more sensitive. Pregnancy must always be thought of, especially if intra-uterine treatment is under consideration.

Intra-uterine tumors may be palpated with the sound, or directly with the finger after dilatation of the cervix. The inflamed uterus is elongated, especially the cervix, which is contracted in virgins and everted in multipara. In cancer small pieces may be removed and examined microscopically.

If the case is simply one of endometritis, the increase in volume and the hypersensitiveness of the entire organ are not marked.

Treatment.—Prophylactic. — During menstruation: rest in bed (not all the time); avoid everything inducing congestion (excitement, especially sexual; heating drinks; constipation; colds). During the puerperium: Ergotin, warm or cold applications, abdominal massage; hot vaginal irrigations (117° to 127° F.) or warm general baths (95° to 100° F.) in the second week.

Special treatment of the hyperemic stage—absorptive: hot injections and baths, with or without salt or lye.

The hyperemia is controlled by constricting the vessels: Ergot or ergotin, hydrastis, stypticin; hot vaginal injections; scarifications of the cervix (every three or four days, ⅓ to 2 fluidrams, especially before the period) relieve

Tab. 39.

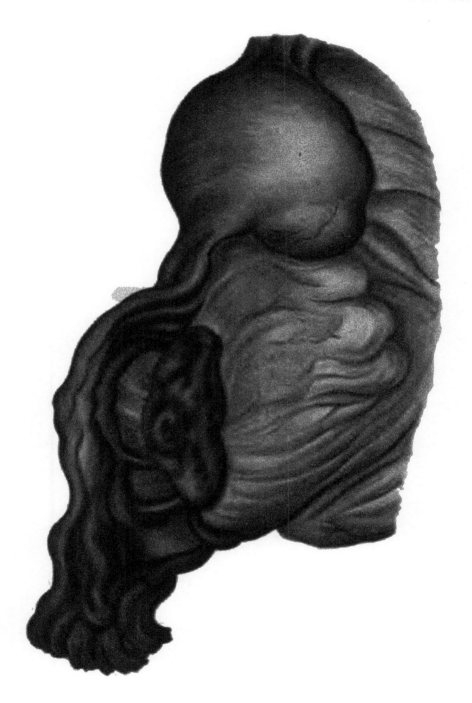

Tab. 22.

congestion and pain. Compression by means of vaginal tamponade and sand-bags or shot-bags laid upon the abdomen.

Glycerin tampons are used as derivatives, and the secretion is further stimulated by astringents and caustics. The applications are to be repeated every week, but only in the first stage. Curetment, followed by chlorid of iron or iodin (Playfair's aluminum sound).

The application of steam to control hemorrhage (menorrhagia) is, according to the author's experience with *atmocausis*, a most valuable addition to our therapeutic measures. It was first employed by Snegirew, the instrumentarium being perfected by Pinkus. My own observations show that it is as effective in obstinate endometritis as it is in inflammations of the myometrium. It is not advisable for one unskilled in gynecologic practice to make use of this method, especially if he is without assistance. It is as little adapted for ambulatory treatment as is curetment.

The instrumentarium is as follows : A tested boiler with safety-valve and thermometer; a rubber tube (tightly screwed to the boiler), rather thick and well wrapped ; and a two-way intra-uterine catheter with a discharge-tube for the steam returning from the uterine cavity. The catheter is covered with gauze or celluloid to protect the cervix from injury and subsequent stenosis. The pressure and temperature of the steam and the duration of its action must be gaged to suit the individual case. A cureted uterus or one having a small cavity must be treated more mildly, probably using only the zestocautery : *i. e.*, the *closed* catheter, 105° to 112° C., for from ten to twenty seconds ; with a large cavity and a thickened endometrium, 110° to 115° C., for fifteen seconds. If obliteration is desired, steam at 115° to 120° C. for from one-half to two minutes is to be employed. This may be repeated, whereas ordinarily the application should not be renewed until the next menstrual period has passed. Narcosis is not necessary, but is usually desirable ; the same is true of assistance. The cervix must be dilated.

The methods of treatment just named are symptomatic and palliative. If pain and a sensation of fullness are present : frequent scarifications and glycerin tampons ; abdominal belt and pessary to remove tension from the uterine ligaments.

For the menstrual disturbances : Previous scarifications, warm sand-bags upon the abdomen or warm alcoholic fomentations (narcotics). In menorrhagia : ergotin, tamponade, application of ferripyrin or introduction of ferripyrin-gauze tampons, gelatin injections, atmocausis.

Operations for the Purpose of Reducing the Size of the Collum Uteri and Removing the Diseased Mucous Membrane.

These results, together with the removal of scars from lacerations, are best accomplished by means of *wedge-shaped excisions* (or amputation of the cervix, removal of conic pieces of tissue—operations of Sims, Hegar, Simon, Schröder). The following operations are to be particularly recommended :

Schröder's Operation.—The inner circumference of the os with its diseased mucous membrane is completely excised. The remaining outer half of the cervical wall is turned in and sewed to the remains of the cervical mucosa.

A. Martin's Operation.—The entire vaginal cervix is excised in the shape of a cone. The cervical mucosa is then drawn down and stitched to that of the vagina.

Kehrer's Operation.—Wedge-shaped pieces are excised from both lips of the os uteri. Their base is formed by the cervical mucosa, and they extend through the entire cervical wall.

After the Operation.—Glycerin or iodoform-gauze tamponade (one day) ; then vaginal irrigations ; for secondary hemorrhage firm gauze tamponade with ferripyrin, solution of sesquichlorid of iron, or suture ; if catgut has not been employed, removal of sutures in eight days.

₹ 15. SEPSIS.

(Acute Vulvitis, Vaginitis, Endometritis, Myometritis, Salpingitis, Parametritis and Perimetritis, Peritonitis.)

The acute inflammations of the endometrium and myometrium present practically the same clinical pictures. They are due to the invasion either of gonococci or of septic germs. It is to the inflammations caused by the latter that attention is now directed.

Etiology and Clinical Aspect.—Invading pyogenic organisms (streptococcus pyogenes ; staphylococcus aureus, albus, citreus, etc.) excite septic inflammations ; the avenues of infection are either the skin or mucous membrane of the genitalia, or the peritoneal covering.

The opportunity for invasion through the lining mucous membrane is given by trauma, by faulty technic in operations and examinations (sounds, dilators), or by the puerperal process.

By virtue of the peculiar quality of the secretion and of the wound surface, which is particularly adapted for the multiplication of invading organisms, the puerperal infections are of the greatest importance. The secretions may stagnate in closed spaces, at body-temperature, and in direct communication with numerous lymphatic channels.

The " gynecologic " infections take the following courses, according to their point of introduction, the infection depending not only upon the place of entrance, but also upon the virulence of the germ and upon the general and local power of resistance of the individual.

Vulva (*Phlegmone Vulvæ*).—The infection usually remains local and leads to abscess formation. The perineal infections, especially when near the rectum, lead to thrombophlebitis and general infection.

Vagina (*Colpitis Crouposa et Diphtheritica, Phlegmone Vaginæ, Abscesses, Paracolpitis, Paraproctitis*).—The infection remains local, at most spreading to the adjoining

PLATE 40.

Fig. 1.—Acute Catarrhal Parenchymatous Salpingitis (Due to Gonococci and Streptococci). The tubal catarrh is the first consequence of the invasion of the cocci in the endosalpinx, and it produces a hypersecretion of mucus. The endosalpinx commences to proliferate; the connective-tissue papillæ (1), covered with columnar ciliated epithelium, form dendritic ramifications that fill the lumen of the tube (2). The stroma of the papilla is infiltrated with young round cells (6). The submucosa (4) and the muscularis (5) are still healthy, but there is a commencing perivascular (3) round-cell infiltration. (Original drawing from a specimen.)

Fig. 2.—Hematosalpinx. In gynatresias (see Figs. 7–11 in text) the menstrual blood remains in the uterus and finally dilates the tube (2); the epithelium (1) desquamates after the papillæ (3) have been flattened by pressure; the vessels (5) of the submucosa (4) are dilated from stasis; there is a reactionary round-cell accumulation (7) about the blood-vessels in the muscularis (6). Tubal hemorrhages occur during the periods, in heart disease and kidney disease, in cases of myomata and ovarian cystomata, and in extra-uterine pregnancy. (Original drawing from a specimen.)

Fig. 3.—Pyosalpinx. The ostia being closed, the pus distends the tube. The epithelium (1) is completely destroyed; the papillæ (2) are flattened; the stroma (3), rich in round cells, is bathed in pus; and the elasticity of the tubal wall is destroyed because the muscle-fibers (4) are separated and replaced by connective tissue (6). The submucous capillaries are dilated from stasis; the vessels of the muscular layer show a chronic inflammatory thickening. Such pus sacs contain different varieties of microbes, the virulence of which depends upon the age of the abscess at the time of its rupture. (Original drawing from a specimen.)

---

connective tissue. Contrary to what is the rule in puerperal cases, the process very rarely extends to the uterus.

Uterus (*Endometritis et Metritis Acuta*).—The course is doubtful, and if progressive, it may be a very chronic affection.

Symptoms. — Bloody and mucopurulent discharge; enlargement and hypersensitiveness of the uterus (expe-

Tab. 40.

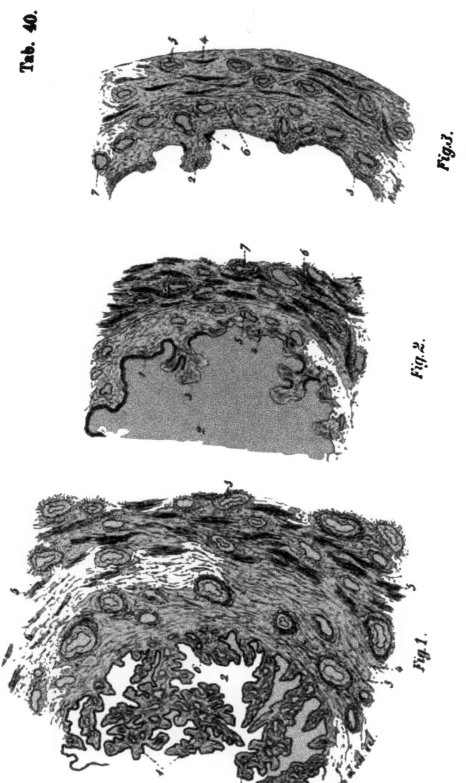

Fig.3.

Fig.2.

Fig.1.

Lith. Anst. F. Reichhold, München.

rienced by the patient as a dull pain in the pelvis, increased by movement, coughing, straining, etc.); strangury; diarrhea with violent tenesmus; fever (rarely, abscess formation).

The patients soon show evidences of a severe infection. They are pale and hollow-eyed; no appetite; meteorismus—pulse-rate and temperature increase; the abdomen becomes sensitive. These are all symptoms of beginning parametritis and perimetritis.

Vaginal examination (to be most gently carried out) reveals hypersensitiveness of the vaginal vault and resistance behind the uterus. Rectal examination shows a tumor behind or beside the uterus, the differentiation of the two being impossible by palpation. Anatomically, it may be a pyosalpinx, oophoritis, perimetrosalpingitis, peri-oophoritis, or parametritis.

The process may remain stationary at this point. The intestinal coils, which roof in the pouch of Douglas, become adherent and wall off the exudate from the general peritoneal cavity—peritonitis exsudativa saccata. The inflammatory products may undergo absorption, may perforate into the rectum, or, rarely, may perforate into the vagina. Chills are present. Permanent resistance beside the uterus may be demonstrated.

As sequels may be mentioned dysmenorrhea, sterility, and deviations of the uterus, the intra-uterine treatment of which, as well as the periodic congestions, may produce febrile exacerbations.

If the inflammation proceeds, a general peritonitis occurs with marked meteorismus, great abdominal pain (which may be absent or intense only at times), compression of the rectum, hindered passage of flatus, threatening symptoms of obstruction, vomiting (even fecal), and sometimes profuse fetid diarrheas. The pulse is rapid, small, and irregular.

The patient may die, the fever being no more pronounced than the anatomic changes. The patient may recover slowly, the pus being absorbed ; or rapidly, the pus emptying externally or into some hollow viscus.

Diagnosis.—Ulcers of the vulva, vagina, and cervix are seen most frequently in the puerperium, occurring elsewhere only in children and in severe acute infectious diseases, such as croupous diphtheria and gangrenous vulvitis. The diagnosis is made by the fetid discharge, pain, slight elevation of temperature, and the gray, green, or yellowish covering of the wound. Ulcers situated near the perineum may be due to injuries or ulcerative processes of the rectum ; or to inflammations of the glands of Bartholin, which in rare cases are not of a gonorrheal nature.

Acute colpitis and endometritis, with their concomitants, myocolpitis and myometritis, may be brought about not only by gonorrhea and puerperal infection, but also by a cold followed by menstrual suppression, by septic operative measures, or by acute infectious diseases (influenza and others).

The main symptoms are fever, purulent secretion, hemorrhages, and pain in the interior of the uterus. The cervix is swollen, and the external os is ulcerated, eroded, and covered with purulent ovula Nabothi. (Plate 37, Fig. 2.)

The deeper the process penetrates into the perivascular and interstitial connective tissue of the muscularis, the more violent will be the febrile invasion. This is accompanied by chills, by hypersensitiveness of the enlarged, hyperemic, softened uterus, by dull pelvic pain, and by vesical and rectal pain and tenesmus. If abscesses form later, their presence is detected by fluctuation.

Parametritis seems, to the touch, like a lateral extension of the uterus. In the beginning it has a doughy consistency. The inflammation has invaded the connective tissue surrounding the uterus, and may spread anteriorly alongside of the bladder to the extraperitoneal connective tissue, and even to the connective tissue of the thigh. It may extend laterally between the layers of the broad ligament to the hollow of the sacrum; or it may go posteriorly, pushing up the serosa of Douglas' pouch and ascending behind the peritoneum, on the iliopsoas muscles, to the renal region.

The tumor is found in some one of the foregoing positions. It is an exudate in the pelvic connective tissue (phlegmon of the pelvis, pelvicellulitis, parametritis of Virchow), and consists of a mucoid swelling and round-cell infiltration of the connective tissue. (Plate 59, Fig. 1; 61, 2; 41, 2.) The exudate is usually absorbed, but scar tissue is left behind, which later binds down and displaces the uterus.

If abscesses form, the pus may burrow its way into the rectum, into the vagina, into the bladder, through the sciatic foramen, along the inguinal canal, or, lastly, through the abdominal wall, pointing above Poupart's ligament.

The overlying peritoneum is usually in a condition of irritation, as is indicated by greater pain, meteorism, diarrhea, and vomiting. The consequent adhesions of the pelvic organs cause sterility. If the peritoneum allows the exudate to escape, a fatal perforative peritonitis will follow. (Plate 39.)

In circumscribed parametritis there may be localized abdominal pain (from the irritation of the serosa), but the violent general pains, the tympanites, and the intraperitoneal exudate are absent. The space of Douglas also remains free. Alongside of the uterus there is at first a hypersensitiveness, then increased resistance, and finally a parametritic tumor of doughy consistency.

For the differential diagnosis from tumors of the pouch of Douglas see § 35.

The diagnosis of peritonitis is based upon the demonstration of an exudate. (Plate 58, Fig. 1.) As long as the process is limited to the pouch of Douglas and is walled off by adhesions at the pelvic inlet (a pelveoperitonitis), the prognosis is far more favorable than when the entire peritoneal cavity is involved.

PLATE 41.

Fig. 1.—Acute Purulent Parenchymatous and Interstitial Salpingitis. Not only the papillæ are proliferated, but also their stroma (1) and the connective tissue of the submucosa (3), and the muscularis (4 and 5) is infiltrated with round cells. The epithelium is partly swollen and partly cast off, the excoriated papillæ adhering and forming small cysts (2). (Original drawing from a specimen.)

Fig. 2.—Parametritis Acuta of the Broad Ligament. Both the connective-tissue fibers and the areolar tissue are infiltrated with round cells. This first stage of swelling and suppuration passes later into the second stage—the transformation into scar tissue. Contraction occurs. (Original drawing from a specimen.)

Fig. 3.—Chronic Oophoritis with Oligocystic Degeneration. (See Plate 45 and Fig. 35.) The inflammatory disturbances lead to a thickening of the tunica albuginea, producing a cystic swelling of the follicles (1 and 2); the follicular epithelial cells desquamate (10) and the ova die. The older corpora lutea become transformed into corpora fibrosa (8) (or candicantia). Recent hemorrhages and older ones with blood pigment (9) are found in the stroma (13). The tortuosity (5) of the vessels (4) is a physiologic peculiarity of the ovary; in places perivascular round-cell accumulations can be seen (6). The follicles are surrounded by the tunica fibrosa (7); the surface of the ovary is covered with cuboid germinal epithelium (3). (Original drawing from a specimen.)

As an intermediate stage we sometimes observe acute oophoritis or salpingitis in the shape of swollen, exquisitely sensitive adnexa, in the bimanual palpation of which the greatest gentleness must be exercised in order to avoid the rupture of an abscess or the destruction of an existing encapsulation. (Plates 39, 44, 59, Fig. 3.)

General peritonitis may follow an acute or a chronic course; the latter is designated as peritonitis pyofibrinosa, and has a more favorable prognosis.

The onset of the inflammation is marked by a protracted chill, and is followed by diffuse abdominal pain. The abdomen may be so tympanitic and distended that

Tab. 41.

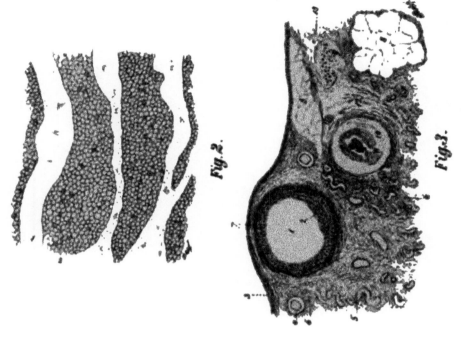

Fig. 2.

Fig. 3.

Fig. 1.

Lith. Anst.v. F. Reichhold, München

dyspnea is caused by the pushing-up of the diaphragm.
Vomiting and constipation are present, giving place to a
profuse fetid diarrhea. Euphoria, together with a rapid
rise of the respiratory and pulse-rates (not always of the
temperature, however), is always suspicious.

Treatment.—All disturbances of menstruation are to
be avoided. Absolute asepsis is to be observed in all
operative measures—therapeutic manipulations (sounds)
and in the care of pessaries. The lighting-up of old
inflammatory residues by exploratory procedures is particularly to be avoided.

Ulcers of the vulva are to be cauterized (formalin) and
treated with iodoform, airol, nosophen, or iodoformogen,
or protected by compresses soaked in oil of turpentine.
The inflammatory edema is to be treated by moist applications (solution of aluminum acetate).

Ulcerations of the cervix are to be cauterized with formalin and treated with irrigations of aluminum acetate, corrosive sublimate, or lysol. Dry powders may be employed
to disinfect the parts, although this method is more troublesome, because of the necessity of daily repetition.

In acute endometritis and myometritis the patients, and
especially the genital organs, should not be disturbed.
The treatment consists of rest in bed, mild laxatives,
warm fomentations, warm vaginal irrigations with potassium permanganate, weak solutions of lysol (0.25%),
normal saline solution, or mucilaginous decoctions, using
about a liter of fluid, carrying the tube high up (gently),
and not elevating the douche bag very much.

If the inflammation increases, the fomentations are to
be replaced by frequently repeated cold applications or by
the ice-bag or ice-coil.

Abscesses should be opened only when they are easily
accessible. They are usually situated in the parametritic
tissues.

Acute parametritis is to be treated with the ice-bag,
calomel, and blue ointment (1.0 applied every two hours

PLATE 42.

Double Pyohydrosalpinx, Chronic Adhesive Perimetritis and Oophoritis. Both tubes are almost filled with pus; the fimbriated ends, walled off both from the isthmus and from the peritoneal cavity, are transformed into cysts. (Original drawing from a specimen of Professor Beck's.)

to the point of salivation), followed by warm fomentations and enemata.

In acute peritonitis several ice-bags upon the abdomen and laxatives in the stage of constipation (infusion of senna; calomel—at first 0.2 to 0.5, later 0.05 to 0.1, at a dose). The diet should be liquid and nutritious. Stimulants, which should contain more alcohol when the patients are accustomed to wine or beer. As soon as free evacuations occur opium is given, or inunctions of blue ointment together with calomel in small doses. Free diaphoresis is excited, and the activity of the skin is increased by cool sponging. [Cases of acute peritonitis should be carefully watched in order not to neglect operative measures. Localized peritonitis with abscess formation always indicates, and promptly responds to, surgical treatment. Acute diffuse peritonitis, however, will usually prove fatal, but that fact warrants early surgical treatment, although most cases succumb.—ED.]

¿ 16. CHRONIC SALPINGITIS.

Etiology.—For definition and anatomy see explanations to Plates 40–43, 44, 46, 59 (Fig. 3), and 74. The most frequent causes are puerperal and gonorrheal inflammations; in every case of endometritis the tubes are not necessarily involved.

(a) Parenchymatous Catarrh of the Tubes (Plate 40, Fig. 1), **with Atresia of the Ostia: Hydrosalpinx.**

The secretion accumulates in the abdominal portion, flattens the papillæ of the mucous membrane and their cylindric epithelium, sepa-

Tab. 42.

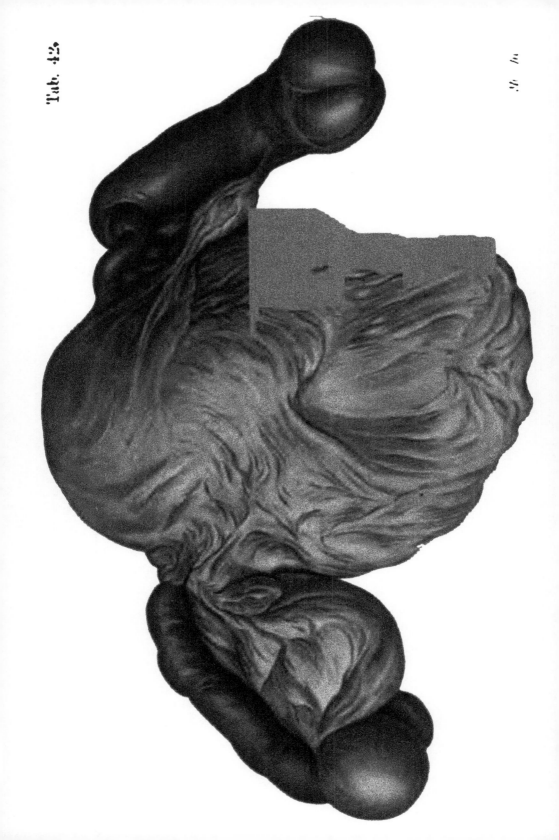

rates the muscle-fibers, and in this way thins and stretches the tubal wall. The tube is held by the serous duplicature of the broad ligament, and presents a spiral appearance with multiple constrictions, as shown in plates 42 and 44. Sometimes the hydrops tubæ (profluens) empties itself periodically into the uterus.

Symptoms.—There are no characteristic symptoms worthy of mention, except anomalies of menstruation, sterility (since the disease is usually bilateral), pressure effects, and perisalpingitic pain.

Diagnosis.—As long as pelvic exudates are absent, bimanual palpation reveals a round, fluctuating, trumpet-shaped tumor, peripherally swollen, extending from an angle of the uterus, and not rarely lying in the vesico-uterine space. The exclusion of a tumor of the ovary is important. (Plate 74.)

Treatment.—In an extreme degree of swelling, celio-salpingotomy, for the purpose of removing the tubal sac; or salpingostomy: *i. e.*, restoration of the lumen of the tube by opening the ostium abdominale and stitching the serosa to the mucosa.

(b) Parenchymatous and Interstitial Purulent Inflammation of the Tubes (Plate 41, Fig. 1), **with Atresia of the Ostia: Pyosalpinx.** (Plate 40, Fig. 3; Plates 42 and 44; Plate 59, Fig. 3; Plate 74.)

The tube is bluish-red and thickened, not only from a passive dilatation, but also not rarely from proliferation of the muscularis. The inflammatory process passes either through the abdominal ostium or through the tubal wall to the peritoneal covering, and thence to the pelvic peritoneum and ovary. It always remains circumscribed, the organs contracting adhesions that often contain purulent deposits. The gonorrheal inflammation is usually bilateral.

We differentiate histologically:

1. *Acute catarrhal parenchymatous salpingitis* with proliferation of the epithelium.

2. *Acute purulent parenchymatous and interstitial salpingitis* with partial desquamation of the epithelium and inflammatory infiltration of the stroma.

PLATE 43.

Chronic Adhesive Perimetritis and Salpingitis with Uterine Myomata. A cross-section shows the marked thickening of the tubal wall and exposes to view the unopened ovarian abscess, which is adherent to the tube. (Original water-color.)

---

3. Chronic interstitial salpingitis, contraction from the connective tissue that replaces the muscularis. The tube loses its elasticity.

From agglutination of the tubal ostia the first class of cases gives rise to hydrosalpinx ; the second and third, to hematosalpinx and pyosalpinx.

Symptoms.—Pain at the side of the uterus, becoming worse at the menstrual epoch and when the intra-abdominal tension is increased. Sterility, from the usual combination with oophoritis. Fever (in gonorrhea, only after exertion or excitement).

Prognosis.—Conception is impossible. The patient is always threatened with peritonitis from perforation. Gonorrheal pyosalpinx does not rupture easily ; the septic form does.

Diagnosis.—By bimanual palpation. (See the differential diagnosis of the retro-uterine tumors under Ovarian Cystomata, and Plate 74, Figs. 1 and 2, and Plate 59, Fig. 3.)

Treatment.—Celiosalpingectomy, stitching the pus sac to the abdominal wall (Hegar, Kaltenbach) and pressing up the uterus from the vagina (Gusserow) are indicated. If the pyosalpinx is not adherent, its rupture can usually be avoided.

If there is distinct fluctuation in the vagina or abdominal wall, free incisions should be made and iodoform gauze drainage established. (See Chronic Pelveoperitonitis.)

§ 17. CHRONIC OOPHORITIS.

Etiology.—Suppurative oophoritis, due to lymphatic

Tab. 43.

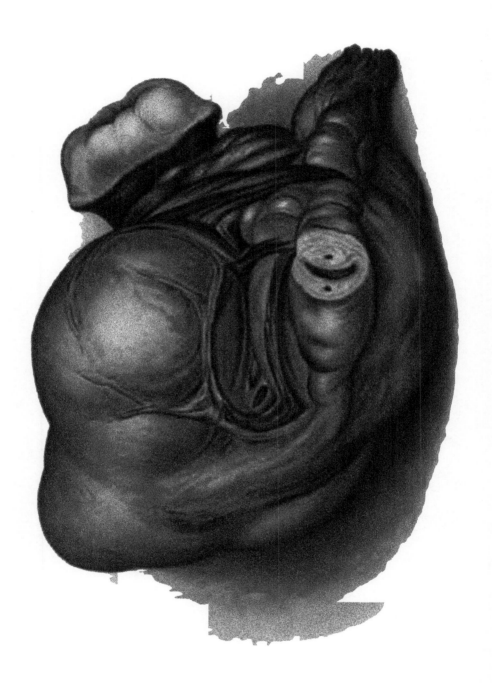

Lith. Anst. F. Reichhold, München

Tab. 48.

absorption from the uterus and tubes, and caused by traumatic or operative septic infection, has been mentioned in connection with peritonitis in a preceding section.

Ovarian abscesses, however, usually follow purulent

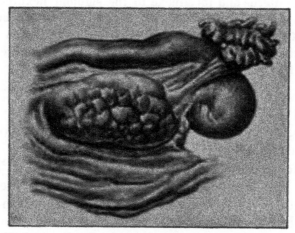

Fig. 34.—Senile cirrhotic atrophy of the ovary.

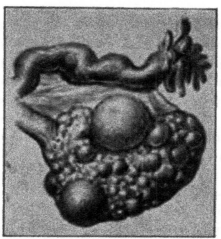

Fig. 35.—Oligocystic degeneration of the ovary.

inflammations of the tubes. (Fig. 36.) This oophorosalpingitis is combined with perimetrosalpingitis, perimetro-oophoritis, and pyosalpinx, forming, together with encapsulated ovarian and peritoneal pus sacs, a large ag-

PLATE 44.

Pelvic Peritonitis, Perioophoritis, Perisalpingitis and Right-sided Pyosalpinx. View of the pouch of Douglas. Pseudoligaments fix the uterus and its adnexa to the sigmoid flexure. The left tube is bent at an angle, the right tube shows inflammatory redness, and is transformed into a pyosalpinx by the agglutination of the abdominal ostium. The globular divisions of the tumor are characteristic. (See Plates 40, 42, 59, 74.) (Original water-color.)

glutinated tumor (pyo-oophorosalpinx). As in purulent salpingitis, the cause is to be found in a septic or gonorrheal mixed infection.

Sclerotic oligocystic ovarian degeneration (Plate 45 ; Plate 41, Fig. 3 ; and Fig. 35), may occur alone, leading to destruction of all the follicles, so that the organ becomes hypertrophic, cicatrized, and dense from the formation of chronic inflammatory connective tissue. (Plate 44 and Fig. 34.)

Symptoms.—These are due partly to the uterine phenomena of dysmenorrhea and partly to hysteria.

The predominant symptom is pain, felt in the lumbar and pelvic regions and radiating to the groins and thighs. This pain increases at the menstrual periods, which are very irregular, sometimes oligomenorrhea or amenorrhea, sometimes menorrhagia, being present. It occurs far less often as intermenstrual pain. It is increased by exertion and constipation, and may present itself as a tubal colic.

Diagnosis.—A hypersensitiveness of the adnexa may be found by bimanual examination ; the tube is swollen, and the ovary is enlarged. These organs should be carefully palpated by the methods demonstrated in Plates 21–23. The ovary is frequently dislocated and bound down behind and below the uterus. (Plate 19, Fig. 1.)

One must not be misled by tenderness of the overlying parts. In lumbo-abdominal neuralgias the belly wall is hypersensitive ; certain hysteric affections (" ovarie " of

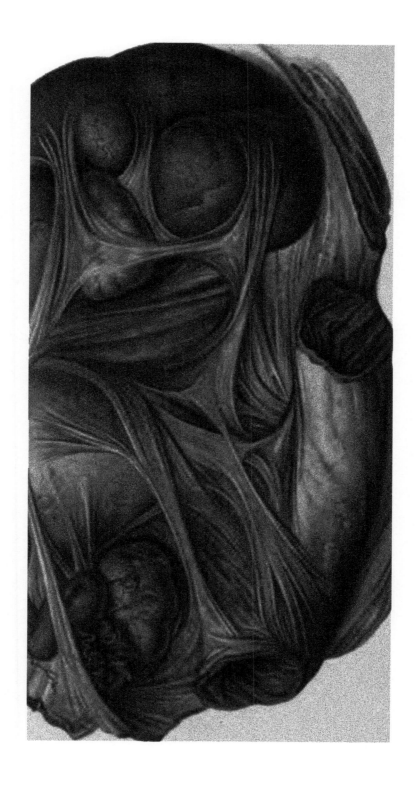

Charcot) may give rise to pain in a healthy ovary, or in the neighboring portions of the broad ligament or vaginal vault.

In perimetrosalpingitic processes the individual organs can not be differentiated.

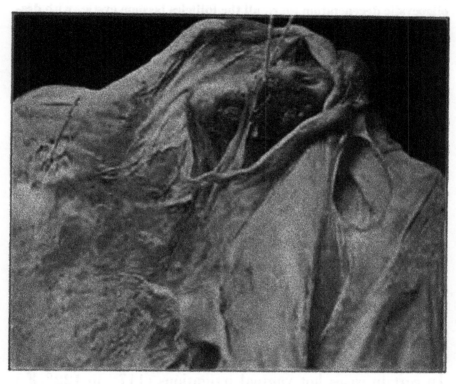

Fig. 36.—Adhesive perioophorometrosalpingitis. The entire posterior peritoneal surface of the uterus and the broad ligaments is covered by adhesions. They form a pocket in which the ovary was completely concealed. It was only by holding up the ovary by means of a thread that it was rendered visible in the illustration. The fimbriated end of the tube is completely occluded and destroyed by the flap-shaped adhesions. An analogous case is described in the "Mon. f. Geb.," 1894, in which the ovary was still more freely movable, and could be distinctly palpated as it slipped in and out of a similar pocket. (Photograph from an autopsy at the Heidelberg Path. Inst.)

Treatment. — Avoid injurious congestions by absolute rest in bed, by sexual continence, and by securing regular evacuations of the bowels and bladder.

PLATE 45.

FIG. 1.—**Pelvic Peritonitis.** The uterus is displaced anteriorly and to the left. Adhesions bind it to the bladder and intestine and fix the tubes and ovaries. The left ovary is enlarged, and shows oligocystic degeneration : *i. e.*, all the follicles become cystic, with desquamation of the germinal epithelium and destruction of the ova. (See Plate 41, Fig. 3, and Fig. 35.) The other ovary is not enlarged, and has a scarred surface from frequent ovulation. (Fig. 34.) These plastic inflammations are due to gonorrheal salpingitis, or to metritis or parametritis from puerperal or operative lesions of the genital mucous membrane. They may start in other organs and sink down into the pouch of Douglas, which is the lowest space in the abdomen.

FIG. 2.—**Left-sided Dermoid Cyst Perforating into the Rectum.** (Original drawing made from the data obtained in palpating a case in the Munich Frauenklinik.) The hair contained in the tumor passes into the rectum through the perforation. Dermoid cysts occur most frequently in the ovary, and contain sebaceous matter, hair, teeth, or even complicated organic structures (brain and nerve masses, portions of the eye, mandible with teeth, etc). (See Plate 79, Fig. 4.)

Removal of the original cause : Treatment of the uterine inflammation, vaginal irrigations, but no intra-uterine treatment.

For the pain : Rest in bed ; the ice-bag, which may be subsequently replaced by warm fomentations and baths. In certain cases hot vaginal irrigations (117° to 122° F.) or hot sand-baths are of value. If the patient is up and about, the organs are to be supported by Mayer's ring (the lever-pessaries press upon the diseased adnexa), or vaginal tamponade (the fornix especially) with iodoform gauze, or depletives, such as potassium iodid, ichthyol, or glycerin, in vaginal suppositories or upon tampons.

If the pain is unbearable or if frequent elevations of temperature occur : Removal of one or both ovaries, usually with the corresponding tube. When the pelvic organs are completely agglutinated, the adhesions consisting of rigid scar tissue, the uterus also is to be re-

Tab. 46

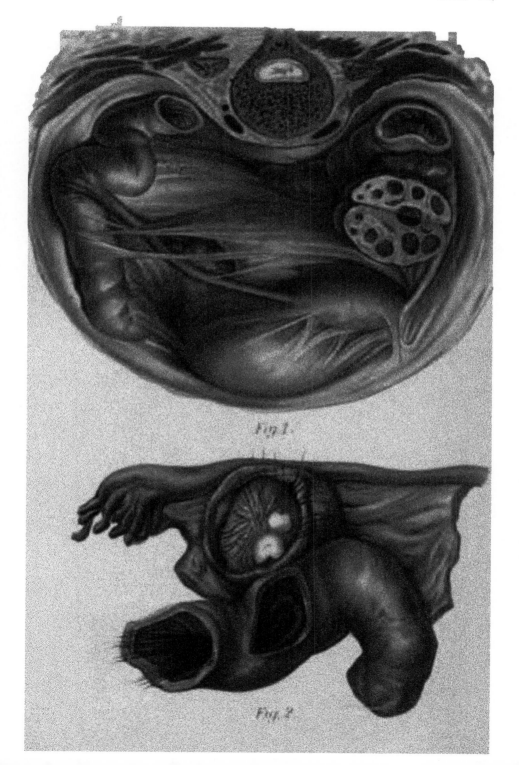

Fig. 1.

Fig. 2.

Tab. 40

moved. Ovariotomy is indicated only when persistent treatment for years has failed.

If all the subacute phenomena have disappeared (occasional chilliness, great pain), massage and compression are useful.

§ 18. CHRONIC PERIMETRITIS, OOPHORITIS, AND SAL-PINGITIS. CHRONIC PELVIC PERITONITIS.

Anatomy.—See explanations to Plates 40–45; 59, Fig. 3; 74, and Diagnosis of Pyosalpinx.

Etiology.—In chronic pelveoperitonitis the tube is by far the most frequent avenue of infection (mostly gonorrheal); small quantities of serum, mucus, or pus escape from the ostium abdominale. The infection may also occur through the lymphatics. Genital tuberculosis is a not infrequent cause.

Catarrhal salpingitis gives rise to perimetrosalpingitis serosa; purulent salpingitis, to purulent pelveoperitonitis saccata. Suppurating tumors (dermoids) furnish an occasional source of infection.

Symptoms and Prognosis.—Sudden violent pelvic pain (from the escape of pus into the abdominal cavity), with chill, vomiting, tympanites, small pulse, and drawn features. The temperature rises and assumes a remittent character. There are rectal and vesical disturbances, pericystitis, and periproctitis. If an abscess breaks through into the bladder, sharp pain and purulent cystitis result.

The fever declines as the exudate becomes encapsulated; the chills reappear, however, as soon as the perforation of a hollow viscus is threatened.

The premonitory symptoms are intestinal tenesmus, vesical pain, and foul-smelling feces and urine.

When perforation has occurred, the process has by no means terminated; from now on there are periods of euphoria, alternating with chills and purulent discharges, the patient becoming gradually weaker—" hectic fever."

PLATE 46.

Genital Tuberculosis of Both Tubes (the Right One Cut Open), of Both Ovaries, and of the Pouch of Douglas. (Original water-color from a specimen.)

Perforation into the peritoneal cavity is rarely followed by immediate death.

In relatively favorable cases the encapsulated exudate becomes absorbed (peritonitis indurata), but from the numerous adhesions, and consequent organic displacements and irritations, there remain serious permanent disturbances of health—sterility (abortion, extra-uterine pregnancy), hysteria, menstrual colic, menorrhagia, and profuse discharge. The gonorrheal inflammation is especially liable to recur.

Diagnosis.—In addition to the hypersensitiveness of the abdomen and of the vaginal vault, bimanual examination causes marked pain, especially on moving the uterus.

The adhesions are recognized from the fact that the uterus has lost its range of motion, being bound down in some pathologic position. (See Displacements of the Uterus and accompanying plates.)

Exudates never exist without peritoneal pain, fever, etc. They are usually found in the pouch of Douglas, and may be palpated from the rectum or from the posterior vaginal vault. The adnexa are embedded in the exudate. (See Retro-uterine Tumors under Ovarian Cystomata.) If the pouch of Douglas is obliterated, the exudate occurs above the pelvic inlet—in the iliac fossae. In other cases the mass may reach as high as the umbilicus.

Treatment.—The acute form is discussed in § 16. In the chronic form every therapeutic manipulation of the genitalia is contraindicated. This includes the introduction of pessaries and of the intra-uterine sound, scarification of the cervix, prolonged bimanual examination, etc.

Tab. 46.

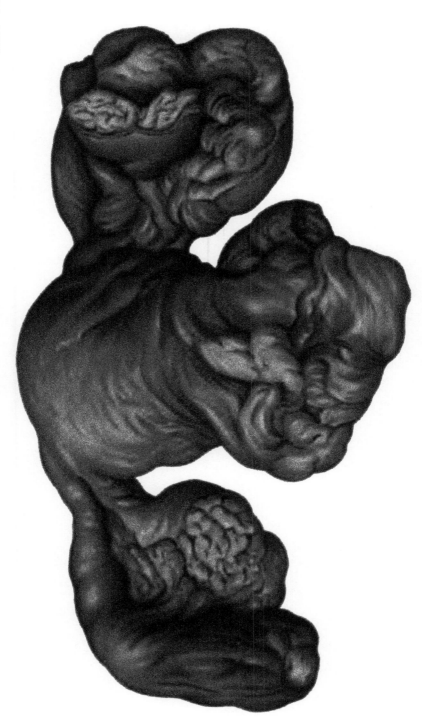

Lith. Anst. J. Reichhold. München

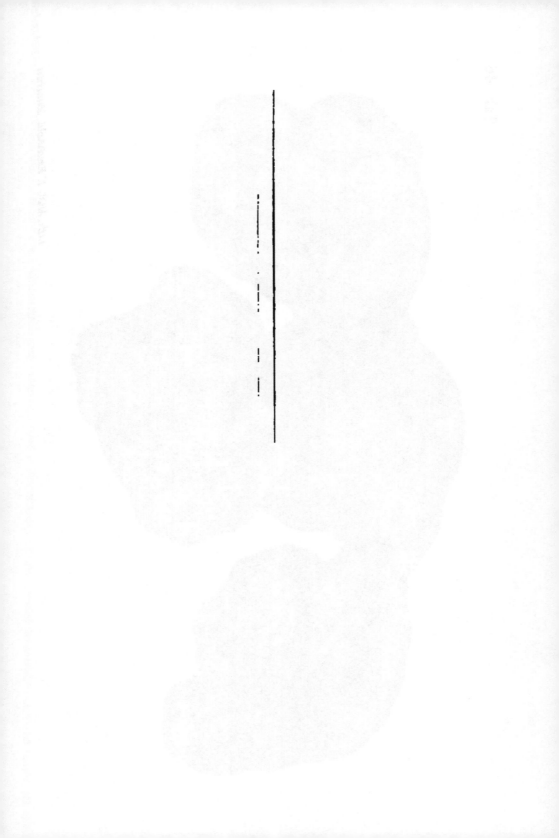

stools are to be secured. For the pain and fever:
zontal position, warm fomentations, lukewarm vagina
jections of mucilaginous or narcotic solutions, introdu
of vaginal suppositories containing anodynes (co
extract of belladonna, morphin). Later, warm sitz-l
(99° F. and gradually cooler).

To stimulate absorption: Compression, hot vagina
jections (117° to 126° F.). Absorbents, such as p
sium iodid, ichthyol, iodoform, glycerin tampons,
baths, salt baths (Kreuznach, Nauheim, Oeynhau
Tölz). Adhesions may be stretched at first by recta
jections (as recommended by Hegar, gradually incre
amount and decreasing temperature); later, if the ┃
are absolutely painless, massage. (See Plates 21–23.

In tubercular peritonitis: Simple celiotomy, wit
without applying iodoform to the serosa. The openin
the abdominal cavity by posterior colpotomy has pr
of value (Löhlein).

In gonorrheal peritonitis: Removal of pyosalpinx
diseased ovaries, as far as enucleation is possible. If p
abscesses cause an increasing impairment of the ge
health, they must be enucleated or freely drained.

The parts may be best surveyed after a celiotomy.
conclusion may then be drawn as to whether it is bett
open and drain the abscess from the vagina, or throug
abdominal wall.

The posterior vaginal vault may be directly incised,
the thickened peritoneum stitched to the vaginal mu
There is danger of infection from putrefactive organ
from the rectum.

If perforation into the bladder occurs, it may be n
sary to establish a vesical fistula, either suprapubi
vaginal.

If the abscess, with or without vaginal fistula, has

PLATE 47.

Cystitis; Ureteritis (Pyonephrosis) as a Result of Lithiasis; Metritis with Endometritis Fungosa; Cervicitis with Marked Dilatation of the Cervical Canal; Vaginitis. The bladder is dissected away and displaced to the left; its hyperemic mucous membrane and thickened walls are exposed to view. On the right may be seen the ureter, cut across near its insertion into the bladder. It shows inflammatory redness at this point, while just above there is an ulceration from which an impacted phosphatic calculus (depicted below) was removed at autopsy. The ureter was markedly dilated above this point, as a result of the obstruction and of the congestive narrowing of the canal at its entrance into the bladder. The endometrium shows marked proliferation and edema; the mucous glands and the uterine cavity are filled with mucus. In the cervical canal a tough mucous plug has been left in position, covering the narrow external os. The internal os is also quite narrow. The vaginal mucous membrane is inflamed. (Original water-color from a specimen at the Heidelberg Path. Inst.)

---

hardened walls difficult of removal through an abdominal wound, vaginal hysterectomy (Landau, Péan); drainage.

§ 19. CHRONIC PARAMETRITIS (PHLEGMON OF THE BROAD LIGAMENTS) AND PARACOLPITIS.

There are two forms :

(a) A chronic process, arising from the acute parametritis just described.

(b) Atrophic chronic parametritis (Freund).

Etiology.—(a) See § 15. (b) Overstimulation of the genital nerves by prolonged and profuse secretion (frequently repeated pregnancies, with lactation during the intervals, sexual excesses). Following upon periphlebitic processes, a connective-tissue change resembling cicatricial atrophy commences in the base of the broad ligament and gradually involves the entire genital tract.

Symptoms and Diagnosis.—(a) An acute parametritis

Tab. 47.

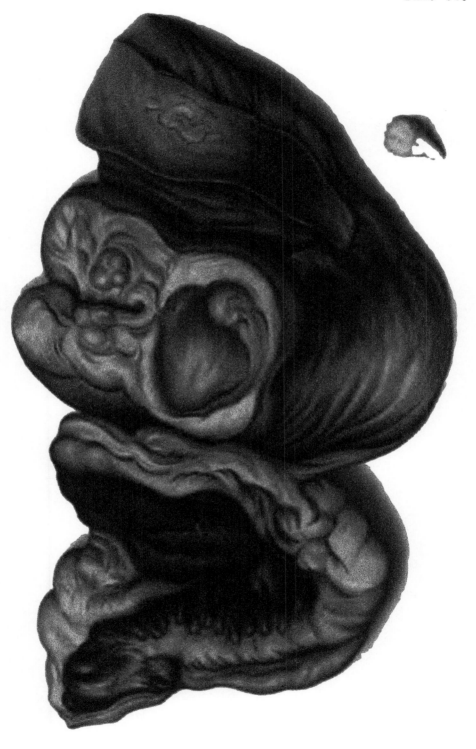

Lith Anon F Reichhold München

that has become chronic may take one of the following courses: The exudate may become thick, remaining for months or years; it may perforate, and, as it has not entirely undergone suppuration, it may discharge from time to time; or, more frequently, it may undergo absorption and cicatricial contraction. These contractions may also follow scars from noninfected interstitial lesions during delivery. They result in displacements and distortions of the uterus and its adnexa. (See §§ 9 to 11 and Plates 23; 41, 2; 55, 1; 59; 62.) These masses of scar tissue are less sensitive than those due to perimetritis. They may be found about the vaginal fornices or alongside of the uterus; the sacro-uterine ligaments may be shortened, limiting range of motion of the uterus.

(*b*) *Symptoms of parametritis chronica atrophicans:* Spontaneous pelvic pain and tenderness of the bladder and rectum if their surrounding connective tissue is involved in the process. Abrogation of the sexual functions: oligomenorrhœa and dysmenorrhea. Nervous irritability, depression, hysteria, and disturbances of general nutrition.

It is difficult to move the organs about in the sensitive and firm connective tissue.

Treatment.—(*a*) *Chronic septic parametritis:* Abscesses are to be incised only when they give rise to fluctuation beneath the skin or mucous membrane, as in chronic pelveoperitonitis. Absorption is to be stimulated by potassium iodid, glycerin, ichthyol, iodoform, hot vaginal injections, Hegar's enemata, mud-baths, and hot sand-baths. Massage is indicated in some cases. Elastic traction on the cervix by means of a bullet-forceps is occasionally of some benefit. No intra-uterine operations should be performed. Secure easy and regular evacuations of the bowels.

(*b*) *Parametritis atrophicans:* Hot vaginal douches and sitz-baths; massage; repeated mechanical intra-uterine stimulation and mild intra-uterine irrigations (soda, Fritsch) are measures to be employed.

PLATE 48.

Chronic Cystitis with Acute Exacerbations. Mucous membrane atrophic, partly necrotic, and thrown into plump, rigid folds by the marked thickening of the bladder-wall. (Original water-color from an autopsy at the Heidelberg Path. Inst.)

---

§ 20. GENITAL TUBERCULOSIS.

Definition and Etiology.—The infection with the tubercle bacillus may be primary or secondary; the latter is the more frequent. On the whole, genital tuberculosis is rare. Gonorrheal, septic, and mixed infections favor its development.

Primary infection may result from cohabitation with a man who has genital tuberculosis, from an infecting digital examination, from infected linen, etc.

Secondary infection may occur by metastasis from the intestines or from the lung, by infection of the tube from the peritoneum (the most frequent cause), or from the adhesion of a tubercular loop of intestine.

The mucous membrane of the tube is by far the most easily infected; the process readily extends from here to the ovaries (by way of the peritoneum, according to Schottländer), or, less rarely, to the uterine mucous membrane, the menstrual changes evidently interfering with the deposit of the bacilli. The cervical and the vaginal mucosa are very rarely affected, the former being protected by its secretion, the latter by its dense epithelium. Here, as in the vulva, fissures form the sole avenues of entrance for the primary invasion of the bacilli.

Tuberculosis of the vesical mucosa, following a general or a genital tuberculosis, is not of more frequent occurrence.

Anatomy.—(1) General peritoneal tuberculosis, which also affects the genital serosa; (2) tuberculosis of the tubes, ovaries, or corpus uteri; (3) the very rare affections of the cervical and vaginal mucosa; (4) the lupous forms seen on the vulva.

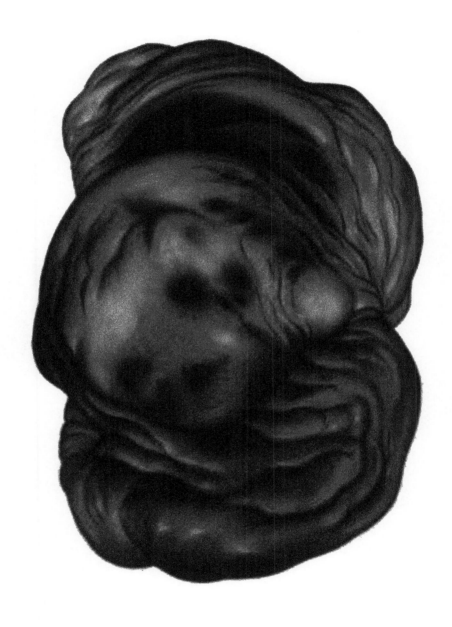

Lith. Inst. F. Reichhold, München

Subacute and chronic inflammatory phenomena (ascites, serofibrinous exudate, formation of pseudoligaments) occur, and the peritoneum becomes covered with tubercles. The tubes are fixed in the pouch of Douglas and their ostia are agglutinated. As the caseous secretion can not be discharged, a pyosalpinx is formed. The walls are reddened, thickened, and infiltrated with yellow tubercular granulations. Caseous areas, very rarely miliary tubercles, are found in the ovaries; they seem to arise most frequently in the stroma. Schottländer also found follicular tuberculosis experimentally; he further found microscopic tubercular changes in the apparently healthy ovaries of tubercular women.

The cylindric epithelium is at first well preserved, only a few cells showing mucoid and granular degeneration. The epithelial layer, however, is finally replaced by a caseous coating, and the muscularis is infiltrated with granulation tissue containing giant cells. The vessels show chronic inflammatory and hyaline changes. Koch's bacilli may be demonstrated, although sparingly present.

In uterine tuberculosis the wall is thickened by the edema of the muscularis; the mucous membrane is totally destroyed and is transformed into a caseous mass; scattered tubercles may be seen. The ulcerative process is sharply limited at the internal os.

Tuberculosis of the vagina and cervix likewise presents irregular ulcerations surrounded by tubercles and a dirty yellow exudate.

Lupus vulvæ usually commences on the labia as small, flat, reddish tumors, which ulcerate. Although they infiltrate more diffusely, they do not extend so rapidly nor secrete so profusely as do syphilitic ulcers. The scars are reddish-violet. The microscope shows no hypertrophy of the papillæ and skin, but a small-cell infiltration about the vessels.

Tuberculosis of the bladder occurs as tubercular infiltration or in the form of ulceration.

The **symptoms** and **diagnosis** of the tubal affections are the same as those of salpingitis or pyosalpinx.

Uterine tuberculosis produces the same phenomena as ordinary metritis, but the organ enlarges more quickly and to a greater degree. The discharge is caseous. The differential diagnosis, from corporeal carcinoma especially, may be aided by curetment, but it is by no means easy: giant cells, tubercles, demonstration of bacilli, or inoculation of the peritoneal cavity of a rabbit with the uterine secretion. An accompanying tubal affection is strong corroborative evidence.

In the beginning of the disease there is amenorrhea, interrupted by blood-tinged or mucopurulent discharges, and a sensation of weight and pressure in the pelvis.

PLATE 49.

Fig. 1.—**Syphilitic Ulcer of the Vaginal Cervix.** Lardaceous exudate; swollen, markedly and sharply cut edges. General inflammatory hyperemia of the cervix. (From Mraçek.)

Fig. 2.—**Syphilitic Ulcers of the Vaginal Mucosa.** Typical |—|-form, the vaginal walls coming in contact. (From Mraçek.)

In vulvar, vaginal, and cervical tuberculosis the bacilli are to be demonstrated, the microscopic changes in excised pieces studied, and the general condition of the patient taken into consideration.

Peritonitis.—Ascitic fluid of a high specific gravity, straw-yellow color—exploratory laparotomy shows confluent tubercles. It must, nevertheless, be remembered that some forms of chronic peritonitis of nontubercular origin show confluent nodules.

Prognosis.—Grave, just as in tuberculosis of the uropoietic apparatus. If an organ is primarily affected, it may be extirpated. We are not yet sufficiently acquainted with the ultimate results from these operations.

Treatment.—Extirpation with a good result is possible (Hegar, Werth, Péan) if the disease is limited to the tubes and uterus; if there are no tubercular peritoneal pseudomembranes; and if the general condition, of the lungs especially, will allow of the operation.

If only the tubes are diseased, they are to be removed, together with the ovaries, by celiotomy. The peritoneal cavity is protected from infection by bringing the tumor outside of the abdominal wound and using elastic ligatures. If the hemorrhage is uncontrollable, incise the posterior vaginal vault and pack Douglas' pouch with iodoform gauze (Wiedow).

If the uterus is affected as well, and is not too voluminous, removal per vaginam should be practised.

If contraindications exist, the pyosalpinx is to be opened from the vagina and drained with iodoform gauze;

Tab. 49.

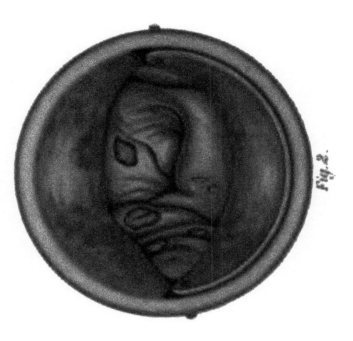

Fig.2.

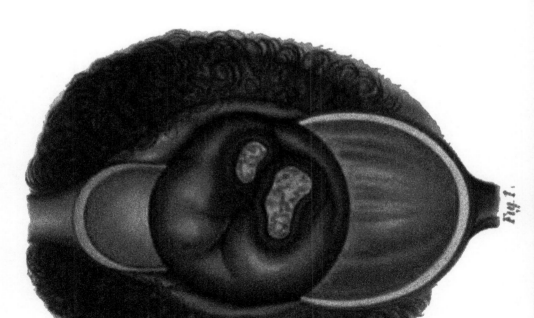

Fig.1.

Lith.Aust   Mündien

the uterus is to be cureted and the raw surface covered with iodoform (iodoform-blower).

Vaginal ulcers and vulvar lupus are to be excised or cauterized with the hot iron, fuming nitric acid, or caustic potash, and dusted with iodoform.

Tuberculosis of the peritoneum is treated by celiotomy.

Ulcers of the bladder: First determine the condition of the kidneys. A suprapubic cystotomy is performed, the ulcers are excised, and the wound is packed with iodoform gauze until it closes spontaneously. [The facility with which circumscribed areas of ulceration may be treated through the endoscope renders cystotomy less frequently necessary.—ED.]

§ 21. VENEREAL DISEASES.

1. Ulcus Molle (Soft Chancre).

Diagnosis.—These round, multiple, sharply circumscribed ulcers occur in from one to four days after exposure, and usually affect the vulva, occurring at the position of a small tear or herpetic ulceration. They are rare in the vagina and upon the cervix. The ulcer is bathed in pus; its edges are undermined, soft, and reddened. It may be the seat of diphtheric inflammation or of a rapid destructive ulceration—ulcus gangraenosum. It may heal at the point of infection (as usual with a scar), yet spread further by serpiginous ulceration.

The infection is a local one, stopping at the inguinal glands, which undergo suppuration (chancroidal bubo) and are very sensitive.

Treatment.—Cauterize the ulcer with fuming nitric acid or chromic acid and treat it antiseptically. Buboes are either to be freely incised or enucleated, and dusted with iodoform.

2. Ulcus Durum (Hard Chancre); Syphilis.

Diagnosis.—The first lesion is a small, single ulcer, in which a papule develops three or four weeks after exposure. Its characteristic peculiarity is that it neither heals nor grows larger, but becomes surrounded by a hard infiltration. Its most frequent situation is upon the posterior commissure, and, next in order, upon the cervix, but it also occurs in the vagina. (Plate 49.)

As a secondary affection, multiple, indolent, inguinal buboes appear, which do not suppurate (differential point from the nonsyphilitic buboes). The infection spreads from here to the abdominal glands. Flat condylomata appear on and about the vulva, extending to the

PLATE 50.

Papular Gummata of the Vulva, of the Anus, and of the Inner Side of the Thigh. Some of them show areas of central necrosis. (From Mraçek.)

thighs and anus. These are secondary proliferations (Plate 50), having the same structure as the primary papule (dense alveolar infiltration of the cutis with cells rich in nuclei; chronic inflammatory thickening of the vessel-wall, with narrowing of the lumen).

Tertiary syphilides rarely occur; gummata are usually situated in the vagina and beside the cervix. They disintegrate rapidly, and strongly resemble the flat ulcerating vaginal epithelioma. (Plate 50.)

The differential diagnosis has been given to insure clinical recognition. The treatment properly belongs to the domain of syphilography.

§ 22. CATARRH OF THE BLADDER AND CYSTITIS.

Anatomy.—Vesical catarrh occurs in an acute and in a chronic form. The latter arises either from the former or from a chronic hyperemia, which produces ecchymosis in the mucous membrane or hemorrhages into the bladder.

In acute catarrh the organ is contracted; the mucosa is reddened, and shows areas that have lost their epithelium. Epithelial debris and emigrated red and white blood-corpuscles may be found between the folds of the wrinkled mucous membrane.

If the inflammation has become chronic, there is a reddening of the entire mucous membrane, or an insular hyperemia (often about the internal urethral orifice, associated with small ecchymoses). Great numbers of leukocytes pass out through the dilated vessels; the mucosa secretes quantities of mucus and casts off its superficial (squamous) epithelium.

If the catarrh decreases, the leukocytes continue to migrate for a long time; in other cases permanent excoriations are established, which are converted into ulcers (most frequently in the trigonum or at the urethral orifice) by the action of bacteria. The muscularis is finally affected.

The original infiltration of the muscularis leads either to an acute extension of the inflammation, to cystitis, and even pericystitis (i. e., inflammation of the vesical subserosa and serosa), or to a chronic parenchymatous hypertrophy of the muscularis. The entire bladder-wall is thick and rigid. (Plate 18.)

The serosa reacts in a like manner and protects the peritoneal cavity from the urine; if it does not, the most acute peritonitis sets in and

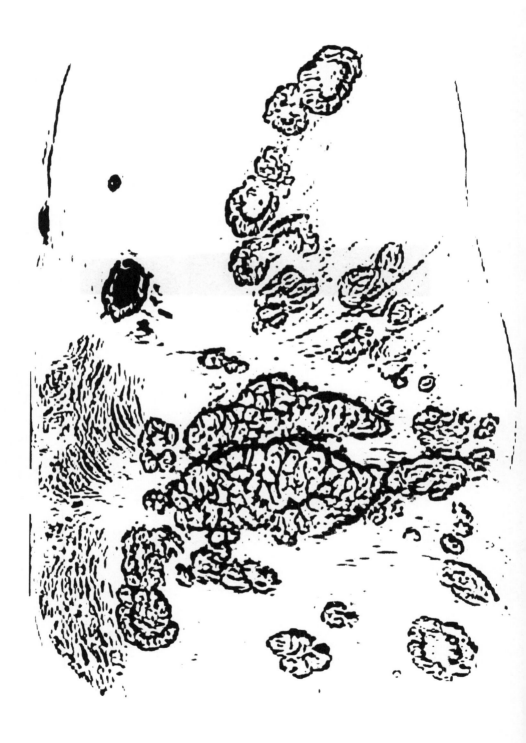

death follows. Such pernicious extension is brought about by progressive gangrene. If the necrosis is limited to the mucous membrane, it leads to casting-off of the same *in toto* or in shreds—cystitis diphtheritica.

Etiology.—The manner of origin differs in many respects from that in the male. The shortness of the urethra allows the infective material to penetrate into the bladder more easily, and yet the same peculiarity prevents the urethritis from becoming chronic and going on to the formation of strictures. Concretions as large as a cherry may pass the urethra, and still larger ones may be removed through it by operative means. The female has no prostate, the hypertrophy of which leads to stasis and decomposition of the urine. The puerperal process gives rise to a series of injurious influences, partly direct pressure effects and partly inflammations. The latter are due either to direct extension from a parametritis or perimetritis, or to the perforation of an exudate or an extra-uterine gestation sac. An analogous predisposition is seen in perforating tumors of the female genitalia (carcinoma, see Plates 85, 86, 88, 89 ; dermoid cysts).

Retention of urine is another cause of catarrh of the bladder. It may be due to incarceration of a retroflexed gravid uterus, to an impacted retro-uterine tumor, or to an inversion of the vagina, with cystocele. The cause may be found in the bladder itself—tumors of the wall or vesical tuberculosis.

The two most frequent causes, however, are direct infection from a dirty catheter and gonorrheal urethritis.

Bacteria are concerned in all vesical catarrhs ; they injure the bladder-wall and cause decomposition of the urine, which irritates the mucous membrane. The catarrh is maintained by irritating urinary ingredients, such as alcohol and cantharides.

Symptoms and Diagnosis.—Increased frequency of micturition, ardor urinæ, vesical tenesmus ; the urine is sometimes bloody and always contains more or less mucus (marked nubecula) or mucopus (thick, white sediment). It is cloudy and has a pungent ammoniacal odor. Slight fever is present.

The microscope shows red and white blood-corpuscles, desquamated epithelium, and, if alkaline fermentation exists, crystals of triple phosphate and acid urate of ammonium.

Diphtheric cystitis is recognized by the great vesical pain, the fever, and the shedding of membranes or shreds. The last-named symptom may render catheterization difficult. If these membranes produce marked ischuria, symptoms of urinary retention (beginning uremia) appear —dyspepsia, nausea, vomiting, alternating constipation and diarrhea, and cerebral congestion.

Hypertrophy of the bladder gradually leads to considerable vesical dilatation from the rigidity of the walls; even the *empty* bladder may be felt above the symphysis. After the muscular hypertrophy disappears the walls of the senile bladder may become almost as thin as paper—atrophy of the bladder. Both forms may be demonstrated by the catheter.

The presence of a cystitis being established, its cause must be diagnosed. The vesical causes are ulcers, tumors (see under Tumors), concretions, and foreign bodies. Vice versâ a whole series of troubles spring from inflammatory irritation, especially of the urethra. The same is true of ulcers (tubercular and others) and fissures at the neck of the bladder, especially those situated at the internal orifice of the urethra and in the urethra itself. These are extremely sensitive, and often arise from catheterization (even with the elastic catheter). These fissures and the catarrh and many of its causes lead to the—

Sequels of Cystitis.

1. Vesical spasm.
2. Paralysis of the bladder—paralysis vesicæ (ischuria, incontinence, ischuria paradoxa, incontinence of retention).

1. Vesical spasm is a neuralgia, and occurs in nervous women, either as a result of vesical catarrh, pericystitis, and all irritations of the bladder (foreign bodies; concretions; hemorrhoids; ulcerations and fissures, especially at the vesical neck and in the urethra; tumors), or as a primary neuralgia from the influence of severe irritations upon an easily excited nervous system. It reminds one of vaginismus, and the two conditions may be associated. It is possible that irritations of the internal genitalia may act as causal factors. Such irritations are overindulgence in sexual intercourse, onanism, interrupted coitus, strong emotions, probably, and colds with subsequent chronic hyperemia. When such primary conditions exist, irritating foods and drinks may bring on an attack. Hysteria also plays its rôle.

Symptoms and Diagnosis.—Violent attacks of pain, lasting from a few minutes to several hours, which radiate from the neck of the bladder, and sometimes assume an extremely painful spasmodic character, especially at the beginning of urination. This spasm may be so violent that the urine can not be voided (ischuria spastica).

If a complicating vesical catarrh exists, the urine is cloudy, containing red and white blood-corpuscles, and mucus. In a pure neurosis it is as clear as water (urina spastica), but is frequently rich in urates and of such a peculiar offensive odor that some abnormal metabolic process (autointoxication) must be considered. The urine is sometimes passed in drops, sometimes in large amounts. The act excites radiating pain in all directions, as well as intestinal tenesmus, nausea, subsequent dyspepsia, ill humor, and sleeplessness, so that the general condition finally suffers. The paroxysms frequently appear irregularly; the affection may persist for years.

Diagnosis.—All causes must be excluded. Bimanual exploration (palpation between the vagina and the symphysis) reveals the presence of calculi, tumors, and vesical hypertrophy. The sound, combined with the palpating vaginal finger, demonstrates sensitive areas (fissures) or small diverticula, the sacculations of which can not be emptied by the catheter, and thus continually reinfect the urine. The interior of the bladder may be digitally explored. Cystoscopy (with or without dilatation of the urethra by means of Simon's specula) allows of inspection of the parts, showing the presence of tumors, ulcers, circumscribed ecchymoses, small foreign bodies, and encysted calculi, and renders catheterization of the ureters possible. The latter procedure is of value in determining the source of pus that does not come from the bladder.

Cystoscopy, as it has been perfected by the instruments of Casper, Nitze, Pawlick-Kelly, and Rose, is the newest aid to diagnosis. In difficult cases it is indispensable. The various methods of its application must be practically learned. The pelvis of the patient is elevated, the urethra is somewhat dilated (previous injection of a few centimeters of a 5% solution of cocain), and a speculum with a beveled end is introduced. The bladder fills with air, and its walls, together with the urethral orifices, may be seen.

In another method of cystoscopy at least 50 c.c. of a boric acid solution are injected into the bladder, and a catheter (not exceeding $\frac{1}{4}$ of a cm. in diameter), armed with a small incandescent lamp, is introduced. By moving the instrument about, the numerous recesses of the female bladder, the interureteric fold, and the trigonum are exposed to view. By means of the operative cystoscope minor operations, such as catheterization of the ureters, may be performed. This method is particularly applicable to determine definitely the source of pus in unilateral pyonephrosis.

It should be mentioned that it is also possible, in the female, to separate the urines from the ureters by means of a double catheter, the dividing partition of which extends to a position between the two ureteral orifices, and is pressed firmly against the bladder-wall.

The ureteral orifices are seen as fine linear fissures, either upon the apex or at the sides of small elevations of the mucosa.

Tubercular ulcers, developing tumors, threatened rupture of a parametritic or pericystic abscess, and encysted foreign bodies (vesical calculi) may be surely diagnosed, and to a certain extent treated, by means of the cystoscope.

2. Paralysis of the bladder may be of a twofold character : paralysis of the longitudinal and oblique muscular fibers—ischuria, retention of urine ; or paralysis of the circular fibers (sphincter vesicæ)—incontinentia paralytica. Both forms may be combined : *i. e.*, the urine dribbles and can not be retained (incontinence) after the desire to urinate has already been lost (ischuria).

If paralysis of the sphincter is not present, in addition to the retention the bladder becomes immoderately distended (without strangury), gradually overcoming the resistance of the sphincter and emptying its urine drop by drop. The bladder suffers no decrease in size, however, and the patient has no suspicion of its dilated condition (ischuria paradoxa, incontinence of retention).

All these conditions (ischuria and incontinence) may follow the puerperal process, from displacements of the bladder, angulation of the urethra, swellings in the urethral region after delivery, or from inflammation of any portion of the genital tract or its serous covering. They may be due to changes in the elasticity of the muscularis (fatty degeneration, atrophy) from cystitis, habitual overdistention of the bladder, advanced age, and acute infectious diseases. They are caused by decreased innervation, as seen in diseases of the spinal cord and other central disturbances, such as apoplexy, neurasthenia, and hysteria (after easy

10

labors, simple operations that do not even involve the vesical region or anterior vaginal wall, emotion, ingestion of irritating foods, new wine and beer, asparagus, strong tea, etc.). Finally, they are seen in weak individuals, in the form of enuresis nocturna, and associated with intoxications.

Symptoms and Diagnosis.—Ischuria paralytica manifests itself by the difficulty of urination, excessive demands being made upon the abdominal muscles to aid in the expulsion of the urine. The cause must, nevertheless, be accurately determined, and the possible existence of urethral tumors especially should be considered. When dribbling is present, the catheter is to be employed in order to exclude ischuria paradoxa and foreign bodies.

Treatment of Cystitis.

Recent gonorrheal urethritis and cystitis are treated as indicated in §12.

In simple acute vesical catarrh (without fever) the bladder is not to be disturbed ; the urine is to be rendered mild and unirritating ; above all, an abundance of tea and milk (add 25.0 of lime-water to $\frac{1}{2}$ of a liter of milk if it is not well borne). Abstinence from all irritating foods, especially alcohol. The diet should be bland, including egg-albumen, milk of almonds, bouillon, and rare meat. The bowels should be regulated by injections and mild laxatives.

Instead of prescribing balsams, as was formerly the custom, urotropin (0.5, three times daily), potassium chlorate, or a solution of sodium salicylate (5 : 150) are given.

The tenesmus is best controlled by rest in bed, warm fomentations, narcotics in vaginal or rectal suppositories (chloral, tincture of opium, morphin, extract of belladonna), or chloral or opium by the month. The vesical mucous membrane itself absorbs nothing. Warm baths.

In chronic cystitis due to infection irrigation of the bladder is to be added to the foregoing measures : physiologic NaCl solution, 1–2% boric acid, ½% salicylic acid, 0.5–1 : 1000 nitrate of silver. To alleviate the irritation of the stronger solution, subsequent irrigations of 0.25% cocain are employed. After solutions of nitrate of silver stronger than 6 : 1000, NaCl solution to precipitate the silver. If the mucous membrane is very sensitive, NaCl or mucilaginous solutions (starch, oatmeal).

The irrigations are carried out with a catheter, or with Küstner's funnel (which I prefer to use, because of the easy formation of a fissure by the catheter) to which a tube and a glass funnel (Hegar's) are attached. The latter should hold from ¼ to ½ of a liter. The apparatus must be rigidly aseptic, and no air-bubbles are to enter the bladder. The funnel is to be filled several times in succession. The temperature should be from 95° to 100° F. The pressure should not be too great, especially with a paralyzed detrusor urinæ. The irrigations are made from one to four times daily; if high fever is present, every two hours.

The quickest results are obtained by permanent drainage of the bladder, which is always to be employed if fissures and severe cystitis are present. As recommended by Fritsch, a rubber tube, 15 cm. long and 0.6 or 0.7 cm. in diameter, is introduced and is held in position by adhesive plaster (or Unna's zinc plaster) or by a suture through the nymphæ. The tube should only be introduced far enough to allow the urine to flow out. The instrument must be changed every three days on account of the incrustation.

Diphtheric membranes must be removed; their presence may be diagnosed from the numerous small incrusted shreds and from the bloody, decomposing urine. The urethra must be dilated by means of Simon's specula. The first three numbers are to be successively introduced, and the irrigation is to be carried out with No. 3. If hemorrhage occurs: Ferripyrin solution (1 : 5), solution of sesquichlorid of iron (1 : 800), or iodoform-ferripyrin-gauze tamponade through the speculum. The after-treatment consists of a bland diet and carbonated waters (such as Wildunger, Vichy) or mild infusions.

Hypertrophy and contraction of the bladder are treated by regular catheterization and lukewarm irrigations, the amount being increased daily (to distend the bladder), cold baths, douches, and vaginal irrigations.

For spasm of the bladder : Removal of the cause (foreign bodies, etc.), bearing in mind fissures at the neck of the bladder or in the urethra ; if these are present, Fritsch's permanent catheter or dilatation of the urethra. Avoid all congestions : injections and mild cathartics ; forbid sexual intercourse ; hot foot-baths ; bland diet without alcohol. For the nervous excitability : Potassium bromid, mild hydrotherapy. During the attack : Chloral internally, by the vagina or rectum ; injections of morphin directly into the bladder, or irrigation with a cocain solution ; or the measures employed for tenesmus.

In paralysis of the bladder the exercise of the will plays an important rôle as far as the sphincter is concerned—enuresis nocturna, for example (wake the patient several times during the night and have her empty her bladder) ; hydrotherapy ; roborants.

Ischuria (detrusor paralysis) is treated by frequent catheterization, cool applications, and abdominal massage.

If the muscularis is already paretic or paralytic (incontinentia paradoxa paralytica), electricity is to be employed. It is also of value in uncontrollable enuresis nocturna. One well-insulated pole is introduced into the bladder, which has been filled with water, and the other pole is applied to the symphysis, lumbar region, or perineum. Ergot is also employed. The treatment of the catarrh—catheterization and lukewarm irrigations—is usually of value in alleviating this condition.

CHAPTER II.

DISTURBANCES OF NUTRITION AND CIRCULATION.
(Exanthemata, Phlebectasia, Neuroses.)

Since the female genitalia, and particularly the vulva, are unusually rich in nerves, glands, blood-vessels, and lymphatics in the shape of cavernous tissue, the affections of one set of structures easily spread to the others, and cause the most varied changes, which usually give rise to a typical symptom-complex : pruritus vulvæ, vaginismus, dysmenorrhea, hysteria.

§ 23. DISTURBANCES OF NUTRITION AND CIRCULATION.
(a) Of the External Genitalia.

By vulvitis pruriginosa we understand an inflammation of the external genitalia, associated with intense itching (pruritus). The parts are dry, fissured, and slate-gray in color.

There are different varieties of vulvitis : simple reddening—dermatitis simplex ; if the corium and subcutaneous tissue are diffusely involved—phlegmone vulvæ with abscess formation ; if partial—furunculosis ; if the sebaceous glands are inflamed (small yellowish projections like acne)—folliculitis ; if an inflammation of the connective-tissue papillæ (small red prominences) also exists—papillary vulvitis. There is a vulvitis diabetica. Bartholinitis has been mentioned in §12.

Cutaneous exanthemata (eczema, herpes, prurigo, miliaria) rarely occur.

Treatment.—*Simple inflammation :* Washings with warm soda solutions and the subsequent application of lead-water, solution of

149

aluminum acetate, zinc ointment, 20% boric-vaselin, 10% carbolized oil, sitz-baths, dusting-powders (bismuth-talcum).

Severer inflammation: Soda solutions, then apply 5–10% solution of silver nitrate, and lead-water compresses.

Abscesses: Incision. In furunculosis: Shave off the pubic hair; Unna's mercurial plaster in the beginning; later, warm sitz-baths, soap plaster, emollient cataplasms.

Diabetic vulvitis: Constitutional treatment, meat diet, laxatives (sal carolinum).

Folliculitis: Remove the grease from the skin by means of solutions of potassium carbonate (a piece the size of a walnut is dissolved in the wash-water) and immediate application of 5–10% solution of nitrate of silver. If pruritus is present, excision of the part, 5% menthol-alcohol, or menthol-lanolin.

Pruritus: Washings with soda solution; application of 10% solution of nitrate of silver and subsequent 10% carbolic acid compresses; applications of ice-water, compresses of 6% menthol-alcohol, or ½–1 : 1000 corrosive sublimate, or salicylic acid; warm sitz-baths with ½ of a pound of wheat bran, oak-bark decoctions, or other astringents (alum, formalin, tannin). Anodynes: cocain (expensive !), eucain B, chloroform, morphin, and belladonna act temporarily in cases having a neurasthenic basis and not rarely appearing after some acute exciting cause (fright).

(b) Of the Internal Genitalia.

By vaginismus we understand a reflex spasmodic contraction of the introitus vaginæ from contact with the marked hyperesthetic, usually thickened and chronically inflamed, hymen, or carunculæ myrtiformes. It is a symptom-complex similar to pruritus, but it also affects the motor elements. The two affections may coexist. Central or hysteric processes are also responsible, as is demonstrated by the fact that the lightest touch with a smooth instrument-handle produces the same result as the impetus coeundi or the introduction of a speculum.

I had a patient in whom the introduction of an irrigation tube was easy and painless when carried out by herself, but accompanied by intense pain when done by any one else. If her attention was engaged, a tampon could be introduced. The thought of a remarriage, with subsequent coitus, also brought on an attack.

There is one form of vaginismus, however, without pain, as is shown by the symptom of the " penis captivus." There are also neuroses of the vagina situated higher up—

painful areas, especially in the posterior vaginal vault and not associated with parametritic processes.

Treatment.—Careful excision of the entire hymen, including the urethral orifice with its caruncles. In the case mentioned the nymphæ (folliculitis) were also removed, on account of pruritus. The patient married, conceived, had an easy delivery, and has now been a mother and wife for four years; in her first marriage, lasting for some years, she was an unhappy, and finally a divorced, woman.

If the hypersensitiveness still remains, the sphincter vaginæ should be forcibly stretched. The actual anesthesia of the parts is now demonstrated to the patient by palpation. Regular coitus and the speedy occurrence of impregnation remove the last vestiges of the trouble.

In other cases conditions of pronounced nervous irritation, and finally nervous depression, or even psychoses, occur.

Masturbation is a frequent cause. In such cases the time of the patient should be completely occupied by absorbing and fatiguing duties, and all irritations of the senses should be removed (lectures, balls, theater, etc.). Other causes are fissures, arising from a resistent hymen, and impotentia cœundi on the part of the male. (See § 5.)

A disturbance of nutrition of the aged, colpitis vetularum (Ruge), leads, as colpitis ulcerosa adhæsiva (irregular areas of round-cell infiltration with desquamated epithelium), to adhesions, scars, and bridges of new tissue.

Examples of vasomotor anomalies of innervation are furnished by phlebectasia of the vulva (Plate 51) and varicocele parovarialis (Plate 53); the latter may give rise to intraperitoneal hematocele or hematoma of the broad ligament.

The disturbances of innervation of the arterial system are usually associated with similar affections of all the contractile elements of the genitalia and their supporting ligaments. This deficient "tonus" is a frequent occur-

PLATE 51.

Fig. 1.—Elephantiasis Vulvæ Originating in the Labium Majus Dextrum and Polypoid Excrescences of the Mucous Membrane at the Urethral Orifice. The elephantiasis starts in the deeper connective tissue and consists of proliferated lymph capillaries (see Plate 29, Fig. 1), partly neuromatous (Czerny) and partly from stasis. The tumors may resemble external papillomata, but their excrescences are usually larger and flatter. (See Plate 24.) Sometimes the tumors grow out from the entire vulva. Their growth is always slow and is characterized by great variations in size.

Polyps of the urethral mucous membrane are seen at the external orifice or at the neck of the bladder. They consist of connective tissue, and rarely contain small retention cysts, arising from atresia of the excretory ducts of Skene's glands (in Fig. 20 the fine orifices of these glands are seen in the urethral wall). Other urethral tumors arise as varices, as vascular proliferations (angioma), as sarcoma and epithelioma. (Original water-color ; case in Munich Frauenklinik.)

Fig. 2.—Phlebectasia of the Labia Majora, of the Clitoris, and of the Nymphæ ; the Right Labium Majus Contains a Hematoma (Thrombus Vulvæ) ; and Hemorrhoids. This condition is most frequently found in parturient or puerperal women, the varices being due to venous stasis ; the extravasation, to subcutaneous injuries of the vessels during delivery. Hematoma may also occur in nonpregnant women as a result of trauma.

---

rence, and leads to descent and prolapse of the uterus, of the vaginal walls with the bladder and the rectum, and to retroversion and retroflexion of the uterus. It produces a chronic hyperemia of these organs, which becomes the noninfectious starting-point of an inflammation.

These affections have been considered in §§ 7–11 and in §§ 13, 14, and 17. The foregoing common etiologic factor must be borne in mind, as it is of far-reaching importance.

The partly uterine, partly ovarian symptom-complex of dysmenorrhea is described in § 4, under 8.

The hysteric symptom-complex (see § 11, under Symptoms, and § 17, under Diagnosis) represents a disease of the entire nervous sys-

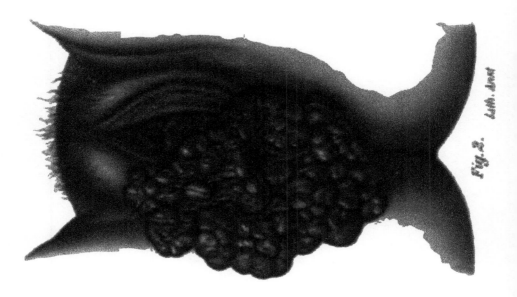

Fig. 2.   lith. Imst

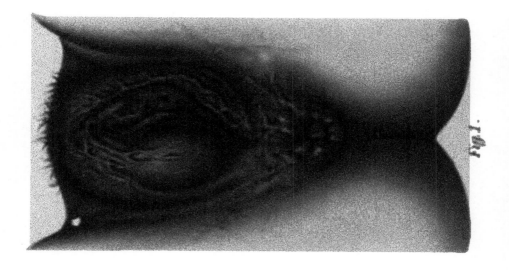

Fig. 1.

tem, with a cerebral origin, and the evolution of certain phenomena, A predisposition either may preexist or may be induced by a too indulgent education. This disease arises from marked sensual or emotional excitement, which individuals with healthy nerves bear without injury, or from a permanent feeling of self-dissatisfaction.

In addition to congenital traits, a general predisposition is furnished by our city life, with its early manifold sensory impressions, its disproportionate mental activity, its luxuries and pleasures, and with its absence of actual invigorating labor, and of precise duties and corresponding strengthening of the will. These pernicious factors must be excluded in youth; amends must be made for them in later years.

Diseases of the genitalia may bring on the disease, but they do not always produce hysteria, nor are they the only exciting causes. As such may be mentioned puerperal diseases, with their infectious irritations and weakening hemorrhages; chronic painful oophoritis and salpingitis; pelveoperitonitic adhesions; retroflexio uteri fixati; spasmodic angulation of a retroverted uterus; inflammations of the uterus; intramural myomata projecting from the os uteri; traction from polyps, etc.

Symptoms.—Ill humor, hypersensitiveness, weakness of will.

Epileptiform spasms and contractions, usually clonic, sometimes tonic, with perfect consciousness and reflex excitability (pupils); of the muscles of the extremities and trunk (Charcot's arch), with accelerated respiration, and, according to the state of mind, paroxysms of shrieking, crying, laughing; of the laryngeal and esophageal muscularis, spasm of the glottis (barking cough), spasm of the esophagus (globus hystericus). Singultus hystericus.

Paralyses: of the extremities, unilateral and bilateral; of the vocal cords, hysteric hoarseness and aphonia (as in a case with retroflexion of the uterus at the Heidelberg clinic).

General and partial hyperesthesias and anesthesias: Tussis uterina, emesis et vomitus, clavus hystericus, spinal irritation, "ovarie" (Charcot).

Vasomotor and trophic symptoms: Palpitation, stenocardia, nervous dyspepsia, meteorismus; anomalies of secretion of the skin (hyperidrosis, anhidrosis), of the kidneys (polyuria, oliguria or temporary anuria, ischuria); nervous diarrhea, etc.

Diagnosis is made from the rapidly changing character of the symptoms. These do not form a clinical picture corresponding to pathologic changes in any definite organ.

Treatment.—*Prophylactic* (see Treatment of Vaginismus).—Psychic influence and education; above all, never criticize the patient's view of her ailment, but demonstrate to her its general nervous character, and change the manner of living, the diet, etc. Regulate the functions as indicated in ¿ 4, under 7. Restricted and bland diet or a more liberal one, as the case may be. Treatment of a genital disease, if present.

Lukewarm baths to render the patient more hardy; gradually lower the temperature from 88° to 72° F., fifteen minutes. Electric baths.

Symptomatic.—Potassium bromid (with heart disease, sodium

PLATE 52.

Edema of the Nymphæ from a Moribund Patient with a Cardiac Lesion. (Original water-color from nature.)

bromid) and monobromated camphor for the excitement, irritation, and palpitation ; phenacetin, lactophenin, heroin, sulphonal, trional, menthol, valerian. Chloroform, morphin, atropin, chloral, and extract of belladonna (by the mouth, by the rectum, or hypodermically) are all used for the neuralgias and as sedatives or hypnotics. They usually do more harm than good. For the paralyses, faradization or massage ; for the spasms and convulsions, cold water in every form known to hydrotherapy.

Charcot's so-called "Ovarie" has been mentioned in § 17, under Diagnosis. In the great majority of cases it has nothing to do with the ovaries or even with the adjacent nerve plexuses. It is generally either a neuralgia of the nerves passing through the abdominal recti muscles toward the hypogastrium, or neuralgia of the posterior vaginal vault, of the pouch of Douglas, and of the contiguous portion of the rectum. The latter cases are usually associated with vasomotor and motor disturbances of innervation of the parts. (See the author's paper in the "Mon. f. Geb.," January, 1898.)

Coccygodynia is a local hyperesthesia of the plexus coccygeus.

Treatment.--Hydrotherapy, or, in extreme cases, extirpation of the os coccygeus.

Sometimes confusion may arise from a pain, which is experienced in the coccygeo-anal region, but the location of which may be shown to be considerably higher—in the posterior vaginal fornix or about the pouch of Douglas; not rarely varicoceles in the broad ligament and hemorrhoids high up in the rectum may be demonstrated. In the puerperium, immediately after delivery, and sometimes even occasionally during pregnancy, an analogous pain is experienced, which is falsely ascribed to the coccyx, to pressure on its plexus, to periosteitis, to luxations, etc. Careful palpation from the rectum and externally excludes these conditions.

Tab. 62.

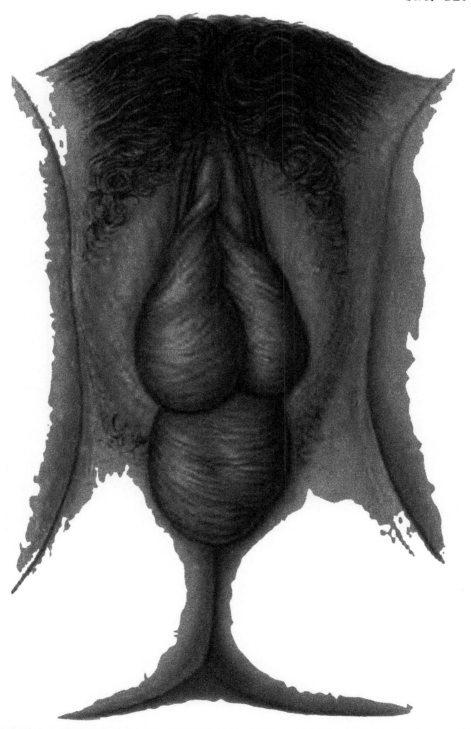

GROUP IV.

INJURIES AND THEIR CONSEQUENCES.

CHAPTER I.

DEFECTS WITH CICATRICIAL CHANGES.

All varieties of genital lesions arise by far most frequently during delivery. The effect they produce is dependent upon their location. Cicatrices in the vulva rarely cause atresia; on the contrary, they produce a gaping. Lacerations of the external os may heal with ectropion; nevertheless, here, as in the vagina and cervix, stenosis and atresias are more likely to occur.

§ 24. INJURIES OF THE VULVA (INCLUDING FISSURES) AND PERINEAL DEFECTS, INCONTINENTIA VULVÆ.

Definition.—The solutions of continuity, which are now to be considered, have the character of incised, of lacerated, and of lacerated and contused wounds. A natural division, based upon the depth of the injury, is as follows:

1. Fissures: Slight linear solutions of continuity of the surface, occurring at the frænulum perinæi and productive of specific results when involving the hymen, the neck of the bladder, or the urethra. (See §§ 22 and 23.)

2. Lacerations of the perineum of the first degree: Tears of the frænulum perinæi and of the mucous membrane of the vestibule.

155

PLATE 53.

Phlebectasia with Phleboliths of the Ligmenta Lata Corresponding to the Ovarian Vessels and the Pampiniform Plexus. The venous stasis in the remaining portions of the broad ligaments is also apparent. (Original water-color from an autopsy at the Heidelberg Path. Inst.)

---

3. Tears of the mucosa of the fossa navicularis, the skin surface of the perineum being intact, but undermined. This important and easily overlooked variety is not rarely produced by the posterior shoulder.

4. Lacerations of the perineum of the second degree: Tears extending to the sphincter ani.

5. Perforations of the perineum (rare): Canal-like lacerations, which pass from the vagina through the middle of the perineum, sometimes involving the anus, the anterior portion of the fraenulum perinæi being left intact.

6. Lacerations of the perineum of the third degree, or complete lacerations: the tear extends into the rectum.

While all these tears are brought about, almost without exception, by incidents of the sexual life (cohabitation, delivery, and the puerperium—urethral fissures from catheterization), the parts of the vulva are also exposed to other traumatisms. These are followed by serious results, especially if occurring during pregnancy, when the parts are very vascular. The region of the clitoris is the most exposed to wounds, which are usually caused by falling astride of some object. It is also the most dangerous region, as patients have bled to death in a short time from hemorrhage from the corpus cavernosum.

Hemorrhages and injuries of this character must be treated immediately by suture.

Lacerations and perforations of the nymphæ are not *productive* of further consequences.

Symptoms and Consequences of Perineal Lacerations.—If primary union is not obtained by immediate suture after delivery, these wounds heal by granulation, the lower portions of the labia being drawn apart and distorted.

Fissures cause only a burning, and may induce infectious ulceration; they may nevertheless be produced in a perineal cicatrix as rhagades (after coitus, difficult defecation).

In perineal lacerations of the first degree (Plate 54, Fig. 3) the tuberculum vaginæ loses the covering and support of the frænulum perinæi. This portion of the anterior vaginal wall prolapses; the urethral orifice gapes; [1] there is a predisposition to urethritis and vesical catarrh.

In perineal lacerations of the second degree the posterior vaginal wall prolapses from above the scar (see Plate 27); and if the entire pelvic suspensory apparatus, including the pelvic fascia and the levatores ani muscles, has lost its "tonus," all those downward displacements described in §§ 7 and 8 and their appurtenant plates may occur. In addition, uterine and vaginal catarrh, cystocele, and rectocele, and their sequels, are produced.

In perineal lacerations of the third degree—the complete variety (Plates 7, 1; 54, 2 and 4; Fig. 26)—fecal incontinence is present, because the voluntary external sphincter muscle is torn. In extreme cases the internal sphincter is also involved.

As is shown in the sagittal section of the perineum (Plate 54, Fig. 1), the transversely striated external sphincter forms a rounded body about the anal pouch (see the corresponding outline of the shading), while the internal sphincter passes vertically upward from it as an elongated mass of fibers. Both sphincters are absent in figures 2 and 4; in figure 3 they are both present. The whole perineum may be destroyed, and yet a portion of the external sphincter may remain intact.

---

[1] In Heidelberg I saw such a case in a peasant's wife. The impetus coeundi had been directed against the prolapsed tuberculum vaginæ and, in this manner, had so dilated the urethra that the finger could be readily introduced. (Plate 19, 2.)

PLATE 54.

FIG. 1.—The normal perineum is a physiologic support for the vaginal walls, and indirectly for the uterus. The intact perineum forms the lowest part of the vulva, being at a lower level than the end of the anterior vaginal wall. It resembles a triangle placed beneath the vaginal ostinm and supporting the tuberculum vaginæ. It also supports the entire posterior vaginal wall, which, in its turn, holds up the upper half of the anterior one. The normal cervix looks backward, resting against the posterior vaginal fornix, and the corpus uteri derives its support from the anterior vaginal wall.

FIG. 2.—**Perineal Laceration of the Third Degree (into the Rectum).** Inversion of the anterior vaginal wall with beginning cystocele; descensus uteri from flattening of the anterior vaginal wall.

FIG. 3.—**Perineal Laceration of the Second Degree.** The loss of support of the anterior vaginal wall is clearly shown.

FIG. 4.—**Perineal Laceration of the Third Degree.** Inversion and prolapse of the posterior vaginal wall; beginning retroversion of the uterus.

There are cases, however, in which solid, and even liquid, stools can be voluntarily controlled. This is due either to an intact portion of the external sphincter, the tear not extending 1½ cm. into the rectum, or to the fact that the lowest portion of the rectum has undergone cicatricial contraction. Such cases are not easy to diagnose, because these rectal scars become pigmented and covered with epidermoid tissue.

The scars may be the seat of neuralgias or pruritus. If fissures form, burning and tenesmus are present. The continual moisture of the prolapsed vaginal walls, with or without discharge or intertrigo, is a constant source of annoyance; there arises a dragging sensation, as if the internal organs would fall out. The deficient closure of the vulva, which increases with the senile atrophy of fatty tissues, allows air to enter the vagina; any increase of the abdominal tension will force this air out in an audible manner—garrulitas vulvæ.

Tab. 54.

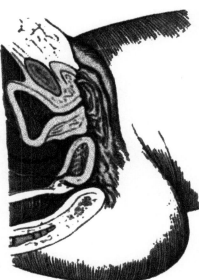

Fig. 2.

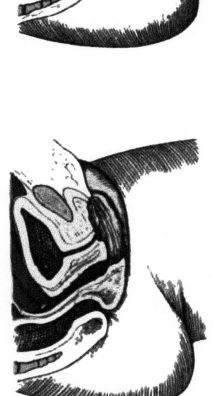

Fig. 4.

Fig. 1.

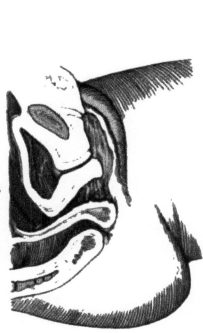

Fig. 3.

Lith. Anst. F. Reichhold. München.

Treatment.—These serious symptoms are best treated by plastic operations, as mentioned in § 8. The success of the operation depends partly upon the preparation of the patient: disinfection of the vagina and cervix by sponging and irrigation, emptying of the bladder, and especially of the rectum (two or three days before the operation). Narcosis. Cotton tampon in the rectum.

The operation may be performed soon after the completion of the puerperium. Not only must the cutaneous bridge between the lower ends of the labia be restored, but the new septum, with its anterior edge (corresponding to the frenulum), must also cover the tuberculum vaginæ and support the anterior vaginal wall.

This new perineal septum must, further, have the same size and shape (triangular in sagittal section) as the normal perineal body, so that a new fossa navicularis will be formed.

The outline of the denudation will vary according to the nature of the defect; if the vagina is injured and deeper, it is hat-shaped (Hildebrandt and Freund); if the chief lacerations are in the lateral portions of the vagina, it is shaped like the wings of a butterfly (Simon and Hegar). In the latter case the area is denuded in that manner so as to form a perineal body resembling the original one. Fritsch pursues the same course, excising the scars in the vagina, with their lateral extensions, and inserting stitches toward the vagina, toward the perineum, and toward the rectum.

Hildebrandt, Freund, and Martin cut one or two or more triangular flaps from the vagina: *i. e.*, either avoid or remove the columna rugarum posterior.

Bischoff, v. Winckel, and Küstner (episioplasty) procure a median vaginal flap or two lateral vulvar flaps of corresponding shape to the outline of the scar, the principal portions of which are rarely in the middle line. This is known as flap-perineorrhaphy.

Simpson, Lawson Tait, Sänger, Zweifel, and v. Winckel perform perineoplasty in as conservative a manner as possible : *i. e.*, without the removal of tissue. This method has been improperly defined as flap-perineorrhaphy. A transverse incision is made in the rectovaginal septum, and its edges are drawn upward and downward by means of tenacula. The original transverse wound is now closed by a vertical row of sutures (deep and superficial), drawing the tissues together in the median line. [In America the importance of repairing ruptures of the pelvic fascia and of the levatores ani muscles is so thoroughly appreciated that Emmet's plan of operating for so-called perineal lacerations has largely superseded all others.—ED.]

The complete perineal lacerations (third degree) are operated upon according to the same principles ; here the edges of the rectal tear must also be freshened and must be united by sutures.

After-treatment.—It is best to leave the wound uncovered ; it should be frequently irrigated, and the most rigid cleanliness should be maintained. The knees are to be bandaged together. The sutures are allowed to remain as long as possible (from ten to twenty days) ; the best materials are silver wire and silkworm-gut.

On the third day, or soon thereafter, the bowels should be moved by castor oil in capsules ; high injections may be used, if necessary. In most cases opium is unnecessary for the production of an artificial coprostasis if the intestinal tract has been previously thoroughly evacuated and the patient is kept upon a nutritious liquid diet. If individual sutures cut through, they are to be removed. Should a rectovaginal fistula occur, the entire septum is to be divided, all granulation tissue removed, and the wound surfaces united as before.

The patient is to be kept in bed for two or three weeks.

§ 25. LACERATIONS OF THE VAGINA AND CERVIX.

(a) **Simple injuries of the vagina** (*i. e.*, without opening neighboring organs) occur most frequently during delivery. They are also the result of accidental trauma or of unskilled or rough manipulations, such as forced coitus, especially in elderly women or where the disproportion between the size of the genitals is great ; rape ; clumsy operative procedures or examinations ; the introduction of specula that are too large ; attempts at abortion ; and cauterizations.

Symptoms.—Often union per primam ; sometimes severe hemorrhages or septic infection. The author observed, two hours after a tear of the fornix with most profuse hemorrhage (illegitimate coitus of an English woman forty-nine years of age, who had had a child twelve years before, and who suffered from vaginismus), a temperature of 101.3° F., a pulse of 120, and an acute urticaria covering the entire body, which lasted twelve hours.

Treatment.—Disinfection, removal of necrotic shreds, ligation or suture of vessels, coaptation of fresh wounds, tamponade with ferripyrin, alum-iron chlorid, iodoform, nosophen, or itrol gauze. Old vaginal scars producing stenosis or atresia are to be excised, stretched (manually or by tamponade), or treated by plastic operations. This will make the treatment tedious, and if conception has already occurred, complicated methods of delivery may be necessary.

(b) **Tears of the cervix** lead to commissural or to star-shaped defects (Plate 55), to scars of the os uteri, and, secondarily, to ectropion. (§ 13 and Plate 56.) If they extend into the vaginal vault and the paracervical connective tissue, they produce torsions and fixed displacements of the neck of the uterus. (See § 11 and Plate 55.)

These lacerations, instead of undergoing simple cicatrization, many persist for a considerable time as yellowish-gray, fissured ulcers with reddened edges. Both processes occur most frequently at the commissures of the os uteri, because these portions of the tissues heal poorly. The ulcers are immediately followed (even in the puerperium, see § 15) by endometritis, metritis and parametritis, and secondary ectropion ; the scars cause direct ectropion and a secondary uterine catarrh.

The distortions produced by the scar tissue cause radiating pains in the lower extremities and nervous reflexes similar to the epileptic and epileptiform attacks associated with scars elsewhere.

Treatment.—Emmet first directed attention to these fissured ulcers and their consequences, and recommended their treatment by the following procedure : The lips of the ectropion are fixed with tenacula, the commissural scar

11

PLATE 55.

Fig. 1.—**Torsion of the Cervix Produced by Scar Tissue.** It extends posteriorly from the commissure of the os uteri into the base of the left broad ligament.

Fig. 2.—**Star-shaped laceration of the external os,** resulting from difficult labor with a rigid cervix, or from an operative delivery before the external os is sufficiently dilated. Tears occur in the lips of the os uteri just as frequently as in their lateral commissures; while the former usually heal well, the cicatrization of the latter is affected by the poorer vascular supply of the sides of the cervix, and results in a greater degree of contraction. The lips of the os gape and the cervical mucosa gradually protrudes (ectropion).

---

tissue is excised, going into the vaginal vault if necessary (not too deeply, however, on account of the large vessels), and the surfaces of the wound are united. The Martin-Skutsch modification is described on page 89, and the excision of the proliferated mucous membrane in § 14. Sänger designed a hysterotrachelorrhaphy. By these methods the normal shape and size of the cervix are restored.

§ 26. TRAUMATIC STENOSES AND ATRESIAS OF THE VULVA, OF THE VAGINA, AND OF THE UTERUS.

The congenital stenoses and atresias are described on pages 22 to 29, 33, and 36 to 38.   ·

PLATE 56.

Fig. 1.—**Laceration of the Left Commissure of the Os Uteri, with Marked Ectropion and Ovules of Naboth on the Projecting Hypertrophied Cervical Mucosa.** (See Plates 28; 29, 4; 30; 90, 3.)

Fig. 2.—**Old Ectropion and Congestion of the Cervix.** The mucosa becomes wrinkled from the minute cicatricial contractions of the newly formed connective-tissue fibers (endometritis interstitialis chronica, see Plate 31, Fig. 2).

Tab. 55.

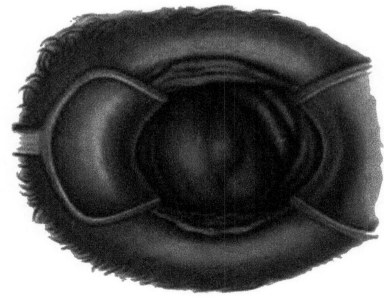

Fig 1.

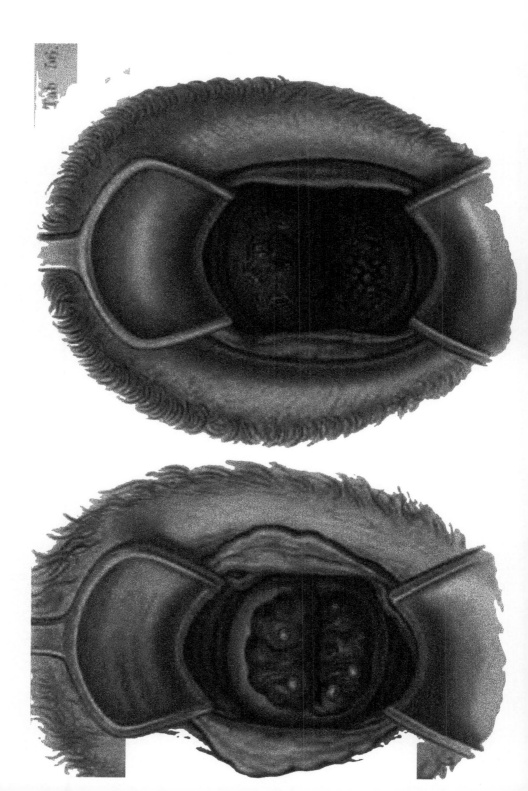

Anatomy and Etiology.—Narrowings, and cv .i a-
tricial adhesions, are brought about by chronic inflammatory
tory processes, circumscribing ulcers with marked contraction, too severe cauterizations, and injuries. They are
seen in advanced life and in connection with acute infec-
tious- diseases.

The ulcerated labia become adherent; the urethral
orifice even may be temporarily occluded. There is a
retention of blood and of the secretions of the entire
genital canal.

Actual obliteration occurs in the vagina, chiefly from
cauterization and in advanced age.

The external os is the most frequent location for these
agglutinations. It is either contracted to a small, round,
cicatricial opening, or subdivided by a bridge of tissue, or
retracted by scars into a funnel of mucous membrane. The
stenosis may be short and circumscribed or long and tubular, leading, correspondingly, to a membranous or to a cord-
like atresia. Atresias of the internal os from too severe
cauterizations are rarer; those of the ostium tubæ are still
more infrequent. For the anatomic changes see § 1 (6).

Symptoms and Diagnosis.—Stenosis results in dysmenorrhea and sterility (see § 3), with primary or secondary inflammation. The stasis produces either tension and
nausea or colic.

In atresias the more pronounced phenomena first become apparent at puberty (see § 1, 6–8 (*d*)). The diagnosis
is made by examination with speculum and sound; in
hematometra, hydrometra, pyometra, and lochiometra bimanual examination demonstrates a tense elastic tumor
occupying the position of the uterus. In time, perimetritic
changes take place.

Treatment.—To the operative enlargements by forced
dilatation, and by incision of the commissures of the os
uteri, described in § 3 (3, 4), may be added a variation of
v. Winckel's, which is employed if thickening of the
cervix is present. If the cervix is thickened and elon-

gated, it is removed by the elastic ligature; if it is, however, only thickened and the os narrowed, the operation
of Sims (p. 37) is performed, and then small wedges are
cut out of the four wound surfaces produced by the commissural incisions. The wedge-shaped defects are sutured
as in Sims' method. Lastly, excision of the cervix, according to Kaltenbach, may be performed.

The acquired atresia with hematometra is naturally
much more dangerous (from septicemia) than the congenital form. A free incision must consequently be made
as early as possible, the uterine cavity carefully washed
out with a 2 % carbolic solution, and drained by iodoform
gauze or by a tube. (See p. 29.)

Hematosalpinx and hematometra with a uterus bicornis
are to be removed by celiotomy.

Acquired atresia of the vulva is treated by dividing the
adhesions and packing with iodoform gauze, or the raw
surfaces may be separately sutured.

CHAPTER II.

FISTULAS.

Fistulas are most frequently the result of trauma during delivery. They may be the immediate result of lacerations, or they may arise secondarily from the sloughing of contused parts. Other fistulas are due to pessaries (especially the winged pessary of Zwanck), operations, foreign bodies, accidental traumatism, and perforating ulcerative processes—such as occur in malignant tumors (see Plates 85, 86, 88, 89), diphtheric inflammations of the puerperium, syphilis, vesical calculi, and to the perforation of a perimetritic or parametritic abscess, of a hematocele, or of an extra-uterine gestation sac.

Several fistulas may exist in the same case, as is shown in figures 40, 42, 43, and 48 to 51.

§ 27. CLASSIFICATION OF FISTULAS.

For a more exact study of the more recent works see the classic dissertation of Fritsch in Veit's "Handbook."

A. Fistulas of the Urinary Organs.

Anatomy.—According to the location of their orifices, these fistulas may be divided as follows:

1. Urethrovaginal fistulas (Fig. 37), opening below the tuberculum vaginæ.

2. Vesicovaginal fistulas (Fig. 39), the most frequent. Every portion of the posterior [1] bladder-wall, as high up as the vertex, may be involved; they are more frequent as the vaginal vault is approached. If the fistula extends to the edge of the external os, it is designated as a:

3. Superficial vesicocervicovaginal fistula. (Fig. 38.) This form is of especial importance, because its cicatricial dragging upon the lips

---

[1] The original reads "anterior."—TRANSLATOR.

165

of the os uteri gives it a particular influence upon the uterocervical
canal. If the os uteri is also torn, we have a :

4. Deep vesicocervicovaginal fistula with destruction of the anterior
lip. (Fig. 40.) Both 3 and 4 are small, and are found in the median
line, because they arise in contracted pelves, from contusion against
the symphysis.

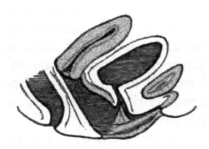

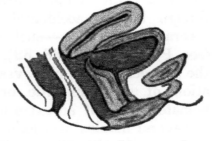

Fig. 37.—Urethrovaginal fistula.   Fig. 38.—Superficial vesicocer-
                                          vicovaginal fistula.

5. Vesicocervical fistulas. (Fig. 41.) They represent narrow canals
which, from the peculiar anatomic relations of the cervix and vaginal
vault, may be combined with vesicovaginal fistulas, since the vesical
end may fork (Fig. 42) or two fistulas may coexist.

The tear may be laterally placed, involving the vesical orifice of
the ureter. If the other opening is in the vaginal wall, we have a:

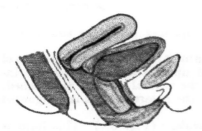

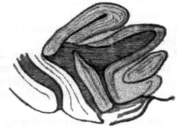

Fig. 39.—Vesicovaginal fistula.   Fig. 40.—Deep vesicocervico-
                                    vaginal fistula with a defect of the
                                    anterior lip of the os uteri.

6. Vesico-ureterovaginal fistula. (Fig. 43.) Such a fistula will be
found laterally along the course of the ureter or posteriorly in the
vaginal vault.

Simple ureteral fistulas arise when the injuries are situated high
up; even then they may pass to the vaginal vault as:

7. Ureterovaginal fistulas. (Fig. 44.) As in all ureteral fistulas,
the orifice is so minute that its recognition is difficult. Its position is

the same as in 6; they frequently empty, as does the urethra, upon a reddened prominence.

8. Ureterocervical fistulas. (Fig. 45.)

There are also uretero-intestinal and uretero-abdominal fistulas.

9. Vesico-abdominal fistulas. (Fig. 46.) These urinary fistulas are peculiar in their origin. They include different degrees and locations

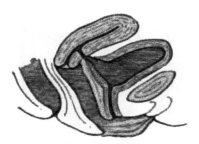
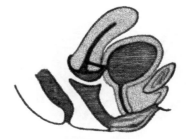

Fig. 41.—Vesicocervical fistula.

Fig. 42.—Vesicocervicovaginal fistula with colpocleisis.

of the defect. Their occurrence is very rare; they are usually of a congenital nature, rarely the result of perforation into an inflamed adherent bladder.

We designate as fissures:

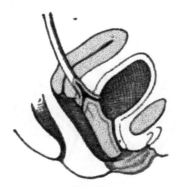
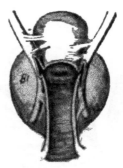

Fig. 43.—Vesico-ureterovaginal fistula.

Fig. 44.—Ureterovaginal fistula—bilateral (inflammatory adhesions). *Bl*, bladder.

(*a*) The *fissura vesicæ inferior*—a cleft beneath the united symphysis, often combined with a fissured clitoris.

(*b*) The *fissura vesicæ superior*—a cleft above the normal symphysis.

(*c*) The *fistula vesico-umbilicalis:* i. e., the persistent urachus. This is an actual fistulous tract.

(*d*) *Eversio* (exstrophia, ectopia) *vesicæ*—clefts of the bladder, with or without a fissured symphysis. (See § 1.) These are extreme congenital defects.

10 . Ileovesical or *ileo-ureterovesical fistulas.* (Fig. 51.) Of the communications between the bladder and intestine due to trauma and ulcerative perforations, that with the small intestine is the more fre-

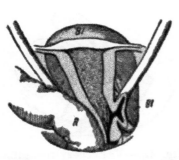

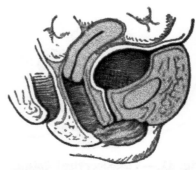

Fig. 45.—Right-sided ureterocervical fistula : *R*, rectum ; *Bl*, bladder.

Fig. 46.—Vesico-abdominal fistula (persistent urachus).

quent. There are also fistulas connecting the bladder with the stomach.

11. Rectovesical or *recto-ureterovesical fistulas* (Fig. 50) arise from perforating pelvic abscesses.

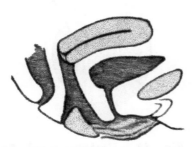

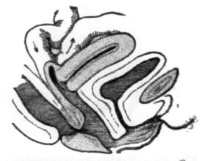

Fig. 47.—Central perforation of the perineum.

Fig. 48.—Ileovaginal fistula. Rectovaginal fistula (most frequent variety).

B. Intestinal Fistulas.

1. Rectovaginal fistulas (Figs. 48 and 49), or *rectovestibular fistulas* (when outside of the hymen).

2. Ileovaginal fistulas (Fig. 48) : an opening in the small intestine empties (usually) into the vaginal vault in such a manner that the greater portion of the feces passes on through the intestinal canal. If the upper end of the ruptured bowel is united with the vagina throughout, complete defecation occurs through this canal. This communication is designated as an :

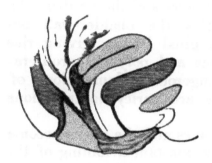

Fig. 49.—Ileovaginal preternatural anus. Rectovaginal fistula.

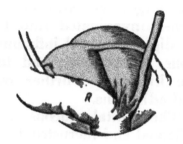

Fig. 50.—Vesico-ureterorectal fistula. Sinistropositio uteri. *R,* Rectum.

3. *Ileovaginal preternatural anus.* (Fig. 49.) Both varieties are very rare, occurring in both the anterior and posterior peritoneal pockets.

Fistulas vary greatly in shape and size. At first they are usually wide; later, they undergo cicatricial contraction; they may pursue a direct or a tortuous course. Vesicovaginal and rectovaginal fistulas are the largest. The length is dependent upon the mode of origin; they may be long and multiple, for example, when they follow the perforation of an abscess into two hollow viscera. If the tissue has undergone necro-

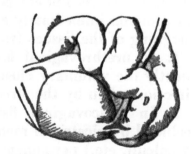

Fig. 51. — Ileo-ureterovesical fistula. *D,* Ileum in the vesico-uterine pouch.

sis from contusion, the surrounding scar tissue is quite extensive; a clean-cut fistula is surrounded by much healthier walls. In the beginning every fistula is characterized by secretion, and forms granulations.

The concomitant injuries may be so great that it is impossible to find the uterus in the cicatricial mass.

If the urine is constantly emptied through the fistulous tract, the normal passage becomes contracted—or even obliterated, in the case of the ureters and the urethra. In the larger vesicovaginal fistulas the bladder-wall becomes invaginated into the vaginal lumen, giving rise to slight catarrhal inflammations and polypoid proliferations, which may lead to dangerous inflammations of the kidneys. Further results are pericystic irritations and adhesions.

The genital mucous membranes and the vulva become inflamed and incrusted from the constant dribbling of the decomposing urine.

Inflammations of the rectum develop in a similar manner. In perforating ulcerations the fistula pursues an oblique course, the larger primary orifice being the higher. (Fig. 49.)

Symptoms.—Incontinence of urine, varying according to the nature of the fistula and the position of the patient ; if the vulva is swollen, the urine may be retained in the vagina in the recumbent posture. This incontinence does not come on immediately after the injury, but follows the sloughing of the tissues from pressure necrosis.

1. In urethrovaginal fistulas the sphincter, and consequently the voluntary closure, may be maintained, but the direction taken by the stream of urine is different.

2. In vesicovaginal fistulas (with large orifices not occluded by cicatricial membranes or temporarily blocked by calculi, etc.) permanent incontinence is present.

3. In vesicovaginal fistulas emptying into the fornix and in vesico-uterine fistulas the patient, when erect, can hold her urine until the lower portion of the bladder has become filled ; the uterus, in addition, may act as a lever or as a valve—the body drops forward, distorting and displacing the fistulous tract and the cervix may directly occlude it (in vesico-uretero-uterine or vesico-ureterovag-

inal fistulas). In the recumbent posture the urine trickles directly into the vagina.

4. In fistulas of the ureter the emptying of the bladder is voluntary, as only a small amount of urine can escape through the narrow canal ; the lesion may be unilateral, only affecting the urine from one kidney. Some of the urine passes through the vagina during urination.

5. In the smaller rectovaginal fistulas only flatus and liquid stools escape involuntarily ; in the larger ones there is incontinence of well-formed fecal masses.

The maceration of the tissues by the urine gives rise to a penetrating odor and to catarrhs of the genitalia with ulcerations of the vulva ; sleeplessness and loss of appetite occur ; the patient feels that her presence is annoying ; she isolates herself, becomes unable to work, and falls into a melancholic state. The same is true of fecal fistulas. The general condition passes from bad to worse, and the patient finally succumbs after years of discomfort.

Diagnosis.—Fistulas situated in the anterior vaginal wall are the easiest to recognize. If they are as large as the finger-tip, simple digital examination may suffice. A sound or catheter may be passed through them from the bladder.

Small fistulas—especially lateral ones or those emptying into the cervical canal—may be demonstrated by the injection of colored liquids (milk, solution of potassium permanganate) into the bladder and careful inspection of the suspected location through the speculum. The suspicious area is fixed by tenacula and the course of the canal is determined by fine sounds. In vesico-uterine fistulas the external os must be everted, dilated, or incised ; stenoses must also be previously removed.

If urine, but not the colored liquid, flows through the genitalia, we have to do with a fistula of the ureter. The uretero-uterine fistula is differentiated from the corresponding vaginal one by the vagina remaining dry after firm tamponade of the os uteri. The exit of the fistula may be more definitely fixed by giving the patient methylene-blue (0.1) several hours before the examination, and thus coloring the urine.

If doubt exists, the cystoscope may be employed or the urethra may be dilated with Simon's specula and the interior of the bladder palpated. This procedure also gives a clue to the existence of other varieties of vesical fistula (ileovesical, etc.). As a last resort, Trendelenburg performs a suprapubic cystotomy.

In intestinal fistulas conclusions may be drawn from the nature of the fecal mass (ileum or colon-rectum).

Treatment.—Operative closure of the fistula is made possible by modern advanced technic. Minute exactness is of even more importance than in colporrhaphy or perineoplasty.

If stenosis of the urethra exists, it must be dilated before the fistula is closed.

Cervical fistulas are operated upon after incising the lips of the os uteri. Ureteral fistulas are closed by means of oval flaps, which are sutured over a catheter introduced into the ureter (after an artificial vaginal fistula has been made—colpocystotomy, to allow of the introduction of the ureteral catheter) (Simon, Schede). The free ureteral end with its surrounding mucous membrane may be excised and implanted into the bladder (Mackenrodt). If the operation is not possible through the vagina, a lateral abdominal section may be made, the peritoneum stripped up, the ureter dissected out along the linea terminalis and sutured into the bladder. The intraperitoneal operation is hazardous.

If the typical operations fail to close the fistula, transverse obliteration of the vagina (colpocleisis, Simon) may be performed : *i. e.*, the vaginal cavity is converted into a reservoir connected with the bladder, an artificial atresia being produced in its upper portion ; the lips of the os uteri may be freshened and united by suture (hysterocleisis). Vesicocervicovaginal fistulas may be closed in an analogous way, either by the lips of the os or by the body of the extremely anteflexed uterus. The condition brought about by colpocleisis is not very promising; in some cases catarrhs, incrustations, and the like demand the removal of the obliteration. In such a case, nevertheless, the fistula was subsequently permanently closed by v. Winckel.

After-treatment.—Antiseptic irrigation of the bladder immediately after the operation (test the completeness of the closure by milk or potassium permanganate). Later, it is necessary to catheterize only if voluntary urination is impossible. A catheter may be introduced and permanently retained. Rest in bed for several days only. Silk sutures are removed on the fifth, silkworm-gut on the eighth, day. Vaginal irrigation only when a fetid discharge exists. If subsequent operations are necessary, they may be performed four weeks later.

Rectovaginal fistulas are in most cases also to be operated upon either by circumscribing them by an oval incision, and uniting their edges by deep sutures, or by the use of vaginal flaps. Very small fistulas, or those combined with anal defects or following perineoplasty, are closed by means of division of the entire rectovaginal septum. Laxatives are previously given for several days; both organs are thoroughly irrigated with antiseptic solutions. During the operation the upper margin of the fistula is drawn down by tenacula and the upper portion of the rectum is plugged with cotton. Subsequent liquid diet and mild cathartics on the third or fifth day are indicated.

In an ileovaginal fistula the spur must first be destroyed by clamp-forceps, so that the fecal contents may pursue their normal course after the plastic closure of the fistulous tract.

Cauterizations by means of fuming nitric or sulphuric acids, chlorid of zinc, Vienna paste, caustic potash, nitrate of silver, the hot iron, or zestocausis are uncertain; they are slow in producing results, and as they render the edges of the fistula hard and nonvascular, the tissues are in an unfavorable condition for later operations. They are of

PLATE 57.

Recto-uterine Hematocele in Combination with an Extra-uterine Gestation Sac. In this mass I found an embryo of three weeks (above and to the left, near to the tube). (Original water-color from a specimen removed at the Heidelberg Frauenklinik.)

---

value in long, narrow fistulas with healthy granulations. Their use may be combined with the retained catheter of Fritsch. (See § 22.)

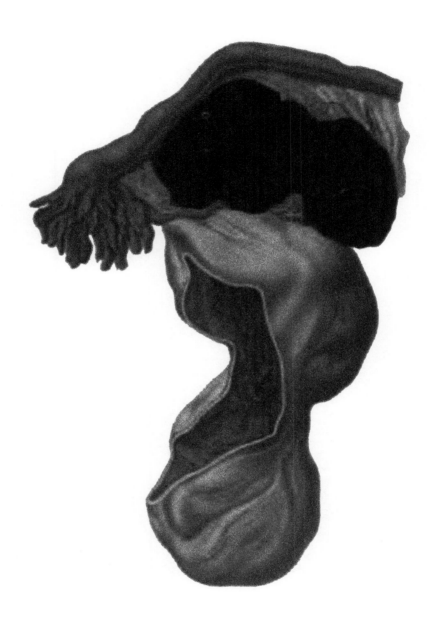

CHAPTER III.

TRAUMATIC EFFUSIONS OF BLOOD.

Traumatic effusions of blood may take place in the connective tissue surrounding the genitalia (hematoma) or into the peritoneal cavity (intraperitoneal hematocele).

§ 28. HEMATOMA: (a) VULVAR; (b) EXTRAPERITONEAL HEMATOMA (RETRO-UTERINE, PERI-UTERINE, OR ANTE-UTERINE).

(a) **Vulvar hematoma** (see Plate 51, Fig. 1) arises suddenly, with irritation and pain, and forms a tense, elastic, fluctuating, bluish tumor in the labia.

Treatment.—Ice-bag and compression; if the skin shows a tendency to break down, incise and pack with iodoform gauze; recovery is slow.

(b) **Extraperitoneal, retro-uterine, peri-uterine, and ante-uterine hematoma** (Plate 58, Fig. 3), especially in the broad ligament and gravitating alongside of the vagina to the pelvic floor. These come on after trauma (such as a fall), with signs of concealed hemorrhage, violent pelvic pain, and disturbances of the bladder and rectum. Fever and peritoneal irritation are absent, unless the broad ligament ruptures and an intraperitoneal hematocele of Douglas' pouch is secondarily formed.

Bimanual palpation shows the pouch of Douglas to be empty; the posterior vaginal vault is pushed down, or a tense elastic tumor may be felt at the side of the uterus.

The internal ligaments may be so slightly lacerated that the effusion of blood can not be discovered by palpation; it may, nevertheless, lead to retroversion and prolapse of the internal genitalia as a result of the acute

175

stretching of the suspensory apparatus. I have frequently
observed such cases in weak individuals after very heavy
lifting and falling backward. The first symptoms are
pain (lasting for days or weeks), discharge, and menstrual
disturbances; they may vanish, if the individual takes
proper care of herself, to recur during the menses or after
colds. Such cases offer a point of diminished resistance
for puerperal or operative infections.

Treatment.—The treatment consists of rest in the horizontal position with the head low. Restoratives (ammonia,
ether) should be administered. Vaginal tamponade and a
sand-bag upon the abdomen are recommended. Incision
may be necessary.

§ 29. INTRAPERITONEAL RETRO-UTERINE HEMATOCELE.

Definition and Etiology.—Intraperitoneal retro-uterine hematocele comes on suddenly without fever, usually
following nonappearance of the menses, as a tense, elastic
tumor, which bulges the recto-uterine pouch into the
vagina and lies in close contact with the uterus. Elevations of temperature may occur later, and brownish
masses of blood are sometimes discharged from the uterus.
The abdominal end of the tube not rarely projects into
the effusion. The mass of blood is surrounded by layers
of fibrin,—probably the result of successive hemorrhages,
—and is walled off from the intestines by pseudomembranes. Extra-uterine pregnancy is the usual, if not the
only, cause (J. Veit); not rarely villi, or even an embryo,
may be demonstrated. In a specimen extirpated at the
Heidelberg Frauenklinik I was fortunate to find an
embryo at most only three weeks old. (See Plate 57.)
The uterus is displaced anteriorly.

The hemorrhage is rarely profuse enough to pass over
the broad ligaments into the vesico-uterine pouch.

Other causes are hematosalpinx (in hematometra from

atresia), ruptured varicocele or phlebectasia of the uterine adnexa, rupture of abdominal organs, and hemorrhagic pelvic pachyperitonitis (perimetritis).

Symptoms.—Sudden appearance of symptoms of concealed hemorrhage, and pain, resulting from the peritoneal irritation. If the extravasted blood is not infected from the bowel, from the tube, or from the parametrium, absorption proceeds, with apyrexia; infection produces violent peritoneal pain and fever.

From the uterus: continued discharge of changed blood (conducted to the uterus through the tube, according to v. Winckel).

From pressure upon neighboring organs: neuralgia and dysmenorrhea (ovaries, see § 23; from the sciatic plexus into the thigh), disturbances of bladder and rectum.

From further hemorrhage (as is especially the case after a previous perimetritis): repeated sudden changes for the worse, until absorption occurs or rupture takes place into one of the hollow viscera (most frequently the rectum) with danger of septic infection. After absorption takes place a scar remains.

Diagnosis.—Bimanual palpation should be most cautious, in order to avoid exciting further hemorrhage, rupturing the fibrin capsule, or pressing infectious material out of the tubes. The posterior vaginal vault is very sensitive to the touch. All manipulations involving the use of the sound or calling for incision are to be avoided.

The uterus is displaced anteriorly; the posterior vaginal vault is pushed down by a tense elastic tumor. The space of Douglas is filled out in such a manner that the contour of the tumor is continuous with the uterine fundus; consequently, confusion with a retroflexed gravid uterus may occur, especially if perimetritis coexists. (For differential diagnosis see Ovarian Cystomata.) The anamnesis and the foregoing symptoms are also to be borne in mind. If the tumor becomes smaller and nodular, with apyrexia, it speaks for hematocele.

12

PLATE 58.

FIG. 1.—**Free Ascites in the Upright Position.** In the dorsal position the fluid (serous or bloody) gravitates toward the spinal column. The anterior border of the dullness on percussion is consequently lower. The border passes back in a line concave toward the chest (while tumors have an almost constant area of dullness, which is convex above). In the lateral position the border again shifts; the fluid seeks the lowest side, and the highest portion of the abdomen is tympanitic (where dullness formerly existed). A wave of fluctuation may be obtained.

Ascites occurs in malignant tumors (malignant papillary ovarian cystomata, cancer of the ovary, of the intestine, etc.), peritoneal tuberculosis, and exudative peritonitis (in addition to the obstructive diseases of the heart, lungs, kidneys, liver, portal circulation, etc.).

If the fluid is an exudate (from an inflammatory process—tuberculosis, for example), it contains red and white blood-corpuscles, cells of various sizes with fatty granules (individual cholesterin crystals), much fibrin and albumin,[1] and coagulates quickly; the specific gravity[2] may exceed 1018—a sign of its inflammatory nature. If the fluid is a transudate from stasis, it contains a few blood-corpuscles, flat endothelium from the serosa, no fibrin, and does not coagulate.

FIG. 2.—**Intraperitoneal Retro-uterine Hematocele.** (See Plate 57.)

FIG. 3.—**Extraperitoneal Retro-uterine Hematoma.** Uterus retroverted and retroflexed. Douglas' pouch is free, but, like the vagina and rectum, it is bulged out by a fluctuating tumor, which can also be designated as a subperitoneal pelvic hematoma. This tumor is due to the tearing of vessels or organs or to the rupture of a phlebectasia.

FIG. 4.—**Large Subserous Posterior Myoma of the Uterus Simulating a Retroflexion.** (Diagnosis made by sound!) This is given for comparison with the other three retro-uterine tumors occupy-

---

[1] Determination of the amount of albumin : From 10 to 50 c.c. of fluid are diluted with ten volumes of water; heat to the boiling-point and add diluted acetic acid until reaction is slightly acid; the precipitate is washed with water, ether, and alcohol; it is then dried and weighed.

[2] The specific gravity is to be measured at room-temperature. If over 1018, inflammatory exudate, because it contains more albumin.

Tab. 58

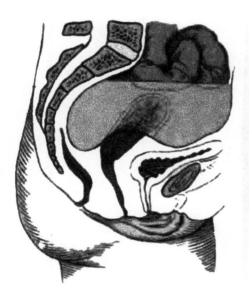

Fig. 1.

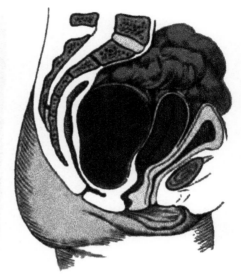

Fig. 2.

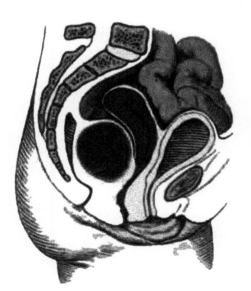

Fig. 3.

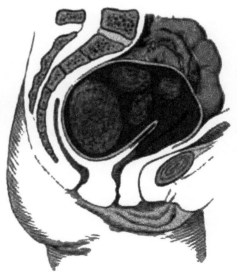

Fig. 4.

Lith. Anst. F. Reichhold. Münc.

ing the pouch of Douglas. Anterior position of the uterus. Bulging of the vaginal vault into the rectum by a firm tumor, which grew gradually without fever. The tumor moves with the uterus; bimanual examination demonstrates the connection.

Treatment.—Absolute rest in bed and the avoidance of all internal therapeutic examinations and procedures. Ice-bag; enemata of opium, morphin, or chloral (to decrease the heart's action). If the collapse continues and there are sufficient grounds for the supposition of an extra-uterine pregnancy (see " Atlas of Obstetric Diagnosis and Treatment "), celiotomy.

If perforation threatens, or if violent pains and elevations of temperature are present, and the tumor remains the same, the most prominent portion is incised through the vagina ; the sac is drained and is irrigated daily under low pressure. Ice-bag, bland diet, enemata, mild laxatives. If perforation into the rectum occurs, no examination should be made, on account of the danger of septic infection.

Absorption is to be aided by the measures indicated in § 18. Rest during subsequent menstruations, when fresh hemorrhages easily occur.

Prognosis.—The earlier and more appropriate the treatment, the more favorable will be the prognosis for a complete absorption in several weeks or months. In perforation it is dependent upon the degree of antisepsis that can be maintained ; rupture into the rectum is the most favorable.

CHAPTER IV.

FOREIGN BODIES IN THE GENITAL CANAL AND IN THE BLADDER.

Foreign bodies in these organs may exert an injurious influence either from the injury attendant upon their entrance or from the inflammation produced by their retention in the viscera.

§ 30. FOREIGN BODIES

owe their introduction into the bladder, vagina, or uterus to a great variety of causes.

(*a*) Retained instruments—pieces of vaginal nozles, glass specula, incrusted pessaries, needles, tampons, laminaria, retained silk sutures, incrusted pieces of catheter (especially the elastic ones).

(*b*) Masturbation, perverse or criminal manipulations: hair-pins, needle-cases, candles, lead-pencils, fir cones, pomade boxes, spools; tampons, sponges, and occlusive pessaries (to avoid conception); knitting-needles and other pointed instruments (to produce abortion).

(*c*) Falls—upon a pointed fence, for example.

(*d*) Causes originating in the body: perforating tumors, such as dermoid cysts (teeth, hair, analogous to Plate 45, 2, into the rectum), extra-uterine gestation sacs, echinococcus-cysts, fistulas from other hollow viscera. Portions of the ovum remaining in the uterus are also to be classed under this heading. Vesical calculi.

The consequences are depicted in §§ 22, 24, and 25; they are mostly inflammations, ulcerations, and fistulas.

Treatment.—The removal of incrusted pessaries is described on page 87.

The genital canal should always be disinfected by irrigation before any foreign body is removed (partly on account of the existing inflammation and fetid discharge, partly on account of the ease with which the mucosa may be injured).

Foreign bodies are to be cautiously extracted with the fingers. If this is not successful, instruments (bullet-forceps or polyp-forceps, tenacula) are to be employed, carefully protecting the vagina from any sharp points. If the foreign body is a long one, it is to be grasped at one end. If this also fails, the object must be made smaller or the parts must be incised. In such cases deep narcosis is necessary.

Foreign bodies in the bladder are diagnosed by the metal catheter, by bimanual palpation, by the cystoscope, or after urethral dilatation.

(See § 22.) The latter procedure is also necessary for their removal : bullet-forceps are introduced alongside of the palpating finger, and the foreign body is seized by one end, if possible, in order to prevent its becoming wedged transversely during extraction. The foreign body may be directly viewed through the speculum. It is sometimes advantageous to fill the bladder with a boric acid solution. If the object is too large, it must be made smaller ; otherwise, colpocystotomy ; in children, suprapubic cystotomy.

From an etiologic, symptomatic, and therapeutic standpoint vesical calculi differentiate themselves not only from other foreign bodies, but also from the same affection in the male. This difference is shown even in childhood. The shortness and the greater width of the female urethra allow concretions the size of a cherry-stone to pass, so that they are rarely able to become calculi by the continued accumulation of uric acid salts.

Etiology and Symptoms.—All foreign bodies, including tumors and particles of mucus and pus in vesical catarrh, become incrusted with deposits of salts of uric, phosphoric, and oxalic acids as well as with cystin. All vesical catarrhs and other affections producing complete or partial retention of urine (vesical paralysis, cystocele, diverticula) are also causes of the formation of calculi. Calculi produce vesical catarrh, so that the symptoms of the latter are components of the clinical picture.

The stone irritates the bladder ; hyperemia, hypersecretion, hemorrhages, pain (local and radiating into the genitalia, sacrolumbar region, lower extremities), spasm. The local rubbing leads to ulceration, to perforating abscesses, and to the formation of fistulas. The urine contains clouds of mucus, pus, blood, ard squamous epithelium.

Diagnosis.—This is made by bimanual examination, introduction of the catheter, cystoscopy, or direct inspection through the speculum, the urethra being more or less dilated and the pelvis raised (Rose's procedure). (See § 22.) The presence of a stone in a cystocele or in a diverticulum may be demonstrated by the cystoscope, or

PLATE 59.

Fig. 1.—**Left-sided and Posterior Parametritis.** An inflammation of the parametrium (or paravaginal tissues—paracolpitis) arises from puerperal or operative infection (laminaria, intra-uterine pessaries), and extends into the broad and sacro-uterine ligaments. A yellowish, doughy, inflammatory exudate is formed (see Plate 61, 2, and Plate 40, 2), which displaces the uterus. Later, cicatricial contraction occurs, causing further displacement and angulation of the uterus as end-results of the process. Contraction of the sacro-uterine ligaments leads to anteflexion of the uterus ; of the septum between the bladder and uterine neck, to retroversion or retroflexion. Other deviations arise if perimetritic adhesions are associated with the parametritis.

Another termination may occur : The inflammation spreads behind the uterus into the pelvic connective tissue and beside the bladder. Abscesses are formed, which rupture into the vagina, rectum, or bladder. They may perforate the abdominal wall above Poupart's ligament or gravitate to the thigh, to the pelvic floor, or through the sciatic foramen, appearing beneath the gluteal muscles.

The acute wound infection may have a fatal termination from severe septicæmia.

Fig. 2.—**Intraligamentous and Retroperitoneal Multilocular Glandular Mucoid Cyst of the Left Ovary.** This consists of a proliferation of the germinal epithelium of the Graafian follicle [1] or of the superficial cuboid epithelium of the ovary, together with proliferation of the vascular and supporting connective tissue (see Plate 72)—cysto-adenoma.

Fig. 3.—**Left-sided Pyosalpinx.** (See Plates 18, 19, and 39.)

Fig. 4.—**Carcinomatous Cystadenoma of the Ovary.** (Diagrammatic drawing from a case in the Heidelberg Frauenklinik.) The uterus is anteflexed and displaced anteriorly by a myxocystoma. The tumor has become malignant ; solid masses have grown into the floor of the recto-uterine pouch and have so surrounded the rectum that a rigid impermeable stricture exists. Ascites, numerous adhesions, and metastases to all organs are seen in such cases. In this case it was necessary to make an artificial anus.

[1] Stefteck demonstrated ovula in the young cysts of cystadenomata.

Tab. 59.

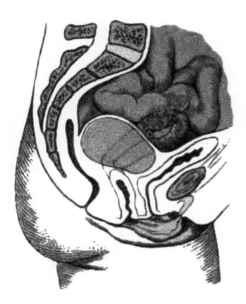

Fig. 1.

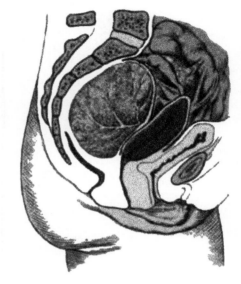

Fig. 2.

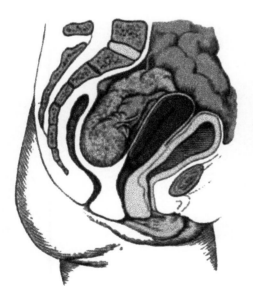

Fig. 3.

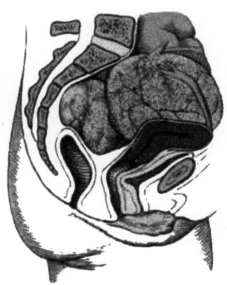

Fig 4.

Lith. Anst F. Reichhold. München.

by means of catheters, after the bladder has been filled with 2% boric acid solution.

Treatment.—(a) **Prophylactic:** removal of causes, such as vesical catarrh, cystocele, foreign bodies, fistula.

(b) **Radical**—removal of the stones:

1. Through the urethra, after dilatation of the same. (See § 22.)

2. By colpocystotomy—opening the bladder by a T-shaped incision in the vagina, the upper transverse arm being situated in the vaginal vault close to the anterior lip of the os uteri. If the stone is too large or the genitalia too small:

3. Suprapubic cystotomy (sectio alta) is to be performed. The intestines are thoroughly evacuated, and 350 gm. of a warm 2% boric acid solution are introduced into the bladder in order to elevate it and its peritoneum above the symphysis. The incision commences at the symphysis and is from 5 to 7 cm. long, directly in the linea alba (or a transverse incision may be made—Trendelenburg). The fascia transversalis is to be divided for

GROUP V.

NEW GROWTHS.

Etiology.—The origin of tumors of the female genitalia, like that of tumors in general, is shrouded in darkness. It is nevertheless striking that organs which undergo such active and variable changes in form, structure, and metabolism, and which are exposed to so many mechanical injuries, bacterial invasions, and nervous irritations, can consequently easily lose their equilibrium of structure: i. e., the normal quantitative relation of the individual tissues.

We observe proliferations in specific infectious inflammations (see §§ 12, 20, and 21) and in chronic congestive inflammations in general. (See Group III, chap. 1 and §22.) We are able, further, to observe that in such inflammatory proliferations the normal relation of the epithelial to the connective tissues is gradually lost; the new formation becomes atypical, and assumes a malignant character. (See Endometritis Fungosa and Erosio Papilloides, § 13 and Plate 30.) In the same manner benign proliferations—myxofibromata, for example—may become sarcomatous; pigmented nevi of the vulva have a great inclination to be suddenly transformed into the most malignant melanosarcomata. Repeated cauterizations, excochleations, and unfortunate subsequent infections have without doubt not infrequently furnished the starting-point for a malignant metamorphosis. As in other epitheliomata, the malignant tendency is particularly liable to appear at the time of the menopause.

A connection evidently exists between the origin of malignant epitheliomata and the liability of certain parts

184

to injury, as is shown both by the predilection of these tumors for the vulva and cervix uteri and by the frequency of their occurrence in multiparæ. This is analogous to the predisposition to mammary carcinoma furnished by the scars of mastitis—whether we suppose the cause to be in the scar itself or in the original infection.

The etiologies of the sarcomata and of the malignant cystomata are unknown; the former are even relatively frequent in childhood or occur congenitally. Dermoid cysts seem to represent a variety of intrafetation.

While the polyps of the mucous membrane are most frequently to be looked upon as circumscribed inflammatory proliferations (endometritis polyposa), there is no etiologic explanation for the proliferation of the muscularis uteri—for the myomata and fibromyomata; indeed, their occurrence is far more common in women who have borne few or no children. Sterility (in spite of regular sexual intercourse) or the causes of sterility are, perhaps, responsible for the tendency of the muscularis to proliferate; secondary proliferation of the mucosa exists often enough, and this may be the cause of the sterility.

It must be remembered that Ribbert and Weigert, and recently Lubarsch also, consider the cause of the proliferation to be a decreased resistance to growth in the surrounding tissues.

CHAPTER I.

BENIGN TUMORS.

By benign tumors, from an anatomic standpoint, we understand those that retain the typical structure of the tissue from which they arise, and that do not "eat up" all the surrounding tissues by a predominant proliferation, nor produce further destruction by metastasis. From a clinical standpoint, certain anatomically benign tumors may, nevertheless, be productive of pernicious results to the organism. This chapter treats only of the absolutely benign tumors.

§ 31. BENIGN TUMORS OF THE MUCOUS MEMBRANES COVERED WITH SQUAMOUS EPITHELIUM (EPITHELIAL TUMORS OF THE BLADDER, VULVA, AND VAGINA, AND TUMORS OF THE STRUCTURES EMBEDDED IN THEM).

The mucous membrane, covered with squamous epithelium, lines the vagina, the vestibule, the bladder and urethra, and, in an extended sense, the vulva. It consists of stratified squamous epithelium resting upon a matrix of cuboid cells, of the connective tissue of the cutis, which forms variously shaped papillæ, and of adipose tissue. The embedded tissues are the lymph-vessels and lymph follicles; blood-vessels, which in the clitoris, the nymphæ, and in the neighborhood of the urethra form erectile cavernous bodies; sebaceous glands—the two glands of Bartholin, lined with cylindric epithelium (see Plates 25 and 26); the similarly clothed small glands and ducts of the urethra (Skene's glands, see Fig. 20) and of the bladder (exceptionally, the vagina has glandulæ aberrantes); and, lastly, muscle-fibers and nerves. The tumors now to be considered may arise in any one of these tissues. We accordingly differentiate:

1. *Papillomata and condylomata*, such as lupus of the vulva (see § 13 and § 20 ; Plates 29 and 50) and, rarely, of the vagina.
2. *Condylomata (caruncle) of the urethra.* (See Plate 51.)
3. *Papillomata of the bladder.*
4. *Fibromata, myxofibromata and fibromyomata of the vulva.*

186

5. *Fibromata, myxofibromata and fibromyomata of the vagina.*

6. *Polyps of the mucous membrane or papillary polypoid angiomata, fibromata, fibromyomata of the urethra.*

7. *Polyps of the mucous membrane, fibromata, fibromyomata of the bladder.*

8. *Lipomata of the vulva* (usually with a pedicle) *and of the vagina.*

9. *Elephantiasis lymphangirelativa vulvæ.* (See Plates 29 and 51.)

10. *Cysts of the vulva* (of the glands of Bartholin; of the glands about the clitoris and urethra; occluded sebaceous glands of the nymphæ; hydrocele of the inguinal canal) *and cysts of the vagina* (which includes—the trimethylamin forming—colpohyperplasia cystica).

11. *Cystic myxo-adenomata of the urethra.*

12. *Cysts of the vesical mucous membrane* (I found them once in the fetus, see v. Winckel's Ber. u. Stud., Munich).

Diagnosis and Treatment.—The new growths of the vulva usually become polypoid, and are consequently easily removed with scissors, the knife, or the galvano-cautery (or Paquelin's cautery), the latter is particularly adapted for the removal of sessile or very vascular tumors.

Fibromyomata of the vagina are rare; they may become so large that they lift the uterus up above the pelvic inlet and disturb the sexual functions as much as similar tumors of the bladder and intestine. If they have a broad base, they are to be shelled out from the surrounding tissues. They sometimes show myxomatous degeneration. In every case it is to be carefully determined whether the tumor is really a vaginal one, or a myoma of the uterus which has been "delivered" into the vagina. The latter tumor may grow fast to the vaginal wall, lose its pedicle, and become a secondary vaginal myoma.

Vaginal cysts vary in size and constitution according to their place of origin. They may be the remains of a duct of Gärtner, having cylindric ciliated epithelium and serous contents; of a vagina septa (see Fig. 20); or of a hematoma which has undergone partial absorption leaving behind a more or less blood-stained fluid.

Treatment.—Enucleation. When that is impossible, a broad piece of the cyst-wall is excised and the cavity is packed.

The tumors of the urethra are very sensitive and

PLATE 60.

Fig. 1.—Polyps of the mucous membrane are circumscribed proliferations of the endometrium, both of the body of the uterus and also of the cervical canal ; they consist of connective tissue containing numerous glands, partly cystic, and dilated, thin-walled capillaries. (See Plate 71, 1.) They form a pedicle by traction (see Fig. 52) and bleed easily on account of their structure. In contrast to polypoid fibromyomata, they are soft. They are livid from the constriction of the os uteri.

Fig. 2.—**Simple Erosion with Ovules of Naboth.** Uterine fibroid on the point of dilating the os uteri : i. e., about to be "delivered." (See Plate 62, 2 ; Plate 90, 4 ; Fig. 55.)

bleed easily. The pain is often associated with itching, troublesome sexual excitement, or dysuria ; it radiates to the surrounding tissues, and may bring on convulsive attacks. Urination is painful, infrequent, or interrupted. If the tumors become larger, they project from the urethral orifice ; in other cases they may be drawn out with tenacula, after incision or dilatation of the urethra.

Treatment.—The latter procedures must be carried out preparatory to the removal of the tumors by ligation and Paquelin's cautery or the ecraseur (wire snare).

Papillomata of the bladder first make themselves

PLATE 61.

Fig. 1.—**Subserous Polypoid Fibromyoma of the Uterus.** (Original drawing from a specimen in the Munich Frauenklinik.) The tumor is composed of masses of concentrically arranged lamellæ.

Fig. 2 –**Myomatosis Uteri.** Parametritic swelling about the neck of the uterus and vaginal vault. Intramural myomata of the fundus ; submucous myoma of the fundus ; submucous polypoid fibromyomata of the body of the uterus. The pedicle is elongated and twisted ; the tumors have dilated the os and have a dark bluish-red color from the constriction. (Original drawing from a specimen in the Munich Frauenklinik.)

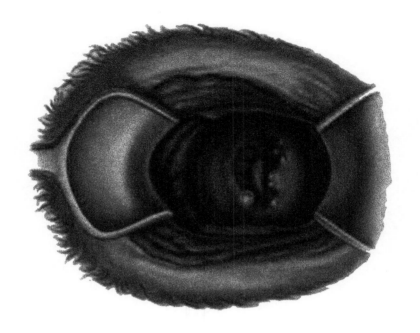

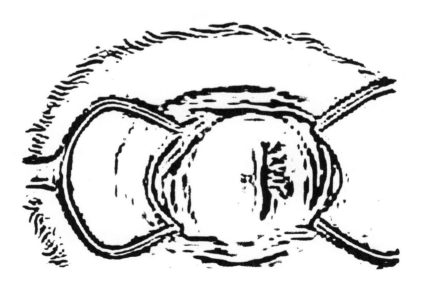

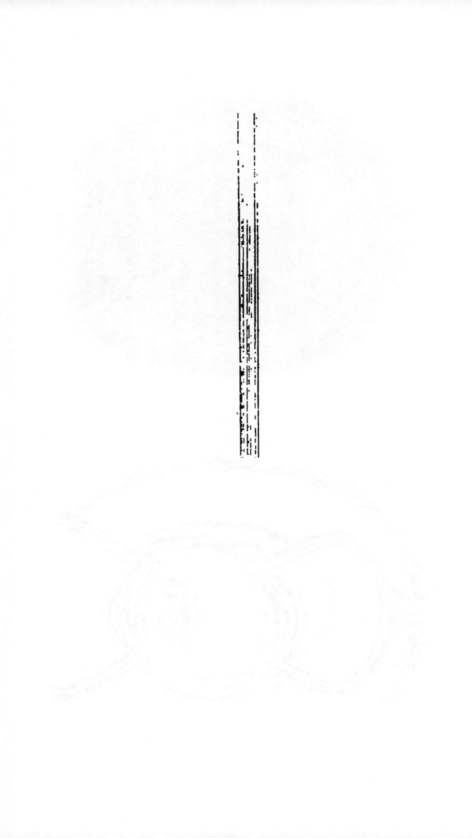

Tab. 61.

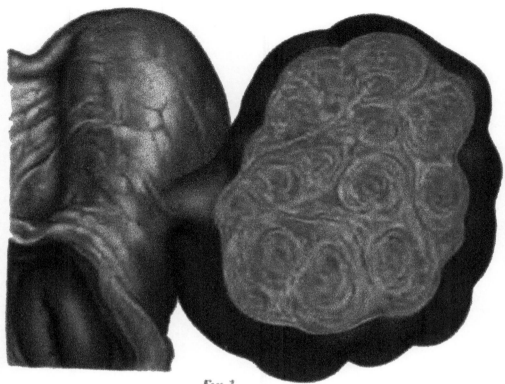

Fig 1

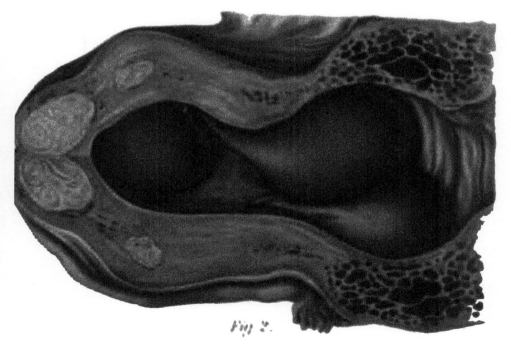

Fig 2

Little Brod & Heastshold Münzen

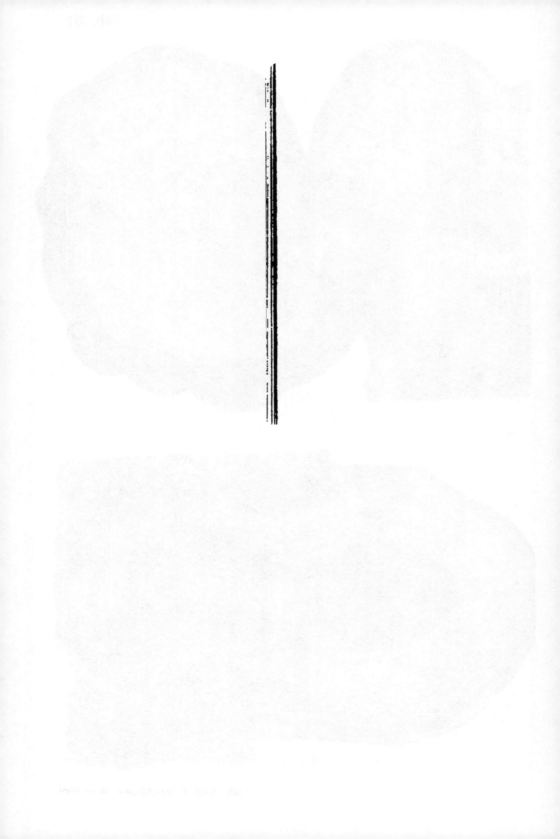

known by an indefinite feeling of pressure in the vesical region and by early disturbances of urination (increased frequency, tenesmus, ischuria). Violent radiating pains subsequently appear. From the ease with which the surface of the tumor may be injured, frequent hemorrhages occur, producing a particularly striking symptom,—hematuria,—which may lead to a blocking of the urethra during urination by a mass of fibrin. The urine then undergoes decomposition and all the symptoms of vesical catarrh present themselves. Particles of the new growth may also occlude the urethra or cause the formation of calculi.

Diagnosis.—When such symptoms are present, cystoscopy or dilatation of the urethra and palpation of the interior of the bladder. Microscopic examination of particles removed by means of the cystoscope. If the tumor is intact, not disintegrated, it is probably a benign growth. Perforating tumors, such as dermoid cysts and extra-uterine gestation sacs, are to be considered.

Treatment.—The urethra is to be dilated ; the left index-finger is then introduced into the bladder, and the tumor is removed by the wire écraseur. If the tumor is sessile or too large, it is either to be incised or crushed bimanually. The hemorrhage is to be controlled by applications of a solution of sesquichlorid of iron or of ferripyrin, by injections of ice-water, by an ice-bag upon the hypogastrium, and by firm tamponade of the vagina. If these methods are inapplicable, colpocystotomy or suprapubic section. (See § 30.)

Prognosis.—The removal of tumors by modern methods is sure, without danger to life, and without permanent incontinence ; the new growth easily returns, however, without showing a malignant structure, evidently because the bed of the tumor has not also been removed.

§ 32. BENIGN TUMORS OF THE UTERUS.

As far as their consequences and removal are concerned, the only *absolutely benign tumors* are the mucous polyps

PLATE 62.

Several Polypoid Myomata of the Fundus, Which Produced Uncontrollable Hemorrhage at the Time of the Menopause. Chronic metritis. Congestive swelling of the ovaries. (Original water-color from a case of total extirpation.)

(*i. e.*, the smaller circumscribed proliferations of the mucous membrane) and the stationary subserous, the smaller intramural, and the small slender pedunculated fibromyomata. Of the remaining varieties of myomata, at least 10 % of the *doubtful, often dangerous tumors* are made up of the flat proliferating polyps of the mucous membrane (molluscum), and the large and broad-based fibromyomata, especially the intramural and submucous varieties.

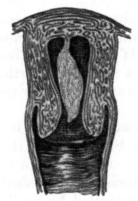

Fig. 52.—Polyp of the mucous membrane of the fundus uteri.

The following are consequently benign :

1. **Mucous polyps (benign adenomata): (*a*) of the lips of the os uteri; (*b*) of the cervical and corporeal mucosa.** (For Anatomy and Histology see Plates 60, 1 ; 67 ; 71, 1 ; 90 ; Fig. 52.) They are frequent, usually multiple, often combined with fibromyomata and projecting from them ; they usually remain small.

Symptoms and Diagnosis.—Slight hemorrhages are frequent. Since many of these adenomata owe their origin to an endometritis fungosa or decidualis (decid-uoma, Küstner), with or without the formation of cysts (ovules of Naboth) (see Plate 90), we have a combination with the symptoms of this disease—above all, anomalies of menstruation.

The adenomata of the lips of the os uteri represent glandular hypertrophies of these tissues, while those springing from the mucous membrane higher up hang

Tab 62.

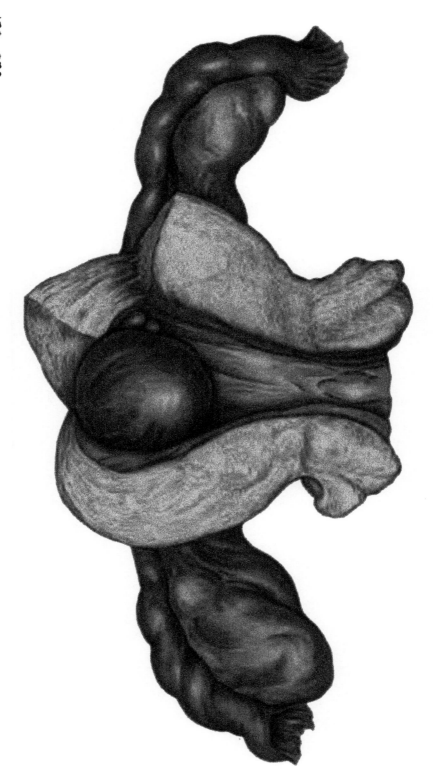

Lith. Anst v. Reichhold, München.

from the latter by a pedicle. Upon this is based the diagnosis by inspection. They are dark red, usually soft, and bleed very easily. As they are forced down against the os they produce a corresponding feeling of pressure and a reflex nausea. Frequently enough, however, such phenomena may be quite overlooked.

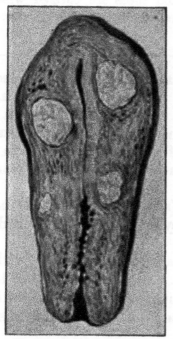 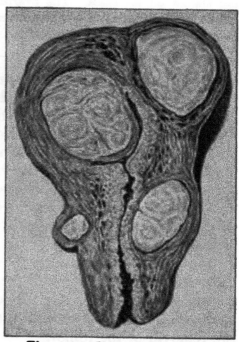

Fig. 53.—Intramural myomata. The myomata of the uterus arise (according to v. Winckel) without exception in the muscularis of the corpus uteri and grow in ous directions. (See Fig. 54.) Cysts are seen in the proliferated cervical mucosa.

Fig. 54.—Intramural myomata arising in the corpus uteri grow out of the wall in different directions: subserous, submucous, and downward into the wall of the cervix. They are all still inserted by a broad base and surrounded by circularly arranged fibrous tissue with widely gaping vessels. The mucosa is thickened.

Treatment.—The easily accessible tumors with a pedicle are to be removed by the wire snare, or they may be ligated and then removed by means of scissors.

If the pedicle of the tumor is difficult of access (Fig. 52),

PLATE 63.

Intraperitoneal Surface of an Amputated Myomatous Uterus (Submucous Myoma). (See Plate 66.) The two surfaces of the incised uterus are drawn apart by the strong elastic retraction of the tumor. The cut surface of the tumors projects above the surrounding tissues on all sides. The ovaries and tubes are covered with small cysts. (Original water-color from a specimen removed by celiotomy at the Heidelberg Frauenklinik.)

---

dilate the os uteri with well-sterilized laminaria or incise the commissures and enlarge the internal os with metal dilators; then hold the lips of the os open with tenacula; profuse hemorrhage is controlled by suture, Paquelin cautery, or applications of solution of sesquichlorid of iron; firm tamponade with ferripyrin-nosophen gauze from twenty-four to forty-eight hours.

Flat tumors are to be cureted (see § 13 (b)); then the gauze tamponade, as previously; cysts are to be punctured. (Plate 90, 3.)

All these tumors must be carefully removed with their pedicles, or they will recur. If the inclination to return is great, the parts are cauterized repeatedly with chlorid of zinc or solution of sesquichlorid of iron after the removal of the tumor.

2. **Fibromyomata with an Absolutely Benign Course.**—Stationary intramural (parietal) myomata, small submucous or polypoid submucous fibromyomata, not causing marked hemorrhage, and small subserous or polypoid subserous fibromyomata. (See Fig. 53, and Plates 14; 15, 4; 18, 1 and 2; 67; 90, 4.)

Anatomy and Histology.—We differentiate histoid and organoid myomata. The histoid fibromyomata consist of nonstriated muscle-cells and of partly dense, partly areolar, connective tissue. (See Plate 71, 2.) They arise in the muscularis of the body of the uterus. They are at first intramural (intraparietal), and grow out in various

directions. (See Figs. 53–55.) They commence in the
neighborhood of vessels, and their origin probably has
some connection with vasomotor disturbances of growth.

The organoid myomata are the adenomyomata (v. Recklinghausen, 1896): *i. e.*, myomata with glandular and
cystic inclusions, which v. Recklinghausen demonstrated

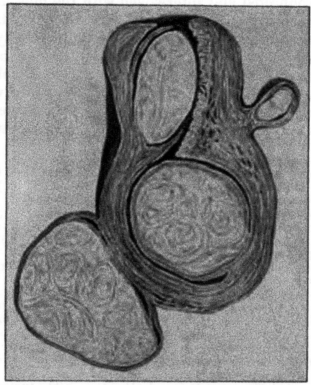

Fig. 55.—The tumors commence to become pedunculated as polypoid subserous and submucous fibromyomata. The myoma of the
cervix, arising from gravitation, begins to shell itself out from its
surroundings. Circular arrangement of fibers within the tumors.

to be partly postfetal from the epithelium of the uterine
mucosa, consequently derived from the epithelium of the
Müllerian ducts (adenomyomata of the mucous membrane), and partly remains of the Wolffian body (paroophoritic adenomyomata). The adenomyomata are most

13

PLATE 64.

Several Bleeding Myomatous Polyps of the Fundus.

(Original water-color from a specimen in the Path. Inst. at Munich—Bollinger.)

---

intimately connected and interwoven with the muscularis; they are not encapsulated, as are the histoid myomata.

The adenomyomata of the mucous membrane may also be due either to a general or local penetration of the mucosa into the uterine wall, or to isolated, misplaced, fetal rudiments of the uterine mucosa (Landau), in which case the presence of a cytogenetic connective-tissue capsule speaks for their origin from the Müllerian ducts.

According to location we differentiate:

1. *Intramural fibromyomata.* (Figs. 53, 57 to 59, and Plate 61, 2.)
2. *Submucous fibromyomata.* (Figs. 54, 55; Plates 63 and 66.) The tumor has a broad base and is still partly in the uterine wall.
3. *Polypoid submucous fibromyomata.* (Fig. 55 and Plates 61, 2; 62, 64.) The tumor has a pedicle and projects into the uterine lumen.
4. *Cervical fibromyomata.* (Figs. 54 and 55 and Plate 65.) The tumor (intraparietal) has gravitated into the cervical wall.
5. *Subserous fibromyomata* (Figs. 54 and 55 and Plates 43 and 65.) The tumor causes a projection of the peritoneum.
6. *Polypoid subserous fibromyomata.* (Fig. 55 and Plates 61, 1; 67.) The tumor is connected to the uterus by a pedicle and projects into the peritoneal cavity. It may form adhesions with neighboring organs and thus have two pedicles; if the primary pedicle becomes obliterated, the new growth seems to spring from the other viscus.
7. *Intraligamentous fibromyomata.* The tumor grows in between the layers of the broad ligament.
8. *Intercorporeal fibromyomata in a double uterus.* The tumor forms the septum.

PLATE 65.

Completely Extirpated Myomatous Uterus.

The posterior lip of the os uteri (very anemic from profuse hemorrhages), as well as its appurtenant cervical wall, is transformed into a myoma larger than a man's fist. Adenomyomata at the insertions of the tubes. (Original water-color from an operative specimen at the Heidelberg Frauenklinik.)

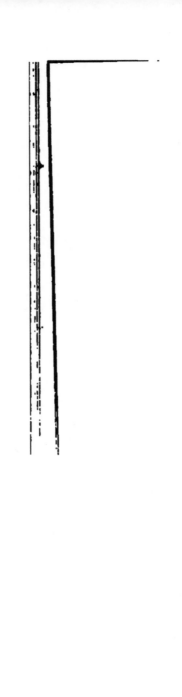

A special group of the paroophoritic adenomyomata is made up of the voluminous juxta-uterine and subserous varieties; for both, although they pass diffusely into the uterine muscularis, may be isolated from it (Landau); they may separate themselves spontaneously and be found as solitary tumors in the broad ligaments.

Isolated glandular and cystic deposits are found in histoid myomata as accidental embryonic displacements of the epithelium, or analogous to the frequent combination of submucous myomata and "mollusca" of the neighboring endometrium (Virchow), since the enveloping endometrium of submucous and polypoid myomata sometimes passes into the muscular tissue in a striated manner.

Symptoms.—As can be deduced from the foregoing statements, these tumors throughout can be looked upon as "absolutely benign" only as long as they are small. Their earliest possible diagnosis and removal is consequently of the greatest importance.

Initial Symptoms.—All the phenomena are independent of the size of the tumors. The most violent boring pains, produced by the tension, are particularly characteristic of the small intramural new growths. These pains are exaggerated by all congestive conditions (menses, cohabitation, constipation) and by exploratory palpation of the uterus, which is neither necessarily enlarged nor displaced. These pains radiate into the surrounding tissues, and cause reflex neuralgias in the sacral and lumbar regions, in the face, etc.; they make up a large part of the hysteric symptom-complex which is present in patients otherwise apparently in good general condition.

Hemorrhage first appears as a menorrhagia; later, as an irregular metrorrhagia.

Cause.—Partly glandular endometritis over the tumor; as soon as the last muscle-fibers between the new growth and the mucosa have disappeared, however, the proliferation of the interstitial tissue causes a fungous endometritis, or multiple adenomatous new growths (Wyder). In other cases the uterus is unable to contract sufficiently to close the

PLATE 66.

Inner Surface of a Uterus with an Incised Intramural Submucous Hemorrhagic Myoma of the Posterior Wall. (See Plate 63.) (Original water-color from an operative specimen at the Heidelberg Frauenklinik.) The anterior wall of the supravaginally amputated uterus is opened, and the entire uterine cavity is filled by a round, tense, elastic tumor, which has been divided into two halves and thrown to each side. By bimanual palpation a deceptive fluctuation was apparent, due to the fact that the muscular tissue was completely saturated with blood.

---

vessels of the myoma (Landau). The contractility of these vessels themselves is evidently insufficient.

These hemorrhages appear early, and, corresponding to their cause of origin, almost without exception in intraparietal and submucous myomata. They frequently continue after the menopause.

If the tumor grows out of the uterine wall, escaping its tension, and is small and of the subserous variety, the initial pains cease and there are no further pressure phenomena; if it becomes submucous, distending the uterine cavity (Fig. 54), new labor-like pains appear and the leukorrhea and hemorrhage become more profuse. These pains bring about a dilatation of the os uteri. (Plate 60.) If the tumor-tissue yields, the pedicle becoming long-drawn-out, the complete "delivery" of the mass occurs.

Diagnosis.—Small intraparietal myomata, as well as diffuse homogeneous substitutions of the endometrium by adenomyomata, are not to be recognized by bimanual palpation. We suspect their presence from the apyrexia, with initial violent boring pains, and, later, menorrhagia and metrorrhagia. These symptoms demand the palpation of the uterine cavity (after dilatation, with or without incision of the commissures of the os), which reveals submucous or polypoid prominences, or different degrees of density of the uterine wall.

Later, the obliteration of the os uteri (Plates 60, 61, and Fig. 55) may be recognized by inspection.

For differential diagnosis see page 219. Above all, pregnancy must be excluded before dilatation of the os uteri (menstruation is not absent, cervix is not so livid nor so soft).

Treatment.— Prophylactic: ergotin subcutaneously (0.05 gm. daily, for months and years) to cause the tumor to contract and disappear. Ergotin also checks the hemorrhage, as does stypticin and hydrastin—the former by exciting the involuntary muscle-fibers in the vessel-wall to contraction, the latter two through the vasomotor nerves.

These measures are rendered more effective by hot vaginal irrigations (117° to 127° F., one or more liters several times daily or every two hours), and, further, by depletives, especially before the period: mild laxatives, salt baths, salt inunctions, applications of alcohol.

If the hemorrhages do not cease, the vagina is to be firmly packed with iodoform gauze or cotton tampons; if this is without avail, cotton is wrapped about Playfair's aluminum sound, soaked in ferripyrin or chlorid of iron solution, and applied to the uterine cavity, or even left there for several hours. Ergotin subcutaneously and by mouth (as extractum secale cornutum[1]). The author uses tampons the size of the finger, saturated with ferripyrin or gelatin emulsion. These are left until extruded by the uterus.

If the uterine cavity is dilated and its walls are relaxed, ferripyrin, solution of sesquichlorid of iron, or gelatin should be injected by Braun's syringe. Great caution must be exercised: the syringe should not contain over two cubic centimeters of fluid; the syringe is to be withdrawn as the injection is made; it is better to inject into gauze (previously introduced) than against the mucous membrane.

---

[1] See Therapeutic Table.

Anemia resulting from hemorrhage is to be treated symptomatically, see § 4, under 7 ; for the dysmenorrhea and neuralgia see § 4, under 8, and, in addition, salt or brine baths (Kreuznach, Tölz) and applications of mud, brine, or hot alcohol to the abdomen.

Fibroid and mucous polyps are to be removed by operation. If the tumors are large, their size is to be decreased by longitudinal or spiral incisions or by the excision of

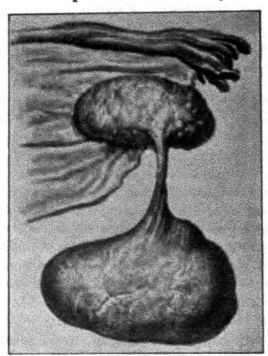

Fig. 56.—Myxofibroma of the ovary with a long pedicle (rare). (Specimen at the Munich Frauenklinik.)

pieces, until the enucleation of the pedicle is possible. The uterine cavity is then to be disinfected and packed with iodoform gauze.

Small submucous tumors are removed after dilatation of the cervix ; the overlying mucous membrane is incised, and the tumor is seized by the vulsella forceps of Muzeux and is shelled out of its bed. If the dilatation is insufficient, the bladder is dissected free and the anterior cervical wall is divided to a point above the internal os. ·

Cervical myomata that have grown into the parametritic connective tissue are removed after incision of the vaginal mucous membrane (Czerny). Vaginal tamponade.

§ 33. BENIGN TUMORS OF THE UTERINE ADNEXA.

The new growths proceed from the visceral serosa of the adnexa, with its subserous connective tissue, and the involuntary muscle-fibers of the broad and round ligaments; from the mucous membrane and muscularis of the tube; from the cuboid germinal epithelium of the ovary; and from the ovarian connective-tissue stroma.

We have the following:

1. *Papillary proliferations of the tube:* circumscribed or diffuse, with or without cyst formation in the tubal mucosa; of an infectious nature.

2. *Fibromata and fibromyomata, including paroophoritic adenomyomata and adenomyomata of the mucous membrane* (Plate 60) *of the tube:* solitary, from the size of a pea to that of a child's head; multiple, as a result of inflammatory proliferation (salpingitis nodosa, combined with hyperplasia of the mucosa and cyst formation) in the uterine isthmus of the tube, which is rich in muscle-fibers.

3. *Small fibromata and fibromyomata of the ovary* may develop from the corpora candicantia or fibrosa. (Plate 40, 3.) Under certain conditions they may become very large; they then lose their benign character, partly because they show a tendency to malignant degeneration, partly because they act as an obstacle to delivery. They may have a cystic or cavernous structure.

4. *Fibromyomata and adenomyomata of the round ligament* are very rarely intraperitoneal;[1] they are more frequent in the inguinal canal.

5. *Fibromyxomata and fibromyomata of the broad ligament* may grow to the pelvic outlet and simulate herniae. The latter must not be confused with intraligamentous uterine myomata and adenomyomata.

6. *Lipomata of the tubes and of the broad ligament* are rare; the former are only the size of a bean, the latter may weigh fifteen kilograms (thirty-three pounds).

7. *Cysts of the tubes and of the broad ligament, of serous origin* (with the exception of the mucous cysts mentioned under 1 and 2), are small and only occasionally of importance, inasmuch as they may become pedunculated (hydatids,[2] such as Morgagni's) and contract adhesions

---

[1] I found such a tumor at autopsy. It was round, as large as a small potato, and in the middle of the broad ligament. This position is very rare ("Samml. d. Münch. Frauenklinik"; v. Winckel's "Ber. u. Stud.," 1884–'90).

[2] This formation of hydatids is a frequent occurrence. I found them 45 times in 130 autopsies; in 8 of these several hydatids coexisted; in 3 cases 2 vesicles had the same pedicle. Several were calcified. Small cysts of the broad ligament were found 15 times; 5 of these were calcified. I have seen them repeatedly in the fetus.

with the intestinal coils. Those cysts situated in the anterior layer of the broad ligament are to be considered as remains of the canals of the Wolffian body; the others, however, are to be looked upon as pedunculated fimbria with epithelial inclosures.

8. *Unilocular cysts of the ovary* are due to dropsy of the follicles. (Plate 68, 1.) The multilocular cysts of the ovary are without significance only as long as they are small.

9. *Parovarian cysts* arise from the remains of the Wolffian duct (probably also from the remains of the Wolffian body between the parovarium and the uterus). These growths commonly remain small, but they may attain the size of a walnut or an apple and cause trouble. They are located between the ovary and the tube, and may be multiple. The cyst is always unilocular; the wall is thin and consists of endothelium and subserous connective tissue with elastic and involuntary muscle-fibres; it is lined with either ciliated or non-ciliated cylindric epithelium.

The contents are clear and are poor in albumin and consequently watery (of diagnostic importance regarding tapping). The fluid contains cylindric cells and has a specific gravity of 1005.

Paroophoritic cysts are found in the course of the uterus as far as the upper portion of the vagina (Gärtner's duct has been demonstrated up to this point in the fetus—Klein). Veit includes in this classification the large vaginal cysts, which extend into the broad ligament.

Symptoms and Diagnosis.—*Ovarian fibromata*, see Ovarian Cystomata and the following section.

Ovarian cysts (unilocular), see Ovarian Cystomata ; also Oligocystic Degeneration, § 17. An ovary may show cystic changes without being enlarged. Nevertheless, pains exist, especially at the menstrual epoch, during palpation, or during defecation, which is usually difficult. These pains are referred to the sacrum, sometimes as the so-called "intermenstrual pain." (See § 17.) Dysmenorrhea follows, or, if the disease is bilateral, amenorrhea and sterility.

This painful affection, usually of an inflammatory nature, gradually stamps itself on the features of the patient—*facies ovarica* (lips pressed together, angles of the mouth drawn down and the surrounding skin correspondingly furrowed, wrinkled and furrowed forehead, sunken cheeks, prominent cheek-bones, and pointed nose).

If the tumor attains the size of a child's head, symptoms arise from the displacement of the uterus and from pressure upon the rectum, bladder, vessels, and nerves (desire to urinate, constipation, hemorrhoids, phlebectasia, neuralgias in the lower extremities, etc.). It is at this point that the ovarian cysts cease to be unimportant.

The diagnosis of ovarian cysts is made by bimanual palpation (also through the rectum). A pedunculated tumor is found beside the uterus ; the tumor replaces the ovary of this side.

Parovarian cysts first give rise to symptoms when they reach to the pelvic inlet. They produce disturbances of the circulation in the broad ligament, and consequently interfere with the nutrition of the ovary. This results in anomalies of menstruation.

They may be recognized as fluctuating tumors at the side of the uterus, distinctly differentiated from it, and upon puncture yield a fluid with the previously described characteristics. They rarely return after being tapped.

Treatment. — Parovarian cysts may be tapped. Those containing a fluid richer in albumin are to be removed by celiotomy. If the tumor has a pedicle, the operation is a simple one. If strong adhesions exist, remove as much as possible and unite by suture. [Celiotomy and complete removal should take the place of tapping.—ED.]

Intraligamentous cysts are to be dissected out from the surrounding connective tissue, or the corresponding portion of the broad ligament is to be excised.

Ovarian cysts not larger than an apple are to be removed only when the disturbances they produce are unbearable. Iodid of potassium is to be given in solution or in vaginal suppositories (as an absorbent) until iodism is produced. To alleviate the disturbances : warm fomentations to the abdomen and applications of iodin ; rest during the periods. If pelvic peritonitis appears, rest in bed and the ice-bag are indicated. Regular movements of the bowels are to be secured. (See also § 35.) [Ovarian cysts presenting symptoms should be removed.—ED.]

CHAPTER II.

TUMORS OF BENIGN STRUCTURE THAT MAY BECOME DANGEROUS UNDER CERTAIN CONDITIONS.

₹34. THE FIBROMYOMATA.

All the large, progressively increasing myomata of the vagina, uterus, and ovary that are not polypoid (intraligamentous and intraparietal growths, and those with broad bases) belong to the group of fibromyomata that are followed by serious consequences (mortality, 10%).

The dangerous results of these tumors are:

1. Extreme anemia and secondary cardiac disease, produced by the continued hemorrhage (later, the dilated, thin-walled vessels may rupture).

2. Hemorrhages may also occur into the substance of the tumor. (Plate 66.) The cause is usually a disturbance of the circulation with thrombosis (this sometimes leads to fatal emboli after operation). These extravasations suppurate easily, and thus cause sepsis.

3. Torsion of the pedicle [1] in large subserous polyps leads to necrosis and inflammation; in the submucous polyps, to ulceration and putrefactive gangrene.

4. Inflammatory adhesions are formed with the intestines.

5. Submucous polyps may lead to inversion of the uterus (Figs. 24 and 57–59) if they proceed from the fundus and if the formation of a pedicle is made difficult by

---

[1] There are cases in which the uterus itself, instead of the pedicle, is twisted about its axis, or even torn open at the internal os. The tumor may become separated from the uterus, and obtain its nourishment through previously existing intestinal and omental adhesions.

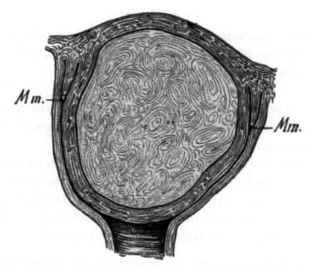

Fig. 57.—Intramural fibromyoma of the uterine fundus, projecting into the vagina. *Mm*, Os uteri.

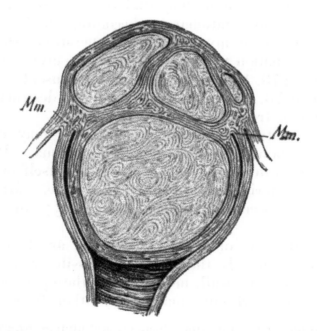

Fig. 58.—Multiple intramural myomata of the fundus. Submucous myoma of the fundus projecting into the vagina. *Mm*, Os uteri.

PLATE 67.

Polypoid Subserous Fibromyoma; Polyps of the Mucous Membrane in the Dilated Cervical Canal. (Original water-color from a specimen at the Path. Inst. at Heidelberg.)

numerous strong muscle-fibers from the uterine muscularis extending into the tumor. Further consequences: pressure necrosis, gangrene.

6. The large size of the tumor (some of them may weigh eighty-five pounds, especially if they are the seat of cystic degeneration) may cause obstruction or distortion of the pelvic organs, [1] or may interfere with delivery. They are particularly dangerous when they are calcified.

Cysts arise from myxomatous degeneration, from absorbed extravasations, or from the edematous softening of muscle-fibers (due to compression or infectious thrombosis of the vessels)

7. Intramural tumors may undergo fatty or calcareous changes, remaining stationary or becoming smaller. They may be the seat of myxomatous degeneration; they then show an inclination to be transformed into myxosarcomata (Plate 87, 2; 73, 1), sometimes with intermuscular pseudo-cysts (Plate 73, 3), which arise from the destruction of round cells or from blood extravasations.

8. The central portions of the tumor may undergo primary metamorphosis into a fibrosarcoma. Primary carcinomatous degeneration of the tumor itself or of the proliferated uterine mucosa may take place. Malignant degenerations occur at the menopause in $4\frac{1}{2}\%$ of all cases (Fehling).

9. The dangers of operative removal are hemorrhage and suppuration. If the tumors are sessile or are located deep in the uterine wall, necessitating the opening of the uterine cavity, peritonitis may occur, either from primary

[1] Occlusions of the intestines, bladder, and ureters which lead to intestinal obstruction, absolute retention of urine, uremia, incontinence with secondary cystitis, pyelonephrosis, etc.

infection or from the later rupture of an abscess of the stump.

Finally, lung emboli are more common than in operations upon other large genital tumors. All these dangers are more pronounced when the patient is profoundly anemic.

Symptoms.— *Vaginal myomata*—only pressure symptoms.

Large uterine myomata (for initial symptoms see § 31). If *intramural*, menorrhagia, and, in addition, pressure

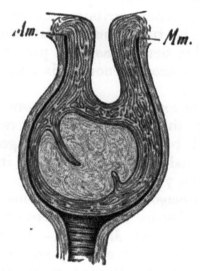

Fig. 59.—Intramural fibromyoma of the fundus uteri producing an inversion of the uterus. *Mm*, Os uteri.

symptoms, as in all these larger tumors. (Plates 63 and 66.)

If *submucous*, menorrhagia and metrorrhagia with violent colicky pains, as the tumors twist the uterus and often occlude the outlet for the discharge. Slight perimetritic pains are present. Sterility or abortion is frequent. The tumors easily undergo suppuration during the puerperium.

If *submucous and polypoid*, all the symptoms of the simple submucous variety, and, in addition, labor-like pains, since the uterus tries to expel the pendulous

When the polyp lies in the vagina, it becomes edematous
and the seat of a foul ulceration. A constant, nonremit-
tent fever exists even when a fetid discharge is not present. This is due to interstitial infection of the tumor.
(Plate 61, 2.)   Catarrhal discharge is profuse because the
irritation of the fibroid polyp causes the mucous membrane to proliferate *in toto.*   Multiple mucoid polyps may
consequently arise.

If *subserous,* the symptoms are few, often not more
marked than the pressure symptoms of the pregnant
uterus (dyspnea ; reflex irritation of the breasts is not
often absent).   The tumor may irritate the peritoneum or
may produce reflex neuralgias from pressure.

In *cervical myomata,* menorrhagia and profuse leukorrhea.   (Plate 65.)

With very rare exceptions the tumors contract during
the menopause ; the climacterium is, nevertheless, not
rarely prolonged by marked hemorrhages.   The author
saw regular periods from this cause in an American
woman, fifty-seven years of age.

In *ovarian fibromyomata* the symptoms are very uncertain : sometimes absence of the menses or ascites.

Diagnosis.—*Vaginal Myomata.*—It must be determined whether the tumor actually springs from the vaginal wall, or is simply adherent to it, as uterine polyps
may contract secondary adhesions with the vagina.

Intramural Uterine Myomata.—The wall of the organ
is hypertrophied and the uterine cavity is elongated.
Metritis and pregnancy must be excluded.   In the former
the wall is not so dense and the sound is not made to
deviate from the straight line by the presence of a tumor.
In the latter the cervix is livid and the entire organ is
strikingly soft ; the increase in size occurs in a typical
way ; the menses are absent.

If one suspects *submucous* or *polypoid myomata,* the
uterine cavity is to be palpated after dilatation of the cer-

vix. The sound is to be passed first; the cavity is enlarged, but the sound passes around the tumor or can not
effect an entrance. At the menstrual epoch the tumor
separates the lips of the os (Plate 60, 2; 61); traction
with the bullet-forceps gives information as to whether the
tumor has a long pedicle or a broad-based insertion.

If such tumors are very large (Fig. 57), and if they
project far into the vagina, it is often difficult to determine
their true origin without bimanual examination through
the rectum and the employment of the sound.

Cervical myomata, especially if they have undergone
suppuration, must be distinguished from epitheliomata of
the cervix. The former have a pedicle leading into the os
uteri; when broken down, they have a loose fibrous
structure and a brownish-red or pale rose color. The epitheliomatous nodules are softer; they crumble and bleed
easily; they are always outside of the external os; they
undergo ulceration without the production of polypoid
excrescences. The microscope shows fibrous tissue in the
one case, epitheliomatous plugs of cells in the other. (Plate
71, 2; 79.) Fibromyoma differentiates itself from sarcoma
by its greater density, slower growth, painlessness, and
absence of foul discharge with particles of tissue. The
transition from myoma to sarcoma is consequently characterized by the appearance of these symptoms and by
ascites. Fibromyomata have been mistaken for placental
polyps, and also for inversion of the uterus. (For diagnosis
of the latter see § 7.) Placental polyps, like polyps of the
mucous membrane, are softer. They contain decidual
cells, glandular epithelium, and chorionic villi.

It is often difficult to diagnose *subserous and intraligamentous uterine myomata* from tumors of the adnexa and
from tumors of the pouch of Douglas. This is partly
owing to the fact that they completely fill the rectovaginal
culdesac, and partly because they may be embedded in the
exudate of a pelvic peritonitis. (For differential diagnosis
see following section, under Ovarian Cystomata.) The

PLATE 68.

Fig. 1.—Unilocular Ovarian Cysts. Two cysts were situated in such a manner that one of them forced its way into the other. (Original water-color from an autopsy at the Heidelberg Path. Inst.)

Fig. 2.—Thin-walled Multilocular Glandular Mucoid Cyst. The pedicle, together with the tube and a hydatid, lies upon the tumor. The furrow is due to the impression of the iliopectineal line, as the smaller portion of the cyst was in the pelvis and filled the pouch of Douglas. (Original water-color from an operative specimen.)

and the uterus, with tumors and adnexa, is removed. If intraligamentous tumors are present, the broad ligament is incised and ligated on both sides in three portions.

The stump may be treated according to various methods :

1. Schröder's Intraperitoneal Method.—Wedge-shaped excision (cauterizing the stump with concentrated liquid carbolic acid, zinc chlorid, or Paquelin's cautery). The mucosa, the muscularis, and the serosa are sutured separately (etage suture) with catgut.

There is danger of secondary infection : i. e., of abscess formation in the stump and rupture of the united serosa. A large stump should consequently be avoided, as portions of it may undergo necrosis.

2. Péan-Heger's Extraperitoneal Method.—Long needles are passed through the stump at right angles, fixing it in the lower angle of the abdominal wound outside of the peritoneum. The serosa of the stump is sutured to that of the abdominal wall. The stump is covered only by the abdominal muscles.

It undergoes necrosis and is cast off, together with the elastic tube, after two or three weeks.

The disadvantage of this method consists in the permanent traction upon the bladder.

Fritsch unites the stump as does Schröder, using sagittal instead of transverse sutures, and sews it into the lower angle of the abdominal incision. On the ninth day he removes the constriction sutures of the stump from the bottom of the wound.

3. Chrobak fixes the stump behind the peritoneum (consequently an extraperitoneal method) by covering it with a peritoneal flap previously excised either from the tumor or from the uterus.

III. Total extirpation guarantees the greatest security against secondary infection of the peritoneal cavity from the secreting or partly necrotic stump obtained by the supravaginal method; [1] it is, however, a more radical operation. In certain cases it is absolutely indicated,

---

[1] At the Heidelberg Frauenklinik, in 1896, thirty myomotomics were performed (the stump being treated by the retroperitoneal method) with two deaths, one from pulmonary embolism, one from severe anemia.

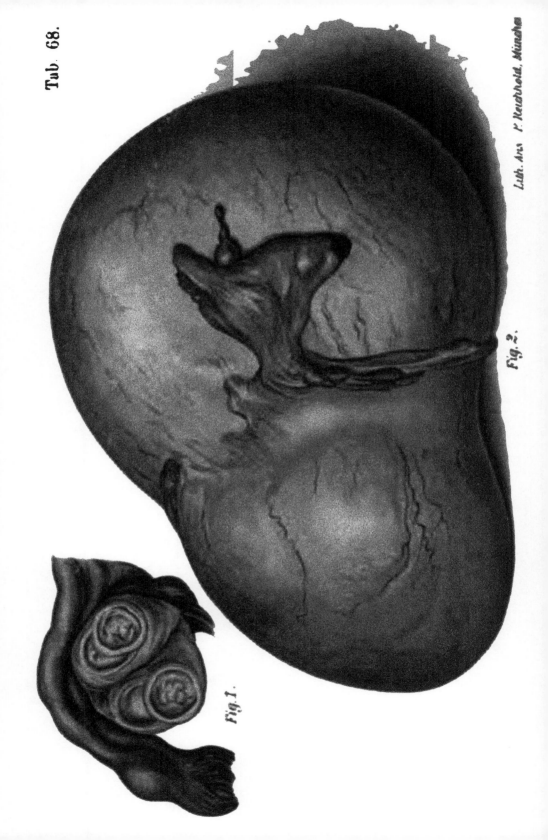

Tub. 68.

Fig. 1.

Fig. 2.

Lith. Ans. v. Leuzhold, München

as in pyosalpinx (Plate 42) and cervical myomata (Plate 65). The ovarian arteries are ligated, transverse incisions are made in the vesico-uterine and recto-uterine excavations, and the ligaments are successively ligated and divided. The neck is amputated in such a manner that a very small portion remains behind with the external os (the orifice may be cauterized). This wound is to be united by some nondraining suture material (silkworm-gut). Catgut ligatures are used in the parametritic cellular tissues and in the serosa.

IV. Hegar's castration is only a makeshift. It is to be performed only when the removal of the myomata must be looked upon as dangerous to life (very large myomata with multiple subserous nodules preventing their removal from the pelvic cavity). The operation has a mortality of 16%, because the ovaries are frequently so close to the tumor that the ligation of the vessels is very difficult. In many cases the looked-for result has failed to appear. The ligation of the uterine arteries from the vagina is a better operation (Gottschalk).

The operative removal of ovarian fibromata is indicated, even if they are of only moderate size and stationary, on account of the danger of malignant degeneration. Hemorrhage, especially from the adhesions, is the chief danger of the operation. The elastic rubber tube is used, and the pedicle is tied off with broad, strong ligatures before the removal of the tumor.

The preparatory treatment and after-treatment in all these celiotomies are the same as in the removal of ovarian cystomata.

§ 35. THE OVARIAN CYSTOMATA.

Definition, Anatomy, and Histology.—The multilocular glandular mucoid cyst arises from a proliferation of the germinal epithelium of the Graafian follicle,[1] together with a supporting and vascular proliferation of the connective tissues (see Plate 72)—cystadenoma.

Five varieties of ovarian cysts may be differentiated:

1. Unilocular cysts (Plate 68, 1)—hypertrophic ovarian follicles (hydrops folliculorum).

2. The *multilocular glandular mucoid cyst*—a nodular complex of many smaller cysts, filled with viscid mucus (greenish-yellow to grayish-black according to the admixture of blood) and surrounded by a single outer wall. (Plate 72.)

---

[1] Stefeck demonstrated ovula in the young cysts of cystadenomata.

PLATE 69.

Multilocular Glandular Mucoid Cyst. As a result of torsion of the pedicle, hemorrhages have occurred in individual cysts (dark-bluish color) and portions of the wall have become necrotic and adherent to the omentum. Subperitoneal disturbances of the circulation have formed cystic spaces (on the left) in the latter. (Original watercolor from a case at the Heidelberg Frauenklinik.)

The tumors show a more or less rapid, progressive, and almost unlimited growth. They become dangerous when they grow larger than a man's head; their weight may exceed that of the patient herself. (Fig. 62.) When the tumor has involved the entire ovary, it is fixed to the uterus and nourished by a pedicle, which consists of the broad ligament, tube, and ovarian ligament. The pedicle is absent in intraligamentous tumors (Plate 59, 2) because the entire growth develops outside of the peritoneum in the subserous connective tissue of the broad ligament. The anterior surface of the ovary is embedded in the broad ligament (by the mesovarium), while the posterior surface, directed toward the pouch of Douglas, is uncovered. If an ovarian cyst develops from the anterior surface, it grows into the connective tissue between the two layers of the broad ligament—it is "intraligamentous"; if the tumor becomes larger, it strips up the posterior lamella, elevates the serosa of Douglas' pouch, and reaches the spinal column—it becomes "retroperitoneal."

The pedicle previously mentioned is pathognomonic of ovarian tumors, and may be demonstrated by the method illustrated in Plate 74. It is usually twisted in a spiral manner in the larger tumors. This torsion of the pedicle is due to intestinal peristalsis, to the variable emptying and filling of the abdominal organs, and to the movements of the body. In left-sided tumors the pedicle is more frequently twisted from 90 to 180 degrees to the right. If it is twisted more than 360 degrees, disturbances of the

circulation and extravasation occur in the tumor, and hematomata are formed in the pedicle; secondary disturbances of nutrition lead to retrograde metamorphoses; both results are serious in proportion to the rapidity of the compression (necrosis; rupture of the mucoid degenerated wall, Plate 72; decomposition; peritonitis). If colloid masses reach the peritoneal cavity, they become organized upon the serosa, constituting "peritoneal myxedema" (pseudomyxoma peritonei, Werth).

The larger tumors always cause fibrinous deposits and adhesions, because the changed superficial epithelium becomes desquamated. In a beginning cystoma the fimbriated end of the tube sometimes becomes agglutinated; if the dividing wall disappears, a tubo-ovarian cyst results.

3. Papillary proliferating cysts. (See explanation to Fig. 61.)

4. Racemose cysts (Olshausen) differentiate themselves from the cystadenomata by the fact that several vesicles are attached to one pedicle; even if they have broad bases, they do not present a smooth globular surface, but look like a mass of small vesicles (resembling a hydatid mole). The vesicles contain a fluid that is not colloid; it is rich in albumin.

5. Dermoid Cysts. (Plates 45 and 79.)

Cystomata may lead to serious consequences:

1. From their increase in size—larger than a man's head.

2. From strangulation as a result of torsion of the pedicle, with hemorrhages, inflammation, suppuration, infection (they may, it is true, undergo absorption and natural cure), septicemia.

3. From intestinal adhesions and the subsequent production of intestinal obstruction.

4. From rupture of the tumor and consequent pseudomyxoma peritonei (Werth).

5. From carcinomatous degeneration.

6. Death from cardiac weakness, uremia.

Symptoms.—(See initial symptoms in § 32.) Pressure symptoms first occur when the tumor reaches the size of

PLATE 70.

Multilocular Glandular Mucoid Cyst.   The middle of the tumor is laid open by an incision.   (Original water-color from an operative specimen from the Heidelberg Frauenklinik.)

PLATE 71.

FIG. 1.—**Histologic Structure of a Uterine Mucous Polyp.** (Original drawing from a specimen from the Munich Frauenklinik.) Circumscribed proliferation of the uterine mucosa (proceeding from the body as well as from the cervix), consisting of glandular and connective tissue in their normal structure and relations (in contrast to the atypical proliferation of malignant adenoma, as seen in Plate 30, Fig. 2). The glandular spaces (1) are lined with ciliated columnar epithelium. Numerous thin-walled, dilated vessels (2 and 4) are seen in the connective tissue (3), and are responsible for the hemorrhage that is so easily produced.

FIG. 2.—**Microscopic Section through the Transition Zone of a Minute Myoma That is Becoming Encapsulated into the Surrounding Normal Uterine Muscularis.**   (Original drawing from a specimen from the Munich Frauenklinik.)   The tumor tissue to the left (1) consists of densely packed and interlaced non-striated muscle-fibers alone, without the admixture of connective-tissue fibers that occurs without exception in the large tumors (consequently called fibromyomata, which always originate in such pure intramural myomata).   The border-line (2) of the normal muscular tissue consists of concentrically arranged parallel lamellæ, which are evidently compressed by the new growth.   To the right, markedly dilated vessels (4) are seen in the muscularis (3), which shows a less parallel arrangment.

FIG. 3.—**Vaginitis (Colpitis).**   (Original drawing from a specimen from the Munich Frauenklinik.)   Round-cell infiltration of the submucous connective tissue, especially in the neighborhood of the numerous normal lymph-follicles (3—surrounded by round cells and lymph-channels).   (1) Normal vaginal tissue ; (2) normal connective tissue.

Tab. 70.

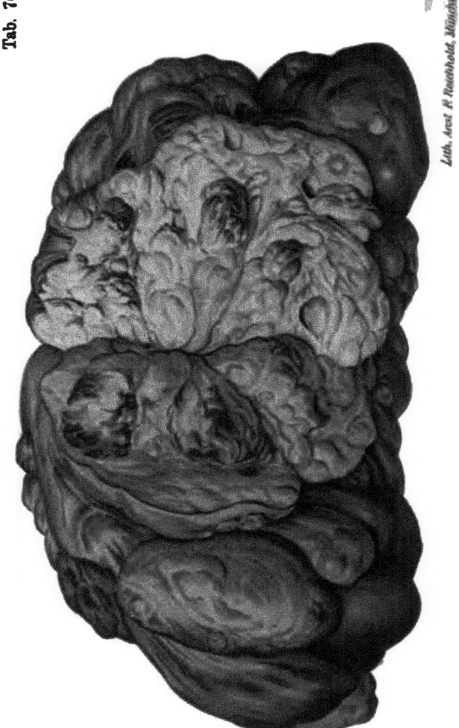

Lith. Arst. F. Reichhold, München

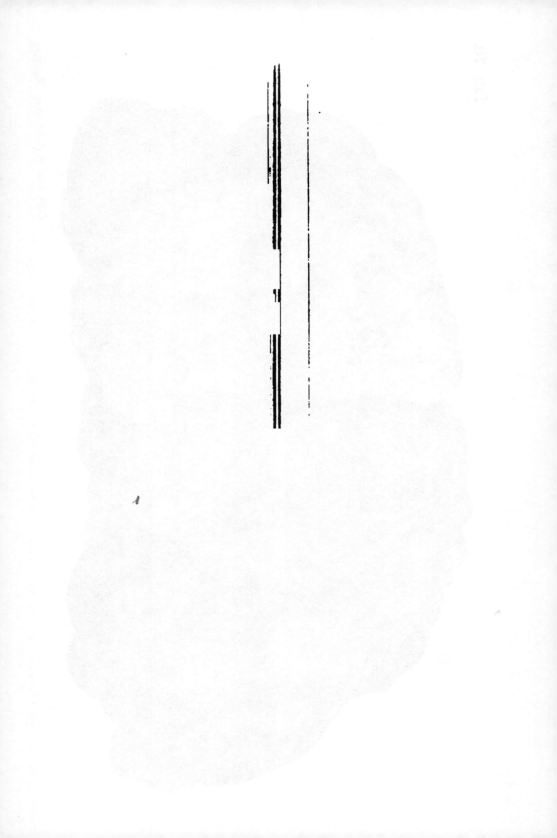

Tab. 71.

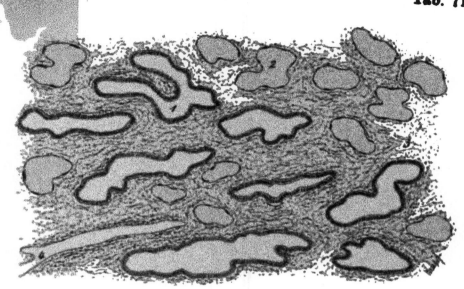

Fig. 1.

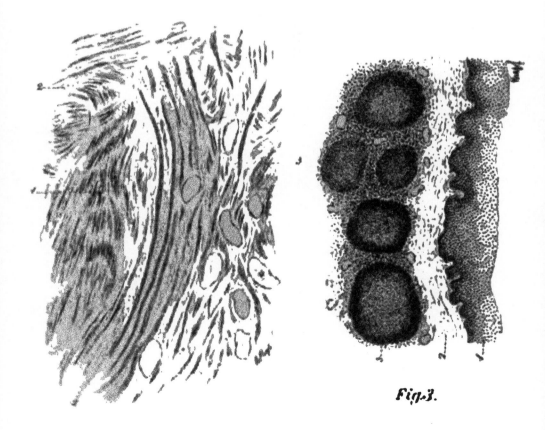

Fig. 3.

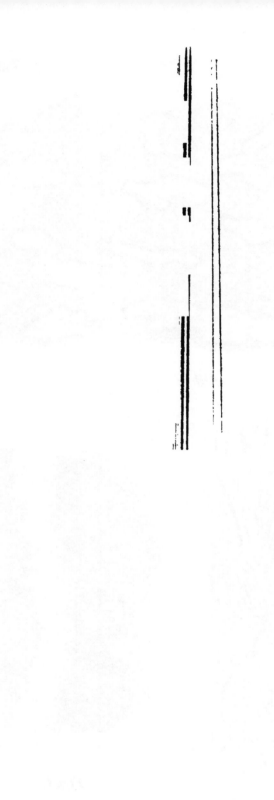

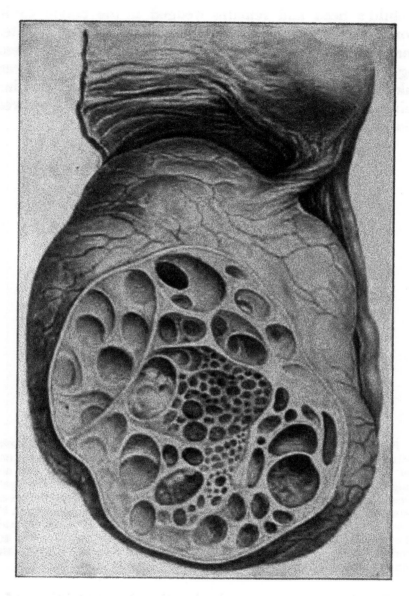

Fig. 60.—Multilocular glandular mucoid cyst of the ovary, with
torsion of the pedicle. (Specimen at the Munich Frauenklinik.)

215

a child's head and remains wedged in the pelvic cavity (constipation, urinary disturbances, neuralgias). Intestinal perforation may occur. (See Plate 45, 2, representing a case treated in the dispensary at the Munich Frauenklinik.) Dyspnea, swelling of the thoracico-abdominal veins, edema, and pressure upon the ureters are observed. The patient is finally confined to bed.

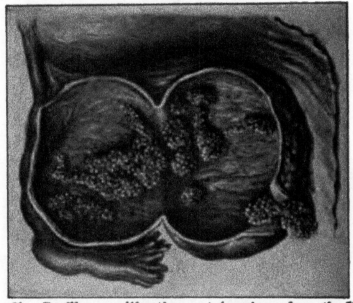

Fig. 61.—Papillary proliferating cyst (specimen from the Munich Frauenklinik), characterized by the fact that the epithelium produces not only glandular—*i. e.*, follicular and cystic—formations, but also conglomerations of papillary formations upon the walls of the cysts. (See also Plate 72, Figs. 1 and 2.) These dendritic proliferations are found either only upon the inner surface of the cysts, or also upon the outer surface; in the latter case they not rarely grow through the wall. They give metastasis to the serosa of the entire peritoneal cavity and produce ascites. Macroscopically, they are not to be differentiated from the similar, somewhat firmer, carcinomatous growths.

The diagnosis is made by the demonstration of a pedicle and the separation of the tumor from the uterus, the method of Schultze being employed. (Plate 74, Fig. 3.) Fluctuation is a further aid. In contrast to ascites, percussion demonstrates an area of dullness which

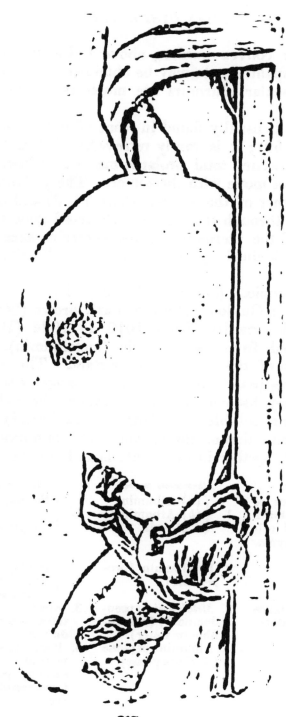

Fig. 62.—Enormous ovarian cyst (from a photograph kindly given to the author by his colleague, Dr. Cohnheim).

217

has an upper convex border; above and at the sides an intestinal tympanitic note may be obtained. Ascites may coexist. Vascular murmurs are much rarer than over myomata.

The uterus is usually found in front of and beneath the tumor (Plate 59); it is rarely retroverted (Plate 16, 4); if pregnancy occurs, total prolapse may take place. The uterus does not move with the tumor. The pedicle arises from one corner of the uterus (Plate 74, 3) and may be best palpated through the rectum. Dermoid cysts usually lie in front of the uterus in the vesico-uterine excavation.

The fluid obtained by tapping has the following characteristics:

(*a*) Microscopic. (See Plate 72, Fig. 5.)

(*b*) Chemic: Golden yellow to dark brown (blood) in color; specific gravity, from 1010 to 1024 (1005 to 1055); colloid from pseudomucin (metalbumin). The demonstration of the latter is important. The albuminous substances pass through a process analogous to digestion until they become soluble in water (the older the tumor, the more soluble the substance—Eichwald). The chemic differentiation of the mucous and albuminous substances found together in cystomata is as follows:

Mucous Series.	*Albuminous Series.*	*Solubility.*
1. The substance of the colloid globules —transformed cellular parenchyma.	1. { (*a*) Albumin. (*b*) Albuminate of soda.	1. { Boiling +. Acetic acid precipitates.
2. Mucin.	2. Paralbumin (propeptone).	2. { Boiling +. Acetic acid precipitates.
3. Colloid substance (soluble in water).	3. *Metalbumin* (pseudomucin) (not soluble in water).	3. Alcohol precipitates, mineral acids do not.
4. Mucopeptone.	4. Albumin-peptone (fibrin-peptone).	4. Precipitated by neutral metallic salts, potassium ferrocyanid, and tannin; soluble in water.

The albuminous series is differentiated from the mucous series by the fact that the former contains nitrogen and sulphur and is precipitated by tannin and neutral metallic salts.

The fluid is boiled, and upon the addition of nitric acid all the albumins, as far as and including paralbumin, are precipitated. These, together with the corresponding mucins, are removed by filtration. Upon the addition of alcohol to the filtrate, the metalbumin is coagulated and sinks to the bottom in white clouds. If acetic acid alone is added to the filtrate, a cloudiness occurs, but no precipitation. Metalbumin is distinguished from the corresponding colloid substance by its insolubility in water, or by its being precipitated by a new test with ferrocyanid of potash.

The reduction test with 10% cupric sulphate solution (Trommer's sugar test) is employed for more exact examinations.

The chemic differential diagnosis between ascitic transudate and peritoneal exudate is given in the explanation of plate 58, 1.

Parovarian Cysts.—Contents clear as water; specific gravity from 1002 to 1006; rarely richer than this in albumin; ciliated epithelium without other formed elements, such as blood-corpuscles.

Hydrosalpinx.—Contents serous, mucoid, or gritty; rich in albumin; cholesterin, red and white blood-corpuscles, cylindric epithelium.

Hydronephrosis.—Much urea is present, demonstrable by partial evaporation, extraction with alcohol, and evaporation; the residue is dissolved in a small amount of water and treated with concentrated nitric acid. Rhomboid plates of urea nitrate are formed. Low specific gravity; little albumin.

Echinococcus Cysts.—(Occur in the genitalia in 4% of all cases, especially in the uterine submucosa and in Douglas' pouch.) Specific gravity from 1007 to 1015; hooklets and scolices; no albumin; much NaCl, and especially succinic acid. The latter is demonstrable by partial evaporation, dilution with water, and extraction with ether; upon evaporation the monoclinic prisms—six-sided plates of succinic acid—are obtained, or the watery solution gives a rust-colored flocculent precipitate with ferric chlorid.

I. Intra-uterine Tumors.

Differential Diagnosis.—*1. Pregnancy.*—Absence of the menses, gradual typical increase in size, and, after the fifth month, fetal movements, ballotement, and audible cardiac sounds. The cervix is livid and soft. Characteristic softening of the lower uterine segment (bimanual through the rectum). The variable signs of pregnancy and secretion from the breasts are worthless, as they also occur with cystomata. The sound and the trocar are not to be used until pregnancy is absolutely excluded.

PLATE 72.

Fio. 1.—**Primary Formation of Cysts from a Multilocular Glandular Mucoid Cyst of the Ovary.** (See also Plates 69-70 and Figs. 60, 62.) The individual cystic spaces (1) are formed because the walls tear, from mucoid degeneration (2, 3), and float about in the fluid colloid contents as free papillæ (2). (4) Smallest cyst. (5) Connective tissue. (Original drawing from a specimen.)

Fio. 2.—**Papillary Proliferating Cyst of the Ovary.** (Original drawing from a specimen from the Munich Frauenklinik.) (1) Broad papilla containing a cyst (2) lined, as is the entire cyst, with columnar epithelium (4), with pouchings similar to glands or folds (5); (3) cross-section of papillæ; (8) fine dendritic papillæ; (6) dense connective tissue of the cystic wall; (7) external wavy elastic layer of connective tissue.

Fio. 3.—**Necrotic Cyst-wall.** Myxomatous degeneration and separation of the connective-tissue fibers (2); vascular space (1). (Original drawing from a specimen.)

Fio. 4.—**Sediment from the Fluid of an Ovarian Cyst.** (1) Cholesterin crystals; (2) red blood-corpuscles; (3) granular columnar epithelium; (4) fatty granular cell; (5) leukocytes; (6) endothelium. (Original drawing.)

Retroflexion of a gravid uterus is to be especially considered. The chief symptom is ischuria.

It is to be further remembered that the product may have died (chilliness).

2. Hematometra, with or without Hematosalpinx.—If congenital, the menses have never appeared; if acquired, they have been absent since a definite time. The patulous condition of the vagina and uterus is to be demonstrated by the sound.

3. Intramural and Submucous Myomata.—Menorrhagia, labor-like pains, slower growth than in cystomata. They are dense, and vascular murmurs are usually present; the uterine cavity is elongated. They frequently coexist with cystomata.

Tab. 72.

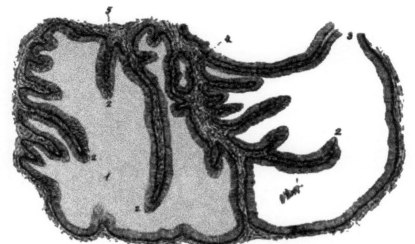

Fig. 1.

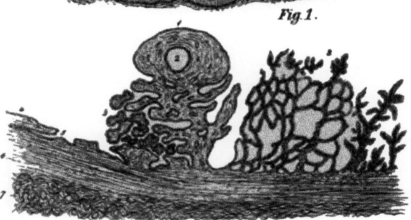

Fig. 2.

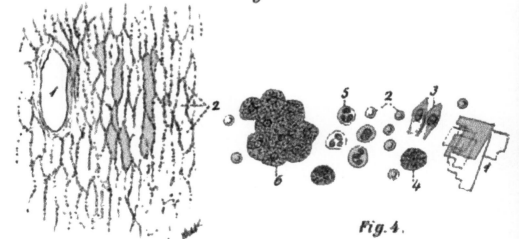

Fig. 3.

Fig. 4.

Lith. Anst. P. Reichhold, München.

II. Pedunculated Tumors of the Uterus and Adnexa.

4. Subserous uterine myomata present symptoms similar to those just mentioned, and, in addition, the cervix moves with the tumor, sometimes being forced in the opposite direction by leverage. With the exception of cystic fibromata and edematous tumors, their consistency is greater (cystomata may also become hard from extravasation of blood after torsion of the pedicle).

5. Intraligamentous Uterine Myomata.—Symptoms as in 3 and 4. They are intimately associated with the uterus, and are to be differentiated from intraligamentous cysts only by their hardness.

6. Hydrosalpinx, Hematosalpinx, Pyosalpinx.—Anamnesis, fever, tenderness and pain, lateral situation and sausage-shaped or horn-shaped, with constrictions. (Plates 41, 44, 59, 74.) Tapping.

7. Parovarian Cysts.—These are round; they show marked fluctuation, and are not nodular, but unilocular. They are close to the uterus and have, at most, an insignificant pedicle. Tapping.

8. Ovarian Fibromata.—These possess a uniform density, a surface covered with small protuberances, and are of slower growth.

III. Tumors of the Pouch of Douglas.

9. Abdominal Pregnancy.—This is characterized by temporary amenorrhea and by pain, and occasionally the decidua is cast off. The sac has no pedicle, and portions of the fetus may be recognized.

10. Intraperitoneal Retro-uterine Hematocele.—Sudden origin, with collapse. The fluctuating tumor fills the recto-uterine pouch. The vaginal vault is tender. No diagnostic incision should be made. (Plate 58.)

The extraperitoneal peri-uterine hematocele (hematoma) leaves Douglas' pouch free and lies to the side of the uterus.

PLATE 73.

FIG. 1.—**Myxosarcoma of the Uterus.** (Original drawing from a specimen from the Munich Frauenklinik.) It arises primarily or from an unusually rapidly growing fibroma (which has undergone degeneration from insufficient nutrition or from infection). (1) Malignant "giant cells." (2) Round-cell proliferation. (3 and 4) Myxomatous connective tissue; the fibers are pressed apart. (See also Plate 73, 2.)

FIG. 2.—**Spindle-cell Sarcoma of the Uterus. With cyst** formation (2); (1) giant cells abundantly present among the spindle cells. (Original drawing from a specimen from the Munich Frauenklinik.) (See also Plate 87, 2.)

By sarcomata we understand tumors of the connective-tissue type with an abnormal predominance of the cellular elements (round, spindle, giant, and stellate cells). They occur as soft, lobulated tumors, which grow rapidly, soon give rise to metastases, and recur upon removal. In contrast to epitheliomata, they arise more commonly in early life. They are found in the uropoietic apparatus, in the vulva, in the vagina, in the uterus, in the ovaries, and in the remaining adnexa.

They occur in the vulva as round-cell sarcomata, spindle-cell sarcomata, myxosarcomata, and melanosarcomata; in the vagina (Plate 73); in the uterus (Plate 87, Fig. 2); in the ovary they present a spindle-cell type, with or without cyst formation.

FIG. 3.—**Malignant Adenoma Growing through a Cyst-wall.** (Half diagrammatic original drawing from a specimen from the Munich Frauenklinik.) The superficial columnar epithelium (1) grows out into an atypically arranged adenomatous mass (6), consisting of cystic glandular spaces (7), with columnar epithelium (6), which is stratified in various places (8). The interstitial connective tissue (9) is scanty. The cyst-wall consists of columnar epithelium (1), dense fibrous connective tissue (2), wavy elastic connective tissue (3), with thin-walled vascular spaces (4), and the endothelium of the serosa (5).

FIG. 4.—**Angioma of the Urethra.** (Original drawing from a specimen.) The blood-capillaries (1) consist of endothelial cells alone, and lie close together in the connective tissue (2). (See also explanation to Plate 51, Fig. 2.)

Tab. 73.

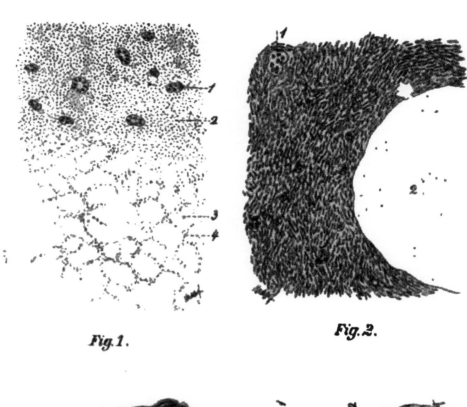

Fig. 1.

Fig. 2.

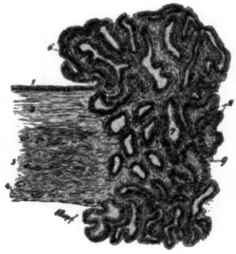

Fig. 3.

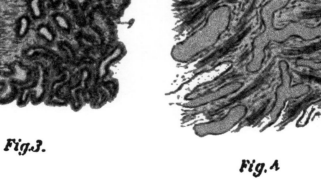

Fig. 4.

Lith. Anst. v. Reichhold, München.

Tab. 73.

11. Fluid Exudative Peritonitis.—This pursues a febrile course, with violent pains, tympanites, and vomiting. Diarrhea is often present. The patient is unable to walk. The tumor is at first fluctuating or doughy; later, it is nodular and the uterus is immobile. (Plate 17, Fig. 1.)

12. Parametritic tumors present characteristics similar to the foregoing. They are to one side or posterior, and above the vaginal vault. Contracted intraligamentous abscesses are connected with the margin of the uterus. (Plate 59, 1.)

13. Rectal tumors are rarer, and are occasionally adherent to cystomata. They are to be palpated from the rectum as they are located in its wall. Stenosis is sometimes present. It is often impossible to establish the true condition of affairs; a cyst may be adherent to the intestine.

14. Tumors of the pelvic bones are immovably connected with them, and grow more slowly. It is very important that the ovaries should be located, since cysts adherent to the pelvis may closely simulate them upon palpation.

15. Anterior sacral hydromeningocele (a hydromeningocele of the dura mater between the body and ala of the sacrum) is a great rarity.

IV. Other Abdominal Tumors.

16. Floating Kidney.—The movable tumor is reniform, firm, and somewhat sensitive. The normal renal dullness is absent, and in its place a tympanitic percussion-note may be obtained. A pelvic pedicle is wanting.

17. Hydronephrosis.—This will have existed for a long time, and grows downward from the lumbar region without a pelvic pedicle. The intestines are in front of the tumor, whereas in ovarian growths they are either behind or above. Tapping.

18. Renal tumors; Hematomata (Plate 77).—Echinococcus cysts of the kidneys, of the liver, and of the pelvis give a hydatid thrill. Tapping.

19. Splenic Tumor.—This extends to the pelvis from

Differential Diagnosis of the Ante-uterine and Retro-uterine Tumors.

A. FLUCTUATING RETRO-UTERINE TUMORS.

See Growth without Fever.
Fundus uteri:

Continuous with the retro-uterine tumor.

(1) Retroflexion of a gravid uterus; (2) intra-uterine cystic myomata; (3) hæmato-metra; (4) echinococcus cysts of the uterus (submucous).

Distinct from the retro-uterine tumor.

(1) Ovarian or præ-ovarian cysts; (2) hydrosalpinx; (3) abdominal pregnancy (variable); (4) subperitoneous cyst of the uterine adnexa and of the pelvis.

Rapid Growth with Fever.
Fundus uteri:

Continuous with the retro-uterine tumor.

(1) Fluid peritoneal exudate; (2) intra-peritoneal retro-uterine hematocele; (3) parametritic exudate and extraperitoneal peri-uterine pouch (Douglas')

B. SOLID RETRO-UTERINE TUMORS.

Fundus uteri:

Continuous with the uterus.

(Both with

(2) Ovarian fibromata more.

C. FLUCTUATING ANTE-UTERINE TUMORS.

Slow Growth without Fever.

Continuous with the tumor.

(1) Physiologic anteflexion of a gravid uterus.

(2) Intra-uterine cystic myomata.

(3) Hematometra.

Rapid Growth with Fever.

Fundus uteri:

Distinct from the tumor.

(1) Ovarian dermoid cyst (usually here; multilocular ovarian cysts rarely here).

(2) Hydrosalpinx (more frequent here).

(3) Abdominal pregnancy (rarely here).

(1) Fluid peritoneal exudate (rare).

(2) Ante-uterine intra-peritoneal hematocele (rarely here).

(3) Anterior parametritic exudates and extraperitoneal peri-uterine hematocele (peritoneal pouch is free).

D. SOLID ANTE-UTERINE TUMORS.

Fundus uteri:

Distinct from the tumor.

(1) Subserous polypoid fibromyomata of the uterus.

(2) Ovarian fibromata and carcinomata (rarely here).

(3) Vesical tumors.

(4) Vesical calculi.

(5) Anterior pelvic tumor.

Continuous with the tumor.

(1) Intra-uterine and (rarely here) broad-based subserous fibromyomata of the uterus.

(2) Consolidated peritoneal exudate (rarely here).

(3) Consolidated parametritic exudate. (Both with a febrile origin.)

15

PLATE 74.

Figs. 1 and 2.—Bimanual Examination of a Pyosalpinx with a Full and with an Empty Rectum. Both bladder and rectum are to be emptied before every bimanual examination, as these illustrations show how easily deceptive ideas of the form and of the size of tumors may be obtained. *Py,* Pyosalpinx; *R,* rectum; *U,* uterus.

Fig. 3.—Bimanual Examination, with Assistance, of the Pedicle of an Ovarian Cyst (according to B. S. Schultze). (Original diagrammatic drawing.) The uterus is drawn downward with the bullet-forceps; the cyst is elevated through the abdominal wall; palpation is made from below through the rectum. In this way the pedicle is made as tense as possible. In the illustration the latter is twisted.

---

the left side of the abdomen, but has no pelvic pedicle. Leukemia.

20. *Tumors of the omentum, subperitoneal hematomata* (Plate 78), *and tubercular and carcinomatous adhesions* have no pedicle extending into the pelvis. Ascites or a tympanitic note may be demonstrated beneath them. The ovaries are normal.

21. *Cysts of the pancreas* have no pelvic pedicle.

22. *Tumors of the bladder* produce characteristic vesical disturbances. The urine should be examined for portions of tumor tissue. Dilatation of the urethra. They may be adherent to cystomata.

23. *Tumors of the abdominal walls and parietal peritoneum* are intimately adherent to the skin, and their outlines are strikingly distinct to palpation. During respiration they move backward and forward with the abdominal wall; intraperitoneal tumors move up and down with the diaphragm and disappear with increased tension of the abdominal muscles. In all positions of the body the tumor holds the same relation to the abdominal parietes. If the tumor is flattened by the contraction of the abdominal muscles, and can be felt immediately underneath their

Tab. 74.

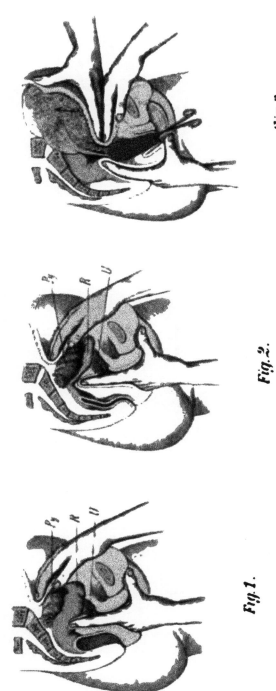

Fig.1.

Fig.2.

Fig.3.

Lith. Anst F. Reichhold, München.

tense fibers, it springs from the serosa or from the transverse fascia; if the tumor becomes more prominent and fixed by the abdominal tension, it springs from the muscles themselves; if the tumor remains movable, it is situated in the subcutaneous connective tissue.

A fluctuating tumor in the lower abdomen may be a perimetritic or a parametritic abscess, or, if tubercular lumbar scoliosis is present, a psoas abscess; if the tumor is right-sided, appendicitis, typhlitis, perityphlitis, and an adherent pus tube in the vesico-uterine pouch must be considered.

V. Conditions Simulating Tumors.

24. Distended Bladder.

25. Ascites. (See Plate 58, 1.)

26. Increased Amount of Fat in the Abdominal Wall.

27. Meteorism.—General tympany is present; the genitalia are normal; localized hardness is absent; so-called "phantom tumors" are to be observed.

Prognosis.—Ninety per cent. of all cysts larger than a man's head are fatal from rupture and peritonitis, from suppuration, or from exhaustion. Malignant degeneration is always possible. Dermoid cysts suppurate easily or undergo carcinomatous degeneration.

Torsion of the pedicle is dangerous. It produces disturbances of the circulation with venous thrombosis, extravasation of blood, or rupture of the tumor. If the nutritional disturbance is gradual, retrograde metamorphoses occur; if it is rapid, necrosis (Plates 69 and 72) and gangrene follow.

Diagnosis of Sudden Torsion of the Pedicle.—Acute increase of pain; the tumor, often the abdomen also, becomes tender, causing the patient to bend forward in walking; reflex nausea; moderate evening rises of temperature, with morning remissions.

Treatment.—(See § 32.) If a cyst is as large as a child's head, it must be removed; pregnancy is no longer

PLATE 75.

Figs. 1 and 2.—Two Different Cut Surfaces of a Sarcoma of the Ovary. (Original water-color from an operative specimen from the Heidelberg surgical clinic.)

considered to be a contraindication to the operation. It is also best, however, to remove smaller cysts by ovariotomy, especially if they produce violent pressure phenomena, severe nervous symptoms, or render the individual unable to work. Since the other ovary likewise may easily undergo carcinomatous degeneration, the age of the patient, the family history, and the marriage relation must be carefully considered in every case, in order to determine whether the immediate removal of this organ is not also advisable.

Tapping should be resorted to only when special indications are present. These are as follows: When the operation is refused; during delivery; when marked dyspnea or other pressure symptoms are present and ovariotomy is contraindicated by malignancy, weak heart with edema, etc., profound anemia, pulmonary tuberculosis, nephritis, or other severe incurable constitutional diseases.

The cyst is to be tapped through the abdominal walls or the vagina by Bresgen's trocar or Potain's apparatus, the most rigid asepsis being observed and the entrance of air being carefully guarded against.

PLATE 76.

Fig. 1.—Sarcoma of the Ovary. (Original water-color from an operative specimen from the Heidelberg surgical clinic.)

Fig. 2.—A Case of Commencing Sarcomatous Degeneration of the Ovary. The albuginea is thickened, and small follicular cysts may be seen through the otherwise atrophic germinal layer. (Original water-color from an operative specimen from the Heidelberg surgical clinic.)

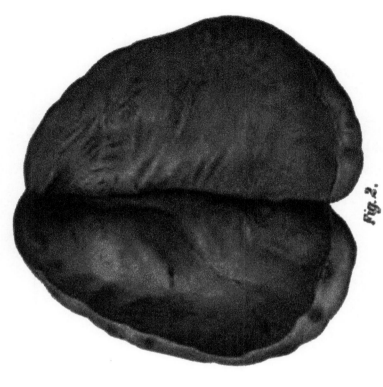

Fig.2.

Lith. Anst. F. Reichhold, München.

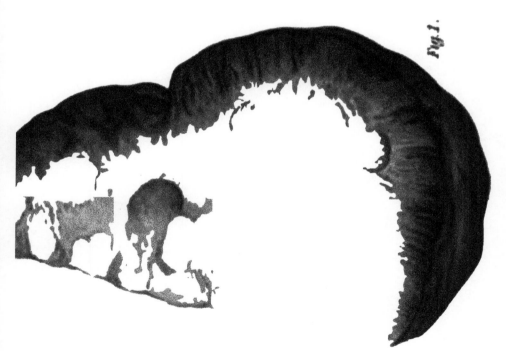

Fig.1.

Tab. 76.

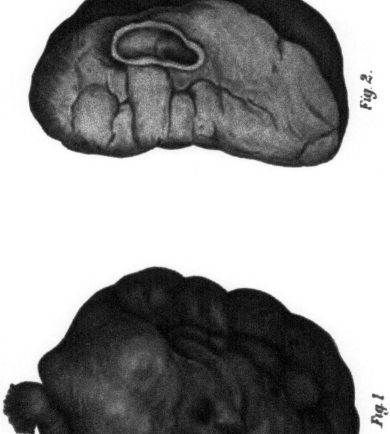

Fig. 2.

Fig 1

Lith. Anst f. Reichhold. München.

The trocar and elastic tube are to be previously filled with sterile water, and the free end of the tube is to be immersed in a receptacle containing the same fluid. This prevents the air from being sucked in by an accidental falling-back of the tumor; this accident is further hindered by sewing the cyst to the abdominal wall, which also renders impossible the escape of the fluid into the abdominal cavity. The cyst is to be evacuated by placing the patient in an appropriate position and not by manual pressure. The fluid is to be slowly drawn off, since a rapid removal is frequently followed by collapse. The puncture is to be closed by adhesive plaster (in the shape of a Maltese cross) or by an occlusive dressing.

Ovarian cysts rarely contract after tapping; they usually refill, and the patient becomes profoundly exhausted. Extirpation by modern aseptic methods has a mortality of only 4½% (Fritsch). At the Heidelberg Frauenklinik, in 1896, there was only one fatal result in sixty celiotomies (severe anemia and multiple myomata); there was not a fatal case from ovariotomy.

It is not within the scope of this book to go into the details of the technic of ovariotomy, but the preparation of the patient and the after-treatment, with its complications, will now be considered. The day before the operation the patient receives a full bath ; the abdominal walls are shaved, scrubbed, and disinfected (soap and brush, alcohol and brush, sublimate solution and brush). During the night a sublimate compress is applied to the lower abdomen (Fritsch). Since infectious germs always exist in the cutaneous glands and in the deeper layers of the epidermis, the disinfection must be repeated immediately before the operation, special attention being given to the navel, old scars, or other uneven places in the skin.

For several days preceding the operation the diet should be liquid but nutritious (bouillon, eggs, milk, oatmeal-water). The bowels must be thoroughly and energetically evacuated, care being taken, however, that this is not carried to excess. Immediately before the operation the bladder is to be emptied ; the vulva and vagina are to be thoroughly cleansed and tightly packed with iodoform gauze in case it is necessary to open the vaginal vault or to perform other operations through the vagina.

Dressing and After-treatment.—Dermatol is to be

PLATES 77 AND 78.

Multiple Extraperitoneal Extravasations of Blood, Especially in the Great Omentum. The largest one was connected with the atrophic kidney by numerous peritoneal adhesions, and simulated a renal tumor. (Plate 77.) The different stages of development are shown in plate 78 in their natural size. Figures 1 and 2, primary extraperitoneal hemorrhages; as the hemorrhage increases a peritoneal pedicle is formed (Fig. 3); the greater portion of the wall is now insufficiently nourished, and undergoes necrosis; the capillary vessels are seen radiating from the pedicle into the tumor; complete necrosis occurs upon torsion of the pedicle. (Fig. 4.) A cross-section shows the bloody contents and the thickening of the wall. (Fig. 5.) (Original water-color from specimens in the Heidelberg Path. Inst.)

---

dusted upon the line of incision ; this is to be followed by iodoform gauze or iodoform collodion, cotton, and an abdominal binder. This dressing is not to be changed for several days unless it is absolutely necessary. The sutures are to be removed on the tenth day ; if vaginal sutures suppurate, they are to be removed earlier, and a compress saturated with a solution of aluminum acetate [1] is to be applied.

Immediately after the operation free diaphoresis is to be encouraged (the bed is to be previously warmed), partly to hasten reaction, partly to prevent abdominal transudation, which furnishes a culture-medium for any micro-organisms which may have accidentally gained access to the peritoneal cavity (Fritsch).

First day : Allow the patient very little fluid in the form of restorative drinks : cold tea especially ; small quantities of wine, cognac, or rum and water are exceptionally allowable ; bouillon, coffee perhaps, and cracked ice and rectal injections of normal saline solution for the thirst. The patient must be kept warm. If reaction is tardy, rectal injections of alcohol, wine, or ether may be given in

[1] See Therapeutic Table.

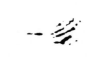

Tab. 78.

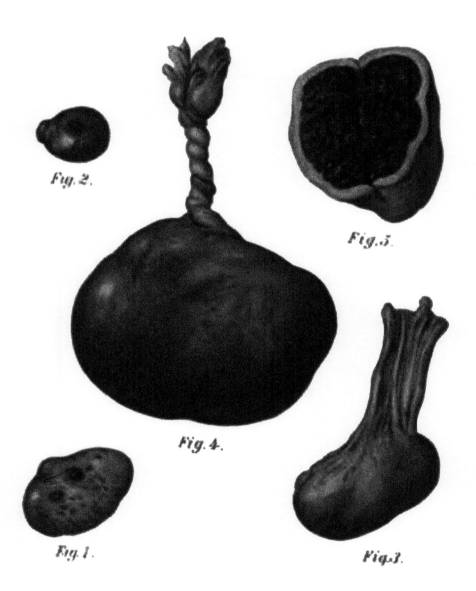

Fig. 2.

Fig. 5.

Fig. 4.

Fig. 1.

Fig. 3.

Lith. Anst f Reichhold München

Vomiting may occur from swallowed chloroform (cracked ice and iced champagne), meteorism, constipation, or peritonitis. The bed is not to be changed until the beginning of the—

Second week: Easily digested solids ; if the condition of the patient is absolutely good, veal, chicken, Zwieback, toast, wheat-bread, etc., may be allowed after the fourth or fifth day.

The patient may get up in the third week.

For meteorism : warm fomentations, oil of peppermint, fennel tea, high introduction of the rectal tube ; if combined with marked vomiting, increased temperature, tenderness, and peritoneal exudate (peritonitis), inunctions of blue ointment, and administration of calomel. (See p. 123 ; § 15.)

If very severe sudden collapse with anemia occurs. (internal hemorrhage), the wound should be immediately reopened. Severe sudden collapse with dyspnea and cyanosis (especially in fibromyomata) indicates pulmonary embolism.

[1] The author is in a position to compare the routine treatments of two clinics for many years. In the one, the opium treatment, placing the intestines at rest, was employed; in the other, the enemata of senna infusion were adopted. The latter treatment is, in his opinion, undoubtedly the better, especially as the subjective condition of the patient more nearly approaches the normal.

PLATE 79.

Fig. 1.—**Epithelioma of the Vulva.** (Original drawing from a specimen from the Munich Frauenklinik.) (Compare with Plate 80, Fig. 2.) The epithelioma originates in the squamous epithelium (4). Numerous plugs of cells (5) are seen dipping down from the surface (4) into the stroma (3) and forming "cell nests," which are surrounded by connective tissue richly infiltrated with round cells. The capillaries are dilated. At the edge of the stroma epitheliomatous "pearls" are formed from the cuboid cells of the matrix (1) and from the polygonal epithelium which proliferates centrally from them. A giant cell is seen among these cells at (2).

Fig. 2.—**Part of an Epitheliomatous Papilloma of the Vaginal Cervix.** (Original drawing from a specimen from the Munich Frauenklinik.) 1, Epitheliomatous papilla: the central connective tissue is infiltrated with round cells and contains thick-walled vessels; the squamous epithelial cells are seen at the periphery. 2, Connective tissue infiltrated with nests of cancer cells. 3, Extravasated blood.

Fig. 3.—**Epitheliomatous "Pearls" from an Ulcer of the Cervix.** The structure is the same as in figure 1. 1, Cuboid cells of the matrix; 2, polygonal cancer epithelium; 3, connective tissue infiltrated with round cells and traversed by dilated vessels; 4, lymph capillaries. (Original drawing from a specimen from the Munich Frauenklinik.)

Fig. 4.—**Dermoid Cyst.** (See Plate 45, Fig. 2.) (Original drawing from a specimen from the Munich Frauenklinik.) 1, Superficial squamous epithelium with connective-tissue papillæ; 2, low epithelium resting upon an even stroma; 3, hair, with sebaceous gland consisting of cuboid epithelium; 4, cross-section of a hair; 5, muscle-fiber; 6, connective tissue.

Dermoid cysts generally originate in the ovary (very rarely also in the vulva). They develop from the same tissue elements as do the cystomata, only with this difference: they assume a cutaneous character and are made up of all portions of the skin, from the epidermis to the subcutaneous connective tissue. There is scarcely a tissue or an organ in the body, be it ever so complicated, which may not also occasionally appear in these tumors (maxillary bones with teeth,

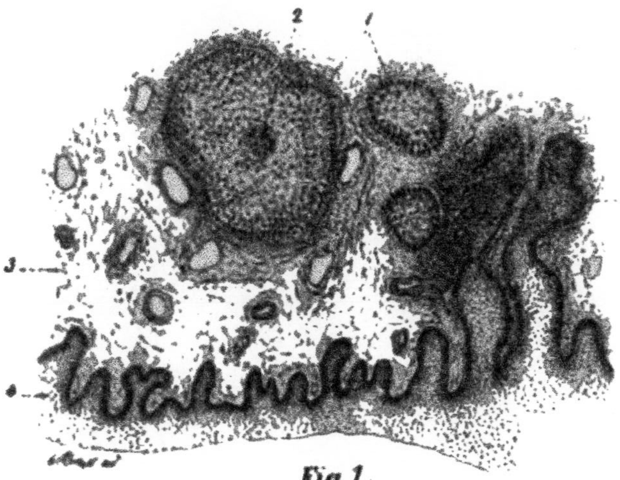

Fig. 1.

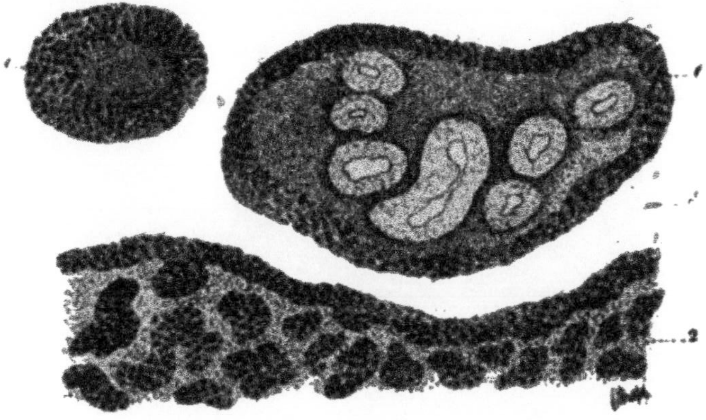

Fig. 2.

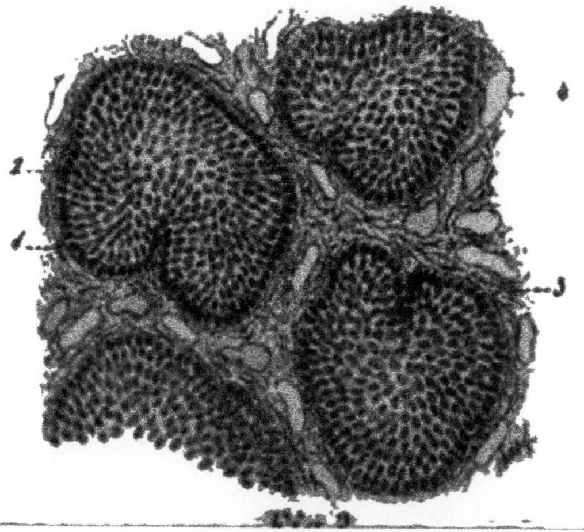

Fig. 3.

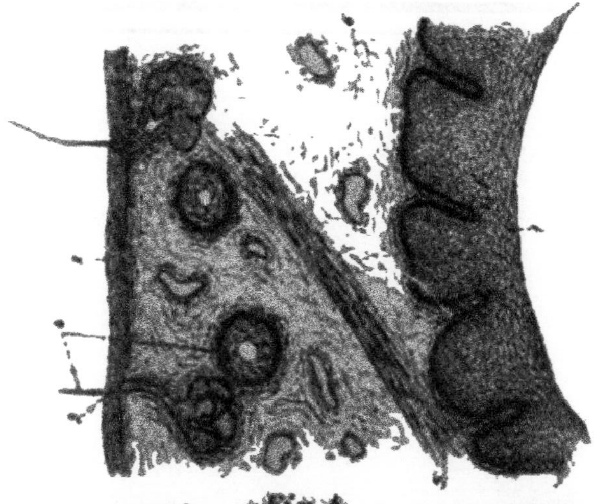

Fig. 4.

Lith. Anst. F. Reichhold, München

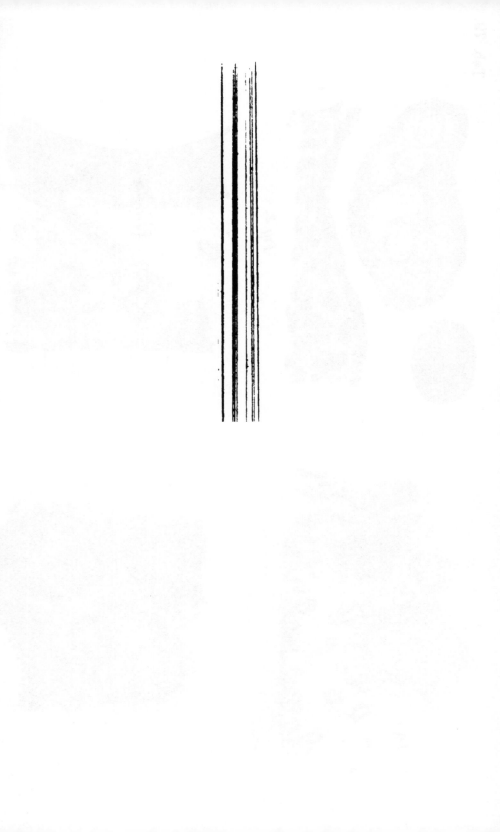

brain-substance, eye, etc.). The cysts are filled with sebaceous matter and blond hair.

These dermoid growths may coexist with ovarian cysts; they may also undergo carcinomatous degeneration. With these exceptions they are always unilocular; they have thick walls and vary in size from that of a man's fist to tumors the size of a man's head.

Their etiology is uncertain; they may be due to "intrafetation," from fission and displacement of the fetal rudiments.

As the peritonitis subsides the exudate undergoes absorption, organization, and encapsulation. (For the treatment see § 18.)

CHAPTER III.

MALIGNANT TUMORS.

The malignant tumors consist of epitheliomata (squamous epithelial tumors), malignant adenomata (glandular cancers), malignant papillary cysts of the ovary (papillary glandular proliferations), sarcomata (round-cell and spindle-cell proliferations, with or without mucoid degeneration or deposits of pigment in the intercellular tissue), and endotheliomata (proliferations of the endothelium of the vessels, or angiosarcomata, since they are a connecting link between epitheliomata and the connective-tissue tumors).

§ 36. MALIGNANT TUMORS OF THE VULVA, BLADDER, AND VAGINA.

These occur:

On the Vulva.—(1) Epithelioma (Plates 80, Fig. 1; 79, Fig. 1); (2) fibrous carcinoma (rare); (3) malignant adenoma of the glands of Bartholin; (4) sarcoma (see explanation of Plate 73, Fig. 3).

In the Urethra.—(5) Epithelioma (very rarely primary).

In the Bladder.—(6) Villous cancer (Plate 88, Fig. 5); (7) diffuse scirrhus of the entire wall; (8) multiple nodular carcinoma; (9) sarcoma (very rarely primary).

In the Vagina.—(10) Papillary epithelioma (Plates 79, Fig. 2; 80, Fig. 2; 88); (11) flat diffuse carcinomatous infiltration (Plates 80, Fig. 2; 88); (12) sarcoma (Plate 73, Figs. 2 and 3; rare).

Symptoms and Diagnosis.—*Epithelioma of the vulva:* pruritus often exists long before the small, flat, reddened nodules make the skin uneven. Later the edges are livid and dense; small nodules are observed in the surrounding skin. Disintegration soon occurs and there is early metastasis to the inguinal glands. The ulcer has irregular

234

edges with hard surroundings. The patient is usually over forty years of age.

Sarcoma of the vulva occurs in younger patients, and may be congenital; the tumor has a fibrous structure. For the anatomy of sarcoma see explanation of Plate 73, figure 2.

Cancer of the bladder: symptoms as in § 31 under Bladder. Urethral dilatation is necessary. The tumor consists of soft, crumbling, polypoid masses, which are readily torn away from the tumor; these do not consist of intact villi, as in a fibrous tumor, but of disintegrated shreds of tissue (microscope). These tumors are usually secondary; metastasis occurs early; embolism is frequent; peritoneal symptoms are observed.

Epithelioma of the vagina: pruritus is also observed here; irregular hemorrhages. Pain, both during coitus and spontaneous. If ulcerated, purulent and offensive discharges and casting-off of fetid, crumbling pieces of tissue. Vesical disturbances gradually appear, and finally fistulous tracts are formed. (See Plate 79.) When a vaginal epithelioma is diagnosed, it must be determined whether it is not a secondary growth from the cervix. (Plate 88.) Papillary epithelioma usually begins anteriorly with a broad base (chronic vaginitis). The nodular form is usually peri-urethral; the nodules quickly coalesce and soon ulcerate.

Sarcoma causes analogous disturbances. (See Plate 73.) Death follows from venous metastases, septicemia, or hemorrhage. Recurrent fibromata or polyps are to be looked upon with suspicion.

Treatment.—All these tumors must be removed as soon as they are diagnosed. This is accomplished with the knife and the Paquelin cautery; the limits of the extirpation must lie outside of the infiltrated zone. Glandular metastases are not to be neglected. As a prophylactic measure at the time of the menopause, every suspicious large or weeping warty prominence on the vulva should be

PLATE 80.

Fig. 1.—**Ulcerated Epithelioma of the Left** [1] **Labium Majus.** (Original water-color.) This tumor at first consists of slightly prominent individual flat prominences and nodules. The edge of the tumor is very dense and is of a bluish color; the central portion soon becomes disintegrated. The tumor creeps along slowly, giving early metastases to the inguinal glands. The vagina is usually spared. Histologically, the tumor consists of squamous epithelium (Plate 88, Fig. 1); it is very rarely a fibrous carcinoma.

Fig. 2.—**Flat Ulcerating Epithelioma of the Posterior Lip of the Os Uteri and of the Posterior Vaginal Vault.** (Original water-color.) This tumor has grown from epitheliomatous nodules. (See Plate 88, Fig. 1.)

---

removed. It is not right first to subject them to prolonged cauterizations.

Urethral carcinoma does not lead to incontinence as long as the sphincter remains intact. If the case is inoperable, the decomposing urine is to be drawn off as quickly as possible and the interior of the bladder disinfected.

In cancer of the bladder (Plate 88, Fig. 5), if it is a circumscribed villous tumor, the affected portion of the vesical wall is to be removed ; if it is diffuse, flat, and consists of nodular formations, excochleation with the sharp curet. Irrigation with solutions of salicylic acid or silver nitrate ; if hemorrhage occurs, ice-water irrigations, ice-bag, and vaginal tamponade. On the following day the coagula are to be removed through a large catheter.

PLATE 81

Fig. 1.—**Nodular Epithelioma of the Vaginal Cervix.** (Original water-color.)

Fig. 2.—**Epitheliomatous Papilloma of the Anterior Lip of the Os Uteri.** (View of the cervical canal.) (Original water-color.)

[1] TRANSLATOR'S NOTE.—The original reads "right."

Tab. 90.

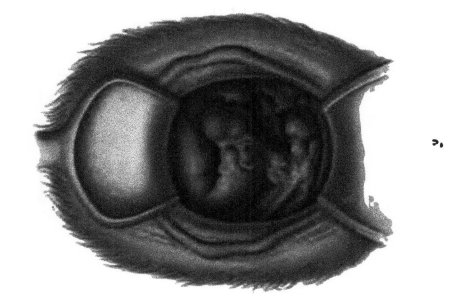

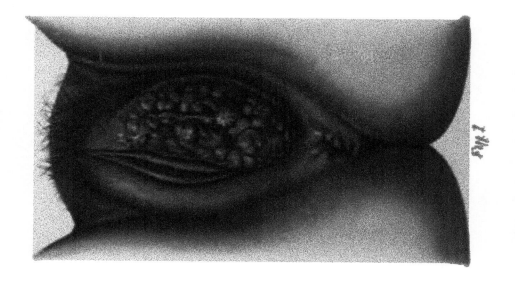

Fig. 1.

§ 37. MALIGNANT TUMORS OF THE UTERUS.

I. Carcinoma of the Uterus.

The individual varieties of uterine cancer are :

1. Epitheliomatous papilloma of the vaginal cervix. (Plates 79, Fig. 2; 81; 84, Figs. 1 and 2 (beginning); 85, 1; 88, 1–4; 90, 2.)

2. Flat epithelioma of the cervix and of the vaginal vault. (Plate 80, Fig. 2.)

3. Epitheliomatous ulcer of the cervix. (Plates 79, Fig. 3; 82; 83; 85, Fig. 2; 86; 89.)

4. Nodular epithelioma of the cervix. (Plates 80, Fig. 2; 83.)

5. Superficial epithelioma of the body of the uterus. (Plate 89, Figs. 3 and 4.)

6. Glandular cancer, malignant adenoma of the body of the uterus. (Plates 30, Fig. 3; 87, Fig. 1.)

Symptoms.—It is of the utmost importance to diagnose these malignant tumors as early as possible, because it is only in the beginning, before metastases have occurred, that the opportunity exists for a thorough removal without recurrence.

The initial symptoms in nearly every case are hemorrhages, discharge (first mucoid, then purulent, and finally sanious with or without crumbling particles of tissue), and pain (sometimes pruritus). Finally, the discharge assumes a most offensive character.

If the hemorrhages and pain are not so pronounced, the case is probably one of cancer of the uterine body.

The irregularity of the hemorrhages at the climacteric period easily deceive both the patient and the physician. These cases must consequently be watched all the more closely.

The pain is inconstant, of a tearing, boring, or lancinating character, and radiates to the sacrum and thighs. In corporeal carcinoma the pain is colicky or paroxysmal and is associated with the discharge of solid tissue particles from the uterine cavity. Other causes for the pain are pressure upon nerves, destruction of the uninvolved soft parts by the foul cancer discharge, the formation of fistulas, and the subsequent vesical catarrh.

PLATE 62.

A View of an Epitheliomatous Ulceration of the Mucous Membrane of the Cervical Canal. The external os is intact. In spite of its apparent insignificance, this case was an inoperable one, as the atypical proliferation, as a matter of fact, extended deep into the parametritic tissues, involving the bladder wall and fixing the uterus. (Original water-color from an actual case.)

All varieties of vesical disturbance make their appearance. Vomiting and headache occur very early, from pressure upon the ureters (v. Winckel), and are to be looked upon as uremic in character. The urine is always decreased in amount.

Later, as the wall of the bladder becomes affected, usually at the trigonum, with closure of the ureters by a dense infiltration, the symptoms assume an unmistakable uremic character. Almost complete anuria exists, the patient becomes unconscious, edematous, and has convulsions. The edema is increased by the firm infiltration of the parametric tissues, which compresses the pelvic veins and produces thromboses. These infiltrations gradually narrow the rectum and cause fecal stasis, hemorrhoids, and tenesmus.

General symptoms occur—cachexia, reflex dyspepsia, and disgust for food. Death follows from exhaustion, uremia, or peritonitis.

Diagnosis.—Inspection of the cervix through the speculum. (See colored plates.) The tumors bleed easily, and are so friable that they tear when seized by tenacula.

In cervical ulceration it is to be noted that the os uteri remains closed and intact, while the cervical canal is transformed into a dilated, disintegrated cavity. This is demonstrated by the sound, as is also the disintegration of the walls of the dilated uterine cavity. These ulcers are punched out, with reddened, swollen edges; they have a lardaceous coating and bleed easily. They are found espe-

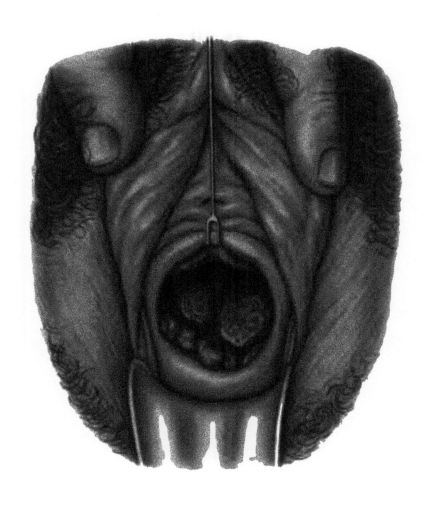

Lith. Anst. F. Reichhold. München

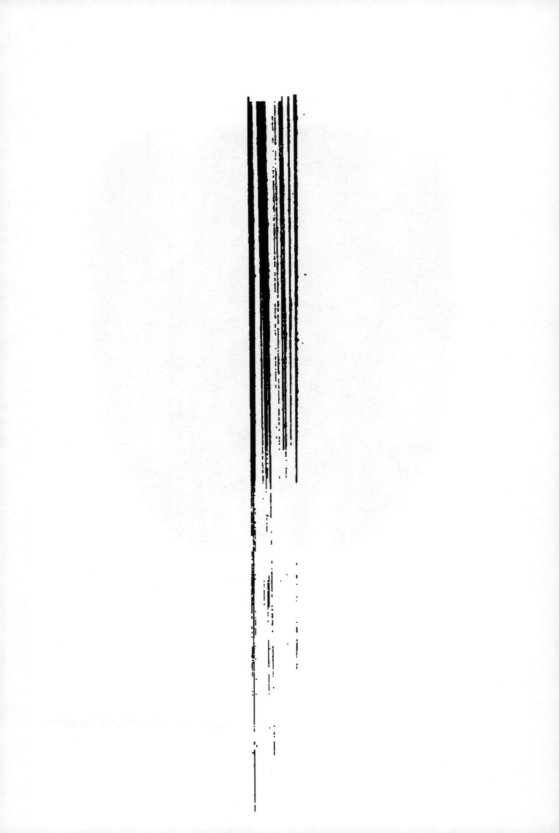

cially in the vaginal vault as extensions from the cervix, as well as in the cervical canal. (Plate 82.)

An absolute diagnosis is made by the microscopic examination of pieces of tissue, which are either cast off or intentionally scraped from the uterine wall. (Regarding glandular cancer, see Plate 30, Figs. 2 and 3.)

An exact anamnesis must always be obtained to avoid errors in diagnosis. In this way a decomposing abortion or retained placenta may be excluded at the beginning; the microscope would, in addition, reveal chorionic villi and decidual tissue. A disintegrating fibromyoma (see § 34, Differential Diagnosis) is recognized by the firm consistency of the pieces of tissue removed for diagnosis and by their histologic fibrous structure. The rare multiple condylomata of the cervix must be considered; they are not yellow, like the epitheliomata, but bluish-red; they have the same etiology as the condylomata of the vulva.

It is also to be mentioned that certain obstinate inflammations of the endometrium occurring at the menopause, and having the microscopic structure of fungous endometritis, are often nothing more than the beginnings of glandular cancers; in the same manner papillary erosions and laceration scars act as predisposing causes of papillary epitheliomata.

Treatment.—The suspected masses, with at least one or two centimeters of the surrounding healthy tissues, are to be immediately removed by operation.

As a prophylactic measure endometritis, erosions, laceration scars, and ectropion are to receive appropriate and early treatment.

If an epitheliomatous papilloma is certainly limited to the cervix (Plates 84, Fig. 2; 88, Figs. 2 to 4; 90, Fig. 2), one or both lips of the os and the affected portion of the vaginal vault may be removed. (Plates 80, Fig. 2; 81; 84, Fig. 1; 85, Fig. 1; 88, Fig. 1.)

If, on the contrary, we have to do with an ulcer of the cervix, it seems to me that its removal can be surely

PLATE 83.

Figs. 1 and 2.—Epitheliomatous Ulcer of the Cerv
(Through the speculum and in cross-section; original water-col
(See also Plate 89, Fig. 2.) The tumor consists of the solitary ;
mary nodules and of their ulcerations. Figure 2 shows the nod:
infiltration of the cervical wall.

---

secured only by the total extirpation of the uter
Schröder's supravaginal amputation of the cervix throu
the vagina, even if the ulcer does not reach to the inter:
os, is frequently followed by recurrences in the body
the uterus, from which metastases may occur. It m
not be a question of metastasis at all, as we have spe
mens which show that beginning carcinomatous degen
ation may simultaneously exist in the body or fundus
the uterus and in the cervix. (Plates 82 ; 83 ; 85, Fig.
89, Figs. 1 and 2.)

Total extirpation may be performed :

1. Through the vagina (Langenbeck-Czerny)—col
hysterotomy.

2. After opening the abdominal cavity (Freund)—cel
hysterotomy.

3. By the sacral method (Hochenegg-Herzfeld-Hega

4. By the parasacral method (Wölfler).

PLATE 84.

Fig. 1.—Epitheliomatous Papilloma of the Anterior Lip
the Os Uteri and of the Anterior Vaginal Vault. (Origi:
water-color.) (See Plates 79, 85, and 88.) The tumor consists
uneven bluish masses, which render the os difficult of recognition
palpation. This form spreads along the surface.

Fig. 2.—Beginning Epithelioma of the Cervix. (Origi:
water-color from a case of v. Winckel's.) Small round nodules devel
at the external os. They are in the cervix, beneath the mucous me
brane, and soon ulcerate.

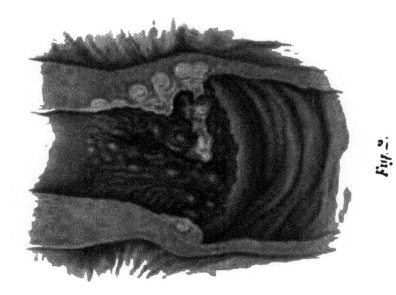

Fig. 2.

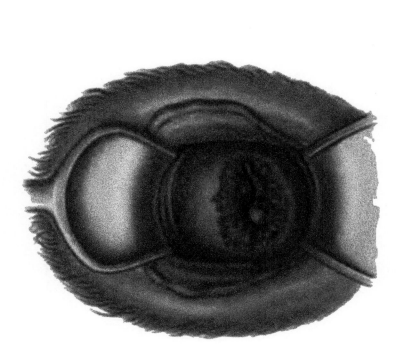

Fig. 1.

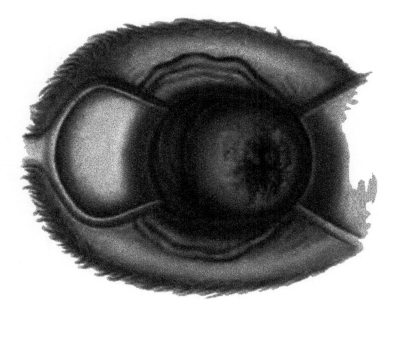

Fig 2.

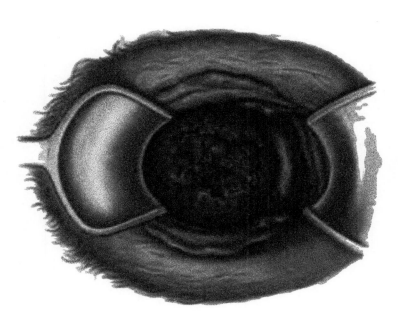

Fig 1.

Lith..Anst Reichhold München.

The patients are prepared as usual (full bath, evacuation of the bowels by laxatives and enemata, bladder emptied immediately before the operation); the vaginal and uterine cavities are to be irrigated several times with antiseptic solutions and then wiped out.

1. Vaginal Extirpation.—The cervix is made accessible by means of Simon's duckbill specula (one posterior, one anterior, and two lateral retractors), and is drawn down by a stout ligature passed through its substance. If the parametritic tissues are infiltrated, the uterus is more or less fixed, and a removal of all the diseased tissue is out of the question.

The stout ligature not only aids in drawing down the uterus, but at the same time it also closes the external os and prevents the escape of the infectious masses of an intra-uterine carcinoma. If the case is one of papilloma of the cervix, as much as possible of the carcinomatous tissue is to be removed by the knife, scissors, and sharp curet, and the remainder is to be destroyed with carbolic acid or Paquelin's cautery before the vaginal vault is opened. The vagina is to be again wiped clean with antiseptics.

After the removal of the uterus from the ligated adnexa, the wound in the vaginal vault is made smaller by several sutures and is drained with iodoform gauze. The ligatures left in the adnexa and about the parametritic vessels usually come away spontaneously. The patient is to be kept in bed for two or three weeks.

2. Total Extirpation by Celiotomy.—This operation, devised by Freund, is still indicated to-day for large dense tumors (or those complicated with fibromyomata) that can not be removed through the vagina. Bardenheuer's modification is the best: the cervix is circumscribed by a vaginal incision; the abdominal cavity is opened, the ligaments are tied off on each side in three sections, the uterus is removed, and the wound is united by suture.

3. The sacral and the parasacral methods may be carried out if adhesions, parametritic cancer nodules, or a large uterus (it may be puerperal) render the median incision ineffectual.

The inoperable cases demand symptomatic treatment.

1. For the putrid suppuration : removal of the carcinomatous masses by means of knife, scissors, curet, and thermocautery. As an eschar, and later a malignant granulating surface, is left behind, the wound should be closed as far as possible by sutures, which exert a certain restraining pressure upon the all-too-rapid proliferation. During this excochleation, avoid creating rectal or vesical fistulas. Atmocausis is to be employed in such cases.

As far as caustics are concerned, especially in cases that can not be cureted, I wish to mention only carbolic acid and formalin. Schröder applied 20% bromin alcohol for

16

PLATE 85.

FIG. 1.—**Epitheliomatous Papilloma of Both Lips of the**
The tumor has ulcerated, invaded the deeper tissues, and spread to
anterior vaginal vault. (Original water-color.)

FIG. 2.—**Epitheliomatous Ulcer of the Cervix.** (Orig
water-color.) The external os and the cervix are intact; the lip
the os and the cervical wall are, however, markedly thickened by
carcinomatous infiltration. The cervical canal is ulcerated and fc
a crater between the external and the internal os, which is es
demonstrable by the sound. The walls contain disintegration c
filled with putrid masses. Solitary cancer nodules are seen in the l
of the uterus. The neck of the uterus is much enlarged, in cont
to the body.

five minutes by means of cotton tampons. These w
held in position by tampons saturated in normal sal
solution. Nitrate of lead (powdered, 30 parts, with
parts lycopodium) is slower in its action—from twelve
sixty hours.

For the fetid odor: potassium permanganate in str
solution (dark reddish-brown), or irrigation several ti
daily with 1%, or 2%, creolin, cresol soap, or ly
Quinin iodid and aristol are to be used as dusting-powd
2. For the hemorrhages the following treatment is pal

PLATE 86.

FIG. 1.—**Epithelioma of the Cervix That Has Perfor**
into the Bladder. (Original water-color.) In spite of the great
struction above it, inspection shows the os uteri to be almost c
pletely unchanged. Greenish-gray putrid masses and necrotic sh
cover the floor of the carcinomatous ulcer. The uterine wall is i
trated with nests of cancer cells. (See Plate 89, 5.)

FIG. 2. **Perforation of an Epithelioma of the Cervix i**
the Bladder and Rectum. (Original water-color from a speci
of v. Winckel's.) The os uteri has become ulcerated and the pro
extends to the vagina. (See Plate 89, 6.)

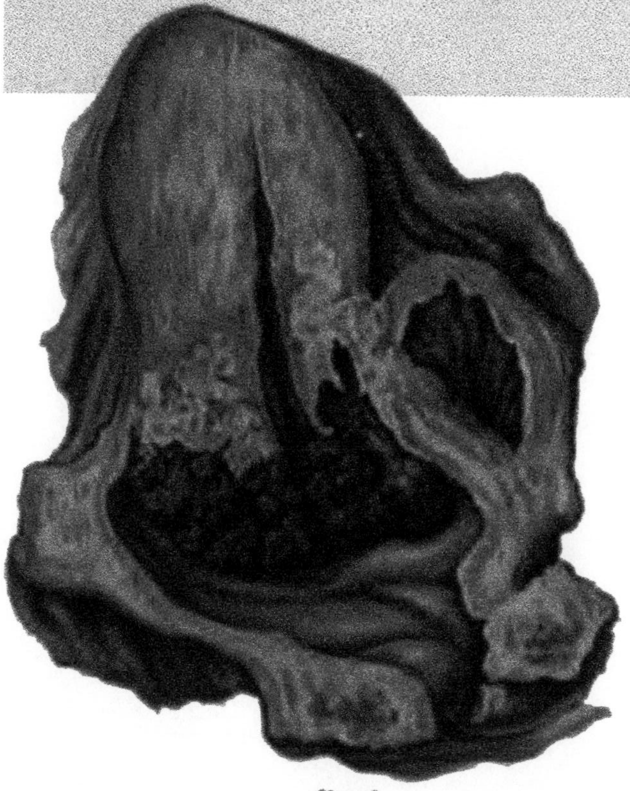

Tab. 80.

Fig. 2. Esch.   F. montevensis, Hildenbrand

Fig. 1.

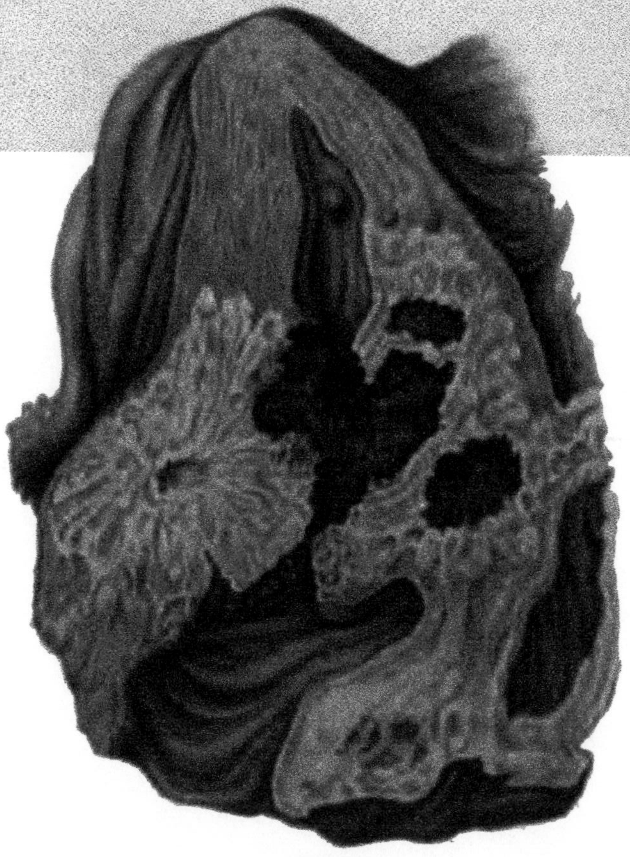

Tab. 86.

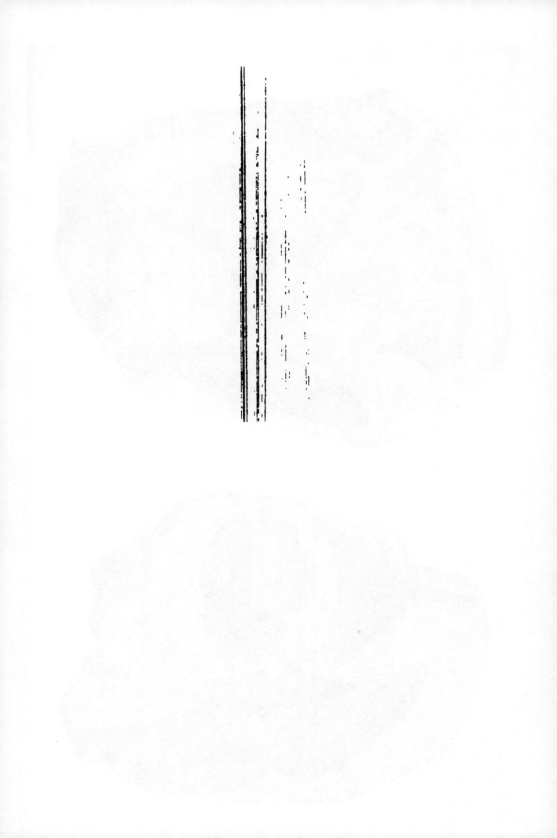

tive : astringent irrigations or vaginal suppositories, vinegar, alum, ferripyrin powder, chlorid of iron ; iodoform gauze tamponade, or packing with gauze soaked in solution of aluminum acetate or in formalin solution.

The general nutrition is to be carefully regulated. Preference is to be given to a light, easily digestible and stimulating diet, with stomachics (compound tincture of cinchona), hematogen, hemalbumin, ferratin, wine of iron peptonate, and the like. Laxatives and high injections, if necessary, with infusion of senna.

3. For the Lancinating Pains.—The following may be used successively as the pains grow more severe : sulphonal, trional, urethan, and chloralamid by the mouth ; antipyrin, extracts of hyoscyamin and belladonna, chloral, and laudanum by the rectum, later also by the mouth ; finally, morphin subcutaneously in gradually increasing doses.

4. For the vomiting : stomachics, decoctions of condurango, cracked ice, cold milk (buttermilk), iced champagne, cold tea.

5. For the headache : cold applications, lactophenin, phenacetin, antipyrin.

Since the two latter symptoms are of a uremic nature, they are also to be treated by warm baths, hot packs, and the induction of profuse sweating.

II. Sarcoma of the Uterus.

For anatomy see Plate 73.

These tumors are as malignant as the carcinomata, if not more so. They occur in the uterine body as primary growths or as secondary deposits from ovarian sarcomata (see Plate 87, 2) ; the patients affected are often in their youth. They usually consist of a round-cell proliferation, sometimes associated with spindle cells. (Plate 73.) They become villous or polypoid, and dilate the os uteri. Metastases take place through the venous system—finally as

PLATE 87.

FIG. 1.—**Carcinoma of the Uterine Body.** (Original wat color from a specimen of v. Winckel's.) Nodular, soft, easily cru bling, bluish-red masses are seen upon the mucous membrane. Th also extend into its depths, either as solid plugs of cells from superficial epithelium, or as a malignant adenoma from the glandu epithelium.

FIG. 2.—**Sarcoma of the Uterus.** (Original water-color from specimen from the Munich Frauenklinik.) The soft, fibrous mas are like tinder. They are mucous, muscular, or subperitoneal, a may arise from the myxomatous degeneration of a fibroma. (See a Plate 73.)

pulmonary emboli. Endotheliomata occur very rarely the cervix.

Symptoms.—The discharge is profuse, mucoid, u

PLATE 88.

FIG. 1 **Flat Cervical Epithelioma of Both Lips of the Uteri Involving Both Vaginal Vaults.** There are two varieties epithelioma of the cervix: 1 the superficial form; (2) the epithel matous papilloma. Both consist of plugs of the proliferating squ mous epithelium See Plate 79

FIG. 2 **Epitheliomatous Papilloma of Both Lips of the Uteri.** (See Plate 85, Fig. 1.)

FIG. 3 **Polypoid Epitheliomatous Papilloma of the Ant rior Lip of the Os Uteri.**

FIG. 4 **Epitheliomatous Papilloma of the Posterior Lip the Os Uteri Filling the Entire Posterior Vaginal Vault.**

FIG. 5 **Villous Cancer of the Bladder in Its Most Freque Position.** In the region of the ureteral orifices It has infiltrat the vesicovaginal septum It causes cystitis; cancer cells and shre of tissue are found in the urine

FIG. 6 **Rectal Carcinoma (Glandular Cancer) Infiltrati the Rectovaginal Septum.** The tumor undergoes a crater-like d integration, so that examination reveals two stenoses, between whi a considerable dilatation is situated.

Tab. 88.

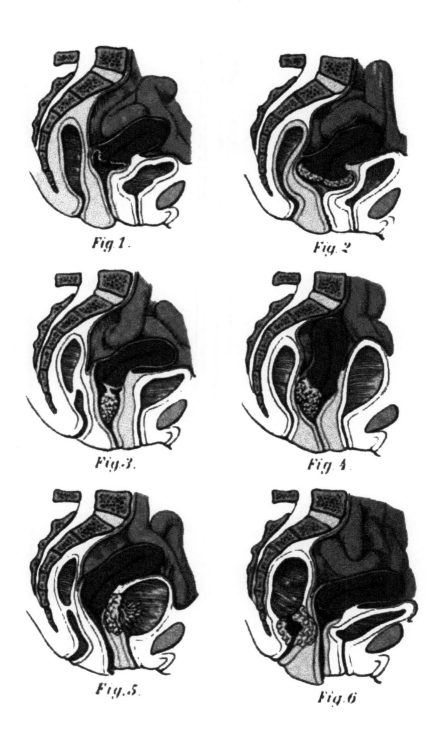

Fig. 1.

Fig. 2.

Fig. 3.

Fig. 4.

Fig. 5.

Fig. 6.

Lith. Anst. P. Herrhold. München

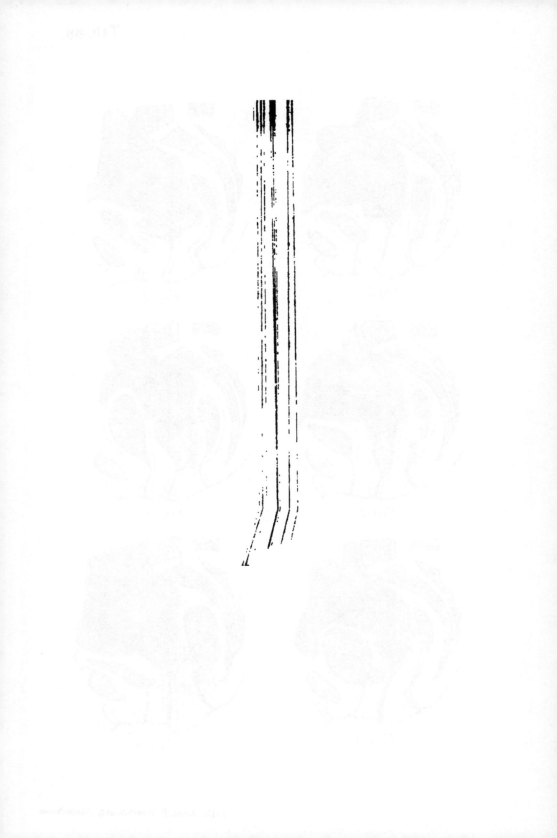

very bloody, and, in contrast to carcinoma, not offensive until late in the disease. Pain first appears with the dilatation of the os uteri. Metastases to the lung cause dyspnea and cyanosis. Anemia is present if the hemorrhages are severe.

Diagnosis.—Enlargement of the uterus (see Plate 87) with or without dilatation of the os uteri. If the os is intact, dilate and palpate the uterine cavity; villous polypoid excrescenses are present. Microscopic examination of cureted pieces. If the fibrous character of the tissue renders its nature doubtful, look especially for "giant cells." (See Plate 73, Fig. 2.) It is to be remembered that a fibromyoma may undergo sarcomatous degeneration. (See Differential Diagnosis, § 34.)

Treatment.—If mucous, excochleation; if the uterus is enlarged, total extirpation. If too far advanced, symptomatic—as in carcinoma.

§ 38. MALIGNANT TUMORS OF THE ADNEXA, ESPECIALLY OF THE OVARIES.

I. Carcinoma.

Carcinoma of the ovary occurs in various forms: (1) Solid papillary; (2) a form resembling the papillary cystadenomata, but more solid; (3) a form resembling the multilocular cystadenomata, but with areas of softening; (4) metastases from a uterine carcinoma, diffuse nodules in the enlarged ovary (very rare).

Anatomy.—The ovaries are disposed to carcinomatous degeneration, not infrequently at the age of puberty (Olshausen).

Symptoms.—Nonappearance of the menses, ascites and peritoneal phenomena, early cachexia, and metastases with disturbances of the circulation in the lower extremities. Stenosis of the rectum. (See Plate 59, Fig. 4.)

Diagnosis.—An enlarged, rapidly growing ovary, or ascites with a previous pure glandular cystoma. Exploratory incision and demonstration of nodules, and multiple,

PLATE 89.

FIG. 1.—**Cancer Nodules in the Cervix, Which Has Not Yet Ulcerated.** The os uteri is closed; the anterior lip is thickened from the carcinomatous infiltration. (See also Plates 80, 82, 83.)

FIG. 2.—**Epitheliomatous Ulcer of the Cervix.** The os uteri is closed. (See Plate 85.)

FIG. 3.—**Epitheliomatous Ulcer of the Cervix Which Has Invaded the Uterine Body.** The os uteri is destroyed.

FIG. 4.—**Carcinoma of the Body of the Uterus Which Has Perforated into the Bladder.** (Plate 86, Fig. 1.) The os uteri is intact.

FIG. 5.—**Epitheliomatous Ulcer of the Cervix Which Has Perforated into the Bladder.** The fundus of the uterus is intact; the os is destroyed.

FIG. 6.—**Epitheliomatous Ulcer of the Cervix Perforating into Both Bladder and Rectum.** (Plate 86, Fig. 2.)

diffuse, papillary, excrescences in and upon the peritoneum.

Treatment.—Extirpation, if limited to the ovary ; if the growth is not so localized, violent pressure demand tapping or the formation of an artificial anus.

Glandular carcinomata of the tubes are very rarely primary, and, as such, are impossible to diagnose.

PLATE 90.

Four Tumor-like Changes at the External Os.

FIG. 1.—**Fungous Endometritis and Ectropion.** (See Plates 30, 31, 56.) Cystic dilated glands in the cervical mucosa.

FIG. 2.—**Epitheliomatous Papilloma of Both Lips of the Os.** (See Plates 81, 84, 85.)

FIG. 3.—**Ovules of Naboth in a Mucous Polyp, Visible at the Os Uteri.** (See Plates 29, 56.)

FIG. 4.—**Fibroid Polyp Separating the Lips of the Os Uteri.** Plate 60, Fig. 2.)

Tab. 89.

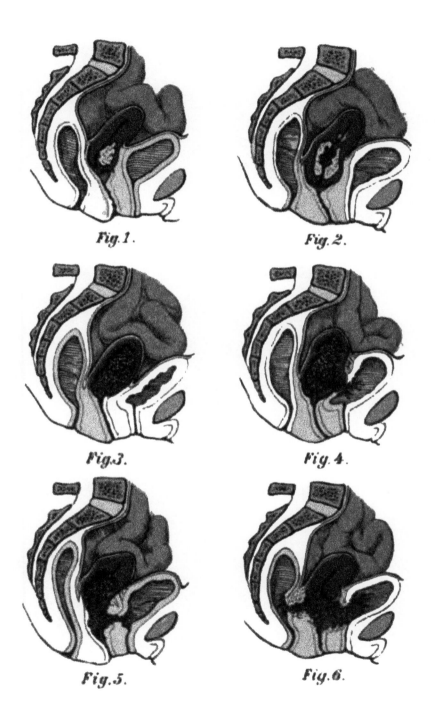

Fig. 1.

Fig. 2.

Fig. 3.

Fig. 4.

Fig. 5.

Fig. 6.

Lith. Anst. F. Reichhold München.

Tab. 90.

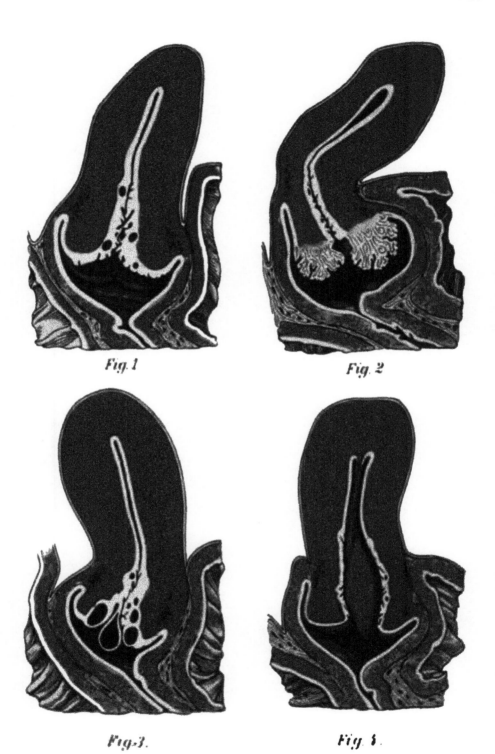

Fig. 1.

Fig. 2.

Fig. 3.

Fig. 4.

Lith. Anst F. Reichhold München

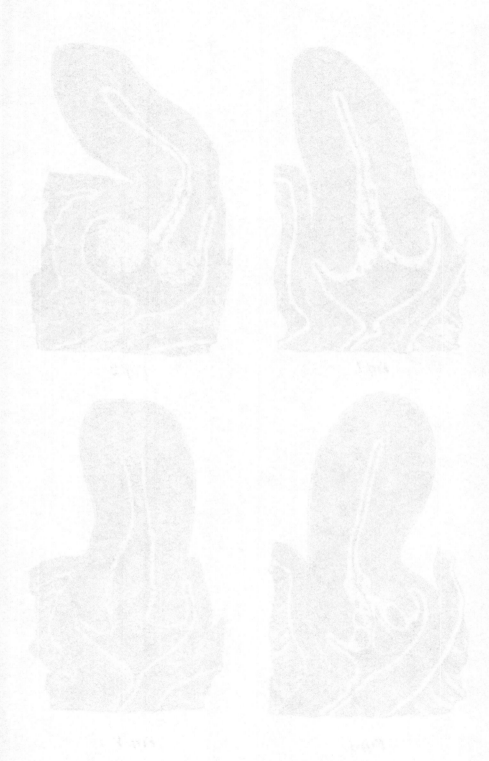

II. Sarcoma.

These are usually spindle-cell tumors in early life, combined with deposits of round cells and degenerations of a myxomatous or carcinomatous character. They grow slowly, and their diagnosis and treatment are the same as those of ovarian fibromata. (See §§ 33 and 35.) Sarcomata also occur in the ligaments.

Endotheliomata (angiosarcomata) may grow to a considerable size and show a decidedly malignant character. They have a cavernous structure; the tissue is usually myxomatous.

The treatment is generally hopeless, as total removal is usually fruitless, even when carried out at the first appearance of symptoms.

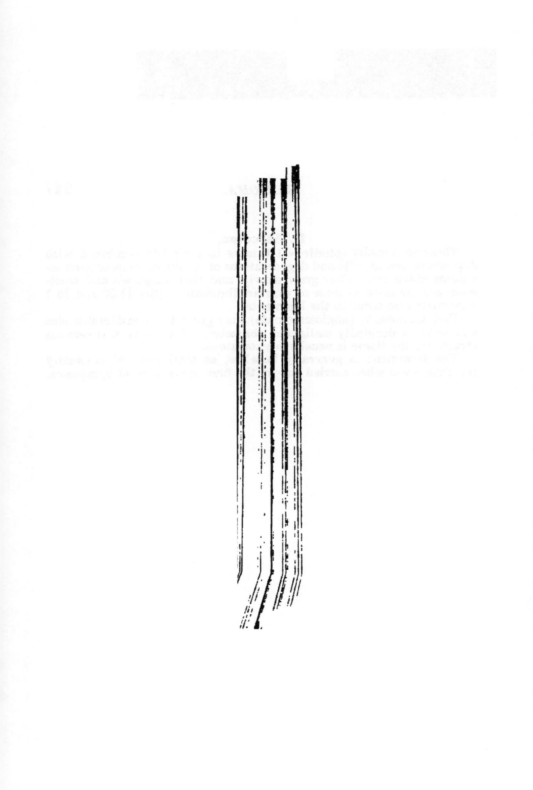

THERAPEUTIC TABLE.

1. **Absorbents.**—Sapo medicatus, potassium iodid, tinct. iodi, iodin glycerin, ichthyol, hot vaginal douches, mud-baths, brine-baths, hot sand-baths.

Acids:

2. **Acetic Acid** (Pyroligneous Acid).—1 : 3 or concentrated. To be applied through the speculum (with 3 to 4% carbolic acid) every two or three days for weeks and months; erosions; cervical catarrha.

3. **Boric Acid.**—2 to 3%. In cystitis, urethritis; 2 to 4 injections daily.

4. **Boric Acid Vaselin.**—5 : 20, for pruritus.

5. **Carbolic Acid.**—½ to 2%, in vaginitis, endometritis. 2 to 5%, in vulvitis. 3 to 5% or concentrated, to wipe out the uterine cavity, multiple recurrent polyps, fistulas.

6. **Carbolic Acid.**—2%. Subcutaneously, ½ to 2 syringefuls in lupus, erysipelas.

7. **Carbolic Acid Glycerin.**—2 to 4%, endometritis, metritis.

8. **Carbolic Acid Intoxication.**—Small doses of opium, morphin, ice, milk, soluble sulphates.

9. **Chromic Acid.**—25 to 33%, as a caustic for condylomata.

10. **Chromic Acid.**—33%, in fistulas, endometritis (every week).

11. **Fuming Nitric Acid.**—As a caustic in lupus, fistulas, endometritis, one drop upon cotton every four to five days. It acts most promptly when immediately followed by the application of liquefied carbolic acid.

12. **Salicylic Acid.**—1 to 5 : 1000, in pruritis, vaginitis, cystitis. 1.0 to 5.0 (gr. xv to gr. lxxv) salicylic acid powder are dissolved in alcohol, and added to one liter of lukewarm water (irrigator); it is not caustic.
    Salicylic Acid Vaselin (Lanolin, Mollin).—1 : 300, for pruritus.

13. **Tannic Acid.**—0.3 (gr. v), intra-uterine pencil for endometritis. (See Intra-uterine Pencils.)

14. **Tannic Acid Vaginal Suppositories.**—0.4 (gr. vj) with 3.0 (gr. xlv) cacao-butter in blenorrhea.

15. **Aloes Extract.**—Ext. rhei comp., aa 3.0 (gr. xlv). Ft. in
No. xxx, two pills daily. Laxative, emmenagog.

16. **Althea Decoction.**—Injection for vaginitis, acute endometi
acute myometritis.

17. **Alum in Intra-uterine Pencils.**—0.3 (gr. v), 4 cm. long, 0
0.4 cm. thick, with gum arabic and glycerin, in endometrit

18. **Alum Solution.**—1 to 3 to 6%, as injection or upon tampon
vaginitis, vaginal inversion. Iodoform gauze is saturated
the solution, and renewed every three hours in acute vag
gonorrhea.

19. **Alum Vaselin** (Lanolin, Mollin).—2 to 4 : 50, in pelvitis, va
itis, vaginal inversion.

20. **Aluminum Acetate Solution.**—10 to 20%, astringent vag
injection. 2 to 5%, intra-uterine application.

21. **Antipyrin.**—0.5 to 1.0 (gr. viij–xv), in pill, every two hours
— 3 —pro die), for menstrual molimina, dysmenorrhea, p
fever.

22. **Antipyrin.**—2.0 (gr. xxx), in solution, as an enema. Also
subcutaneously, 1 : 2; the syringe must be carefully cleaned
each injection to prevent the precipitation of antipyrin crys

23. **Antispasmodics.**—(See Antipyrin, Chloral, Chloroform,]
phin, Opium, Ext. Viburn. Prunifol. Fld.)

24. **Applications and Fomentations.**—"Priessnitz," for paral
of the vesical sphincter, peritoneal irritation, acute corpo
endometritis, oophoritis.
> *Brine.*—In myomata, chronic parametritis, perimetritis,
> tritis, and oophoritis.
> *Hot Water.*—In menorrhagia, dysmenorrhea, combined
> hot alcohol.
> *Lead-water.*—(See Same.)

25. **Argent. Nitrat.**—2% solution, in endometritis, ulceration
the vaginal cervix, urethritis; to be applied or injected (ev
week); or 0.2 to 0.5 : 1000 to be injected from 4 to 6 ti
daily.

26. **Argent. Nitrat.**—1 to 2 to 6 : 1000, in cystitis.

27. **Argent. Nitrat.**—5 to 10 to 20% or solid stick, in pruri
vaginitis, fistulae; applied every week.

28. **Argentamin.**—Specific for older cases of gonorrhea: 1 to
intra-uterine; 5%, in the vagina.

29. **Argonin.**—Specific for gonorrhea: 3 to 5%, intra-uterine;
vesical irrigation; 5 to 10%, vaginal irrigation.

30. **Astringents.**—Alum, aluminum acetate solutions, cupric
phate, decoctions of oak-bark, formalin, glycerin, lead-wa
tannin.

31. **Bathing Resorts.**—Mud-baths (absorbent), Teplitz, Fran
bad, Kissingen, Elster and Mattoni's mixture (5 liters to

bath) in metritis, parametritis, and perimetritis, chronic oophoritis, hematocele.

Brine-baths.—Kreuznach, Tölz, Nauheim, Kissen, Ocynhausen, Hall (upper Austria), Heilbronn, or artificially produced by adding from 10 to 20 pounds of lye or sea-salt to the warm bath. Applicable in myomata, scrofula, vulvitis, metritis, chronic parametritis, and perimetritis (one-half to one and one-half hours in duration, followed by one hour's rest).

For Anemia: Brückenau, Triburg, Elster, Franzensbad, Pyrmont, Schlangenbad, Schwalbach, St. Moritz, Wildbad.

Hot Sand-baths.—Blasewitz near Dresden, Klistritz near Gera. Applicable for same affections as mud-baths. May be replaced by thermaphore.

Iodin Baths.—Kreuznach, Tölz, Hall, in scrofula.

Sea-baths.—In nocturnal enuresis, scrofulous vulvitis, menorrhagia.

For Vesical and Renal Disease: Carlsbad, Wildungen (0.5 (gr. viij) sodium salicylate with 0.015 (gr. ¼) morphin to ½ of a liter, in cystitis), Neuenahr, Assmannshausen, Obersalzbrunn, Vichy, for menorrhagia from nephritis.

32. **Baths.**—Warm baths, 95° to 100° F. (one-quarter to one-half hour), in paralysis of the vesical sphincter, uremia (carcinomatous), oophoritis, acute endometritis, chronic metritis, and subinvolution.

Foot-baths (100° F.), with 1 to 3 tablespoonfuls of salt or mustard once or twice daily in oligorrhea, amenorrhea, anemic dysmenorrhea.

Sits-baths (90° to 100° F.), with wheat bran (½ to 1 pound), decoctions of oak-bark (7 to 10%), one and a half to two hours, in pruritus, urethritis.

Sits-baths, with tannin or alum (2%), sea-salt or lye (1 pound to 2 bucketfuls of water), as before, in dysmenorrhea, amenorrhea, urethritis, pruritis, parametritis, and perimetritis (ten to twenty minutes in the beginning).

33. **Belladonna Extract.**—As rectal or vaginal suppository 0.02 (gr. ⅓) with 3.0 (gr. xlv) cacao-butter, in rectal and vesical tenesmus, dysmenorrhea, endometritis, and myometritis, neuroses of the uterus and vagina.

34. **Belladonna Tinct.**—20 drops t. i. d. (with potassium bromid, 0.3 (gr. v), in nocturnal enuresis.

35. **Belladonna - vaselin** (Lanolin, Mollin).—1 to 2 : 50, in pruritus.

36. **Bismuth Subnitrate.**—Intra-uterine pencils (0.2, gr. iij), in endometritis.

37. **Bismuth Subnitrate Solution.**—2 to 3%, astringent intrauterine application.

38. **Bismuth Subnitrate Ointment.**—10%, in eczema, herpes.

39. **Bismuth Talcum.**—Dusting-powder for profuse secretion.

40. **Bromin Alcohol.**—20%, hemostatic injection in carcinoma

41. **Byrolin-boric Acid—Lanolin-glycerin.**—Good salve for hands.

42. **Caffein Citrate.**—0.1 (gr. iss) (with lactophenin, sacchar. āā 0.5, gr. vij), for hemicrania.

43. **Caffein Sodium Benzoate.**—0.2 (gr. iij), t. i. d., in migr

44. **Calomel.**—0.25 (gr. iv) (with sacchar. alb., 0.5, gr. viij) se times daily, or 0.5 (gr. viij) at one dose, as a laxative, in peritonitis, parametritis, and metritis. To be followed by 15 to 20 drops tinct. opii; later, 0.05 to 0.1 (gr. ¾ to iss).

45. **Camphor.**—1.0 (gr. xv), ol. amygd. dulc., 9.0 (ʒij), subcu ously in collapse.

46. **Camphor, Monobromate.**—0.1 to 0.3 (gr. iss to v) with sac alb., 0.5 (gr. viij), three times daily in hysteric conditions ritability.

47. **Carlsbad Salts.**—1 to 3 teaspoonfuls on rising, in a glass of warm water, as a laxative.

48. **Cascara Sagrada.**—Ext. fld., syr. zingiberis, aquæ, āā (ʒiiss), a teaspoonful twice daily, as a laxative.

49. **Catheter, Permanent.**—15 to 30 cm. long, 0.6 to 0.7 cm. t left in position for three days; it is to be well sterilized!

50. **Catheterization.**—Before every operation, after perineal in paralysis of the vesical sphincter, incontinence of r tion.

51. **Caustics.**—(See Fuming Nitric Acid; Argent. Nitratis, 2 to ? Carbolic Acid, 3%, conc.; Chromic Acid, 33%; Zinc Chlori to 10 to 50%; Vienna Paste; Solution of Mercurous Nit Caustic Potash; Sublimate, 1 : 1000; Formalin, conc.) vagina is to be thoroughly irrigated after cauterizing uterus.

52. **Caustic Potash** —Fistulas, lupus.

53. **Caustic Potash.**—1 : 300, aq., in severe cases of intertrigo.

54. **Chloral.**—By the rectum, 1 to 2 : 15 (with potassium bro āā), in rectal and vesical tenesmus, dysmenorrhea, carcin

55. **Chloral in Rectal or Vaginal Suppositories.**—0.5 (gr. with 3.0 (gr. xlv) cacao-butter, for vesical and intestinal t mus, dysmenorrhea, uterine and vaginal neuroses, carcinor

56. **Chloral Solution.**—5 : 100 (with syr. aurant. cort., 35), t taken for the same affections as above.

    Chloral Solution.—(With syr. aurant. cort., āā), 15 : 175 one teaspoonful 3 or 4 times daily, in nocturnal enur It may be combined with potassium bromid.

57. **Chlorin Water.**—(and aq. dest., āā 50.0 (ʒiss) with 1.0 xv) acid. hydrochlor.) one tablespoonful every two hou meteorism, peritonitis, diarrhea.

58. **Chloroform Narcosis.**—Chloroform, 3; sulphuric ether, 1; absolute alcohol, 1 (Billroth).   Chloroform + ether (1 : 2) = Vienna mixture.

59. **Chloroform and Ol. Hyoscyami,** āā 10.0 (℥ iiss).—Inunction in pruritus; upon tampons for the pain from carcinoma, perimetritis and parametritis, oophoritis.

60. **Cocain Hydrochlor.**—5 to 10% solution or ointment as a local anesthetic, in pruritis (alternating with 10 to 30% argent. nitrat.), vaginismus, uterine and vaginal neuroses, dysmenorrhea.
    Cocain Hydrochlor.—⅓ to 1 : 1000, as injection, in cystitis.
    Cocain Hydrochlor.—0.01 to 0.2% in 0.2% NaCl solution for Schleich's infiltration anesthesia.
    Cocain Hydrochlor.—In rectal or vaginal suppositories: 0.1 (gr. iss) to 3.0 (gr. xlv) cacao-butter, in vesical and rectal tenesmus, carcinoma.

61. **Colocynth. Ext.**—0.005 to 0.02 (gr. ¹⁄₁₂ to ⅓), as a drastic cathartic.

62. **Condurango Decoction.**—12 : 175, in carcinomatous dyspepsia.

63. **Cornutin Citrate.**—0.003 to 0.005 (gr. ¹⁄₂₀ to ¹⁄₁₂), in pill, twice daily, in metrorrhagia.

64. **Cupric Aluminat.**—1.0 to 5.0 : 1 liter of water, in endometritis.

65. **Cupric Sulphate.**—⅓ to 2% injection or upon tampons, in metrorrhagia; 1 : 1000, in endometritis.

66. **Cupric Sulphate Vaselin or Zinc Sulphate Vaselin.**—2 to 3 to 5 : 50 to 75, on tampons, in metrorrhagia.

67. **Dermatol,** as a dusting-powder after plastic operations.

68. **Diaphoretics.**—Ammonium chlorid solution (5 : 200), liq. ammon. acetat. (1 to 2 teaspoonfuls in elderflower or chamomile tea).

69. **Diet in Anemia.**—(See § 3, under 7, Treatment.)

70. **Digitalis Inf.**—2 : 180, syrupi 20, one teaspoonful every two hours (with potassium nitrate 10.0— ℥ iiss), in menorrhagia from cardiac disease.

71. **Disinfection of the Hands.**—(See § 34, under Treatment.)   In office practice the hands must be scrubbed with alcohol and 1 : 2000 sublimate, especially if they have come into contact with discharges. Instruments (specula, sounds) are to be well boiled each time they are used.

72. **Diuretics.**—Potassium nitrate, urotropin. (See under Digitalis in Pelvic Peritonitis.)

73. **Douches, Hot.**—(See Vaginal Injections.)

74. **Dry Cups.**—In oligomenorrhea, dysmenorrhea.

75. **Emollients.**—Linseed decoctions, oatmeal water, althea decoction, starch.

76. **Enemata for Hemorrhage.**—0.6% warm NaCl solution (2 or more); alcohol, wine.

77. **Enemata of Oil.**—In intestinal and vesical tenesmus. Tinct. Opii, Emollients, and Injections, Rectal.)

78. **Enemata (Purgative).**—⅓ to 1½ liters of lukewarm mucilag or oily fluid, or of water with or without salt, soap, glycer senna (5.0—gr. lxxv—to the cup).

79. **Ergotin.**—(See Secale Cornutum.)
2.0 (℥ss) with aq. dest. 8.0. (℥ij) and acid. carbolic gtt. j, one syringeful daily (three to six times a week) (gr. iij), in menorrhagia, metrorrhagia, myomatosis.

80. **Ergotin.**—2.5 (gr. xxxviij) with aq. dest. 15.0 (℥iij) and salicyl. 0.03 (gr. ½); 1 to 2 syringefuls = 0.15 to 0.3 (g ivss), as in above affections.

81. **Ferric Chlorid Solution.**—20 to 50% or concentrated, ap upon cotton to the interior of the uterus by means o aluminum sound; or, upon tampons or injected, in mu recurrent sessile polypi, menorrhagia, carcinoma, Werlhof ease, myomata.

82. **Ferric Chlorid Solution.**—1 : 800, injected into the bladd hematuria—ferripyrin is better.

83. **Ferripyrin.**—In powder or solution, 1 : 5, as a hemostatic.

84. **Formalin (35% formaldehyd solution).**—1 : 2 to 3 par water, 1 tablespoonful to a liter of water, as a vaginal and uterine irrigation. Undiluted as a caustic agent.

85. **Frangula Cortex.**—Add 1 tablespoonful to 3 cups of water evaporate to 2 cups; or—

86. **Frangula Decoctions.**—25.0 (℥vss) : 180.0 (f℥vj) with so salicylate 5.0 (gr. lxxv) and sodium sulphate 20.0 (℥v) wineglass of this mixture is given morning and evening laxative. The fluid extract is given in doses of from 20 drops.

87. **Gelatin Injections.**—Intra-uterine, as a hemostatic.

88. **Hemostatics.**—Ferripyrin, ferric chlorid solution, acetate solution, gelatin emulsion.
Iodoform gauze tampon ; galvanocautery, Pacquelin's cau actual cautery, atmocausis (in operations for carcinoma myoma); bromin alcohol (carcinoma).

89. **Hydrarg., Ung.**—1.0 to 8.0 (gr. xv to ℥ij) pro die, with e part of vaselin, inunctions, every two hours for a week, in tonitis.

90. **Hydrastis Canad. Ext. Fld.**—15 to 25 drops, four times d for months, in menorrhagia (especially if ovarian).

91. **Hydrastinin Hydrochlor.**—0.05 (gr. ⅓) in pill, three times daily; or 10% solution, ½ to 2 syringefuls(subcutaneous)pro die.

92. **Hyoscyami, Oleum.**—As inunction. (See Chloroform.)

93. **Hyoscyami Ext.**—1.5 (gr. xxiij) with aq. amygd. am. 150.0 (f ℥ v), 15 drops, four times daily, in uterine and vaginal neuroses, vesical and intestinal tenesmus, dysmenorrhea.
    Hyoscyamus Injections.—15 : 1000, in vaginitis, dysmenorrhea.

94. **Hysteria.**—Asafetida; ext. cannabis indica; lactophenin, 0.5 to 1.0 (gr. vij to xv); salophen, 1.0 (gr. xv); salipyrin, 1.0 (gr. xv); phenacetin, 0.5 to 1.0 (gr. vij to xv); antipyrin, 0.5 to 1.0 (gr. vij to xv), also by the rectum; monobromated camphor; castoreum; chloral; chloroform; belladonna; cocain; hyoscyamus; potassium bromid; morphin; opium; flor. chamomillæ; fol. menth. pip.; valerian.

95. **Ice-bag.**—In acute oophoritis, peritonitis, parametritis, metritis, hematocele, erysipelas, uremia (carcinomatous).

96. **Ice, Cracked.**—In vomiting.

97. **Ichthyol.**—For the exanthemata seen with amenorrhea.

98. **Ichthyol.**—10% solution in water or glycerin, in vulvitis, pruritus, parametritis, hematocele.

99. **Ichthyol or Ammonium Sulpho-ichthyolate Vaselin** (Lanolin, Mollin, Glycerin).—10%, in chronic perimetritis, parametritis, oophoritis, vulvitis, hematocele; 10% with green soap, upon the abdomen for peritoneal exudate.

100. **Ichthyol in Intra-uterine Pencils.**—0.2 (gr. iij), in endometritis.

101. **Intra-uterine Pencils.**—With gum arabic and glycerin (4 cm. long, 0.2 to 0.4 cm. thick). (See Alum, Bismuth Subnitrate, Iodoform (90%); Itrol; Protargol, Ferric Chlorid Solution, Tannin, Zinc Oxid, Zinc Chlorid.) Iodoform may be added to them all.

102. **Injections.**—*Into the Bladder* (82° to 88° F.), one cup of oatmeal water with 15 to 25 drops of laudanum, in vesical spasm. Into the bladder in cystitis : ½ to 1 liter, 1 to 3 times daily, 90° to 95° F. (See Argent. Nitrat., Boric Acid, Cocain, Limewater, Saline Solution, Tannin.)
    Into the Vagina.—Hot (115° to 130° F.), several liters 2 to 3 times daily, or every two hours in menorrhagia, metrorrhagia, myomatosis (for the hemorrhage and as an absorbent) ; to soften the cervix (in dilatation), in chronic indurated parametritis and perimetritis, chronic oophoritis, chronic metritis (during the menses also). They are also used when the uterus is infantile, or when it is undergoing involution. Into the vagina : 82° to 88° F., several times daily ; astringents, antiseptics (carbolic acid, lysol, potassium permanganate, salicylic acid, sublimate), or emollients in beginning metritis.

Vaginal injections of brine in chronic metritis are best
in the full or sitz-bath (5 to 9 liters, 111° to 118° F.
Into the Uterus.—By means of Braun's syringe (dr
drop), the two-way catheter; or permanent irrigati
means of an elastic catheter, which is held in the n
cavity by a rubber cross-piece.
Rectal Injections.—(See Chloral, Glycerin, Narcotics,
Solution, and also Enemata.)

103. **Iodin Glycerin.**—10 : 200, upon tampons, for above affec

104. **Iodin, Tincture.**—Applied to the abdomen, cervix, and v
vault in corporeal carcinoma, chronic metritis, parame
perimetritis, and oophoritis.

105. **Iodoform Emulsion, or Iodoform Glycerin.**—10%, i
poreal carcinoma, endometritis.
Iodoform Vaselin (Lanolin, Mollin).—10 to 20%, in
tis, pruritus, oophoritis, parametritis, and perim
(upon tampons).

106. **Iodoform Gauze.**—10 to 20%, intra-uterine tamponade
twenty-four hours), vaginal tamponade (at first, for six h
later, from twelve to twenty-four hours), in menorrl
metrorrhagia, hemorrhages from myomata and carcinol
It is also used to dilate the cervix and in endometritis.

107. **Iodoform Intra-uterine Pencils.**—90%, 4 cm. long, 0
0.4 cm. thick in acute (puerperal) and chronic endomet
In puerperal endometritis they are to be made 6 cm. lon
0.4 to 0.6 cm. wide; in inflammations of the vulva and v
in children, they are to be made 5 to 8 cm. long.

108. **Ipecac.**—1.0 (gr. xv) every ten minutes, until vomiting is
duced. Dover's powder, 0.3 (gr. v), several times dail
dysmenorrhea, dyspepsia.

109. **Itrol.**—Excellent dusting-powder for wounds and ulcer
to 5000 for intra-uterine and vaginal irrigation.
used as a bougie (3% to 10%) and as a salve (3%
sepsis (instead of blue ointment).

110. **Krameriæ Ext.**—4 : 50, upon tampons, in vaginitis;
painfully astringent. It is also used in intestinal

111. **Lactophenin.**—0.5 to 1.0 (gr. viij to gr. xv), several t
daily (with 0.1—gr. iss—caffein), in neuralgia.

112. **Laminaria.**—As intra-uterine tamponade, in metrorrhagia,
orrhagia, to dilate the cervix. They are to be previously
fully disinfected for fourteen days in 5% carbolic acid
10% iodoform-ether, or 1% corrosive sublimate alcohol,
are left *in situ* twenty-four hours.

113. **Largin.**—Specific for gonorrhea; used like protargol. (Se
99.)

114. **Lassar's Paste** = Sulph. prec. 50.0 (℥ iss) with β-naphthol 10.0 (℥ iiss) and lanolin, saponis viridis, āā 25.0 (℥ viss). This is to be rubbed into a smooth paste. It is applied for acne.

115. **Laxatives (in the Order of Their Efficiency).**—Enemata (see the same), senna infusion by the rectum ; calcined magnesia, with or without sulphur ; citrate of magnesia ; compound licorice powder ; castor oil ; decoctions of frangula ; wine of cascara sagrada ; calomel ; tamarind (Grillon) ; Carlsbad salts ; tincture of cascara sagrada ; various waters, such as Kissingen, Friedrichshall, Carlsbad, etc.; powdered rhubarb with aloes ; infusion of senna ; compound extract of colocynth by the mouth. Dietetic : Fruit (boiled), kefir, whey, buttermilk, in chronic perimetritis, dysmenorrhea, oophoritis, metritis, and parametritis.

116. **Lead Acetate.**—One teaspoonful to one cup of water = lead-water (2 to 5 teaspoonfuls to a liter of lukewarm water), in pruritus, vulvitis, vaginitis, erysipelas.

117. **Lime-water.**—Used in full strength, for irrigation in cystitis; or 25.0 in 500.0 milk internally.

118. **Linseed Decoctions.**—In vaginitis, cystitis, acute endometritis, and metritis.

119. **Magnesia, Calcined.**—1.0 to 2.0 (gr. xv to gr. xxx), 1 to 3 times daily, as a laxative.

120. **Massage.**—In oligomenorrhea, infantile uterus, chronic parametritis and perimetritis, ovarian adhesions.

121. **Menthol Spirit.**—5% in pruritus of the vulva, urticaria, and pruriginous exanthemata the result of amenorrhea.

122. **Mercuric Chlorid.**—1 : 2000, intra-uterine injection, in multiple recurring uterine polypi, endometritis; 1 : 5000, in urethritis.

123. **Mercuric Chlorid.**—1 to 2 : 1000, in vulvitis, pruritus.

124. **Mercuric Chlorid.**—½ to 1 : 1000, in vaginitis.

125. **Mercurous Nitrate.**—Caustic for catarrh of the cervix.

126. **Morphin Hydrochlorate.**—0.2 to 10.0 (gr. iij to f ℥ iiss) aq. dest., ¼ to ½ to 1 syringeful hypodermically = 0.005 to 0.01 to 0.02 (gr. ₁₂ to ⅙ to ¼) morphin hydrochlorate, in vesical spasm, carcinoma.

127. **Morphin Hydrochlorate (Powder).**—0.01 (gr. ⅙) with sacch. alb. 0.5 (gr. viij), in menstrual molimina, dysmenorrhea, uterine neuralgia, vesical spasm, and as a hypnotic in carcinoma.

128. **Morphin Suppositories (Rectal or Vaginal).**—0.02 (gr.⅓) with 2.5 (gr. xxxviij), cacao-butter, for same affections as the preceding.

129. **Morphin Vaselin (Lanolin, Mollin).**—1.0 to 2.0 (gr. xv to gr. xxx) : 50.0 (℥ iss) in pruritus.

17

130. **Narcotics (in the Order of Their** Efficiency).—Hyoscy (with chloroform) as an injection; ext. belladonna, in rec vaginal suppositories; cocain, to be administered in the manner; laudanum, by the rectum; chloral ($\div$ pota bromid), by the rectum; antipyrin, by the mouth or m morphin, by the mouth, by the rectum, or hypodermi Hypnotics: Sulphonal, trional, potassium bromid, cx chloral, morphin.

131. **Nosophen.**—Antiseptic and desiccating dusting-powde wounds.

132. **Oak-bark Decoctions.**—10 to 20 : 250, in vaginal lavem vaginitis.

133. **Oatmeal Water.**—(See under Injections into the bladd Cystitis; and under Injections into the Vagina in Vagi Acute Endometritis, and Myometritis.)

134. **Obesity Cures.**—Banting, Oertel, Epstein, Mendelsohns when the panniculus adiposus is excessively develop cause of menorrhagia.

135. **Oleum Ricini.**—2 to 3 capsules, one tablespoonful several daily.

136. **Oophorin.**—For menstrual molimina; after removal of ovaries.

137. **Opium.**—Laudanum, 15 to 25 drops, by the rectum or upon inal tampons in menstrual molimina, dysmenorrhœa, cys itis, metritis, parametritis, perimetritis, carcinoma, hæ cele, peritonitis.

   Opium: Extract of opium 0.2 (gr. iij) with emuls. am dulc. 150.0 (f $\frac{3}{5}$ v), one tablespoonful every two h (mixture only keeps a day!), in carcinoma, intest catarrh, acute metritis, pelvic peritonitis.

138. **Phenacetin.**—0.5 to 1.0 (gr. viij to gr. xv) t. i. d., for neura

139. **Potassium Bromid.**—In powder (1.0—gr. xv—once or daily) or solution (15 : 175, 2 to 4 tablespoonfuls daily nocturnal enuresis, uterine neuralgia, dysmenorrhœa, cys tis, hysteria, pruritus.

140. **Potassium Carbonate Solution.**—In folliculitis of the vu 1% solution for boiling instruments.

141. **Potassium Iodid.**—In vaginal suppositories, 0.2 to 0.5 (g to gr. viij), with 3.0 (gr. xlv) cacao-butter, in paramet perimetritis, metritis, uterine and vaginal inversion, oopho hematocele.

142. **Potassium Iodid-glycerin.**—10 to 15 : 200, upon tamp (may add 15 to 20 drops of laudanum), for the affections mentioned above.

143. **Potassium Iodid-vaselin** (Lanolin, Mollin).—3 to 10% in pruritis, vaginismus, acute (puerperal) metritis, and parametritis.

144. **Potassium Permanganate.**—Dark cherry-red solution, as an irrigation fluid in foul carcinomata. Given as an emmenagog, in pill form (0.5—gr. viij—in a pill, 2 or 3 pills thrice daily).

145. **Protargol.**—0.5 to 2.5 (or even 5)%, intra-uterine irrigation; 5%, vaginal irrigation; 1 to 2.5%, vesical irrigation. Protargol with glycerin or salve, 5 to 10% intra-uterine (or as a bougie), in urethritis. Used in vaginal tamponade. *It is a specific for gonorrhea (Neisser).*

146. **Quinin, Compound Tincture.**—20 drops to a half-teaspoonful, thrice daily, in anemia, uremia, dyspepsia.

147. **Quinin-iodin.**—Dusting-powder, in foul carcinomata.

148. **Rhubarb, Infusion of Root.**—5.0 to 15.0 : 180.0 (gr. lxxv to f℥iv : f℥vj) with sulphate of sodium 10.0 (gr. iiss) and elæosacch. menth. piperit., 5.0 (gr. lxxv), 2 tablespoonfuls every two hours as a laxative.

149. **Rhubarb, Powdered Root.**—Used as a laxative.

150. **Sagrada, Wine.**—½ teaspoonful, as a laxative.

151. **Saline Infusion.**—0.6%, NaCl solution, ½ to 1 liter (sometimes more), intravenous or subcutaneous injections.

152. **Saline Solution.**—5%, in cystitis, especially after injections of silver nitrate.

153. **Salol.**—1.0 to 2.0 (gr. xv to xxx), 3 or 4 times daily, in cystitis.

154. **Santonin.**—Troches or pills, 0.025 to 0.05 to 0.1 (gr. ⅜ to ⅝ to iss), 3 times daily, with laxatives to prevent xanthuria; as an emmenagog and anthelmintic.

155. **Secale Cornut., Aqueous Extract.**—15.0 : 175.0 (ℨiv : ℥vas) with dilute sulphuric acid 2.5 (gr. xxxviij) and tinct. cinnamomi 15.0 (ℨiv); 1 tablespoonful every fifteen minutes, for acute hemorrhage.

156. **Secale Cornut., Extract.**—With pulv. secale cornut., āā 2.0 (gr. xxx). Ft. in pil. No. xxx—1 pill every two or three hours, in conditions mentioned above.

157. **Secale Cornut., Ext. Aqueous.**—2 to 4 : 180 (ℨ as to ℨj : f℥vj) aquæ with syr. cinnamomi 30.0 (f℥j); 1 tablespoonful every two hours, in conditions mentioned above and in paralysis of the vesical sphincter.

158. **Secale Cornut. Pulv.**—In vesical or uterine hemorrhage, in metritis (chronic hyperemia), and after reduction of an inverted uterus.

159. **Sennæ Fol., Infusum.**—2 to 4 teaspoonfuls (with 1 teaspoo of fennel) to 1 cup of water, as a laxative.

160. **Sinapisms.**—Mustard plasters and analogous applications; c tharidal plasters; or two parts of cantharides, dissolved in phuric ether, to one part of a solution of gutta percha chloroform, to be applied to the cervix! Tincture of iodi also applied to the cervix. It is painted upon the abdomen dysmenorrhea, and upon the thigh in amenorrhea.

161. **Sodium Salicylate.**—With sacch., āā 0.5 (gr. viij); 1 pow every two hours, or in solution 0.5 : 150.0 (gr. viij : f℥v neuroses, cystitis, erythemata.

162. **Strychnin.**—0.005 to 0.0075 to 0.01 (gr. $\frac{1}{12}$ to $\frac{1}{8}$ to $\frac{1}{6}$) subcu neously, in vesical paralysis.

163. **Stypticin.**—0.05 (gr. $\frac{3}{4}$) (6 to 8 tablets : 20 aq. ci namomi (30 drops 5 times daily), or 1 : 10 of a 1 solution subcutaneously.

164. **Sulphonal.**—1.0, as a somnifacient.

165. **Sulphur.**—2 teaspoonfuls daily; precipitated sulphur, powde rhubarb root, compound licorice powder, āā 7.5 (℥ ij), a laxative.

166. **Suppositories (Rectal).**—2.5 to 3.0 (gr. xxxviij to xlv) cac butter. (See Morphin, 0.01 to 0.02 (gr. $\frac{1}{6}$ to $\frac{1}{3}$); Ext. Bel donna, 0.01 to 0.02 (gr. $\frac{1}{6}$ to $\frac{1}{3}$); Chloral, 0.5 (gr. viij); Coc Hydrochlorate, 0.1 (gr. iss).)

167. **Suppositories (Vaginal).**—2.5 to 3.0 (gr. xxxviij to xlv) cac butter. (See Morphin, 0.02 (gr. $\frac{1}{3}$); Ext. Bellad., 0.03 (gr. $\frac{1}{3}$ to $\frac{1}{2}$); Chloral, 0.5 (gr. viij); Cocain Hyd ate, 0.1 (gr. iss); Potassium Iodid, 0.2 (gr. iij); Tann 0.4 (gr. vj).)

168. **Tamarind Decoction.**—8.0 to 50.0 : 100.0 to 300.0 (ʒ ij ℥ iss : f℥ iiiss to f℥ x) aquæ at one dose, as a laxative. It also administered in the form of tamarind paste (Grillon).

169. **Tampons.**—Glycerin (in vaginal inversion), vaselin, lanolin, mollin with tannin, alum, ichthyol, potassium iodid, chlorofo with oil of hyoscyamus, cupric sulphate, zinc chlorid or s phate.

170. **Tannin Solution.**—0.5 to 1.0 : 100.0 (gr. viij to gr. xv : f℥ iiis in cystitis.

171. **Tannin Solution.**—2 to 4%, in vaginitis, vaginal inversic vulvitis.

172. **Tannin Vaselin** (Glycerin, Lanolin, Mollin).—2 to 4 : 30.0 (ʒ to ʒ j : ℥ iss), for the above-mentioned affections.

173. **Trional.**—0.5 (gr. viij), in powder, as a somnifacient.

174. **Ung. Hydrarg. Ammoniat.**—For pruritus

175. **Ung. Zinci Oxidi.**—For eczema, herpes.
176. **Ung. Zinci Oxidi.**—With amyli ā̄ā 50.0 (℥ iss) and acid. salicyl. 3.0 (gr. xlv) and vaselin (lanolin, mollin), 100.0 (℥ iiiss), for pruritus, wounds.
177. **Urotropin.**—0.5 (gr. viij), 3 times daily, as a diuretic.

178. **Viburnum Prunifol., Ext. Fld.**—1.0 to 4.0 (gr. xv to ℨj) several times daily, as an antispasmodic in dysmenorrhea, threatened abortion; 1 teaspoonful may be given several times daily for one or two weeks.

179. **Washing with Cool Water.**—For nocturnal enuresis.
180. **Weir Mitchell Rest-cure.**—For nervous anemic patients.

181. **Zinc Chlorid.**—5% intra-uterine pencil held in position by a tampon, for endometritis (three days rest in bed).
182. **Zinc Chlorid.**—10 to 50% solution, for intra-uterine application (once a week) after dilatation of the cervix in endometritis; 5 to 10% injection, for multiple recurrent sessile polypi.
183. **Zinc Chlorid.**—½ to 1% injection or upon tampons in vaginitis, vaginal inversion.
184. **Zinc Oxid Intra-uterine Pencils.**—0.3 (gr. v), in endometritis.
185. **Zinc Oxid.**—2 : 40 pulv. amyli, for intertrigo.

INDEX.

272   INDEX.

SAUNDERS'
MEDICAL
HAND-ATLASES

A SERIES OF BOOKS OFFERING
A SATISFACTORY SUBSTITUTE FOR ACTUAL CLINICAL WORK

SPECIAL OFFER

AS it is impossible to realize the beauty and cheapness of these atlases without an opportunity to examine them, we make the following offer: Any one of these books will be sent to physicians, carriage prepaid, upon request. If you want the book, you have merely to remit the price; if not, return the book by mail.

A Descriptive Catalogue of all our Publications Sent on Request

W. B. SAUNDERS & COMPANY
925 Walnut Street
Philadelphia
NEW YORK
Fuller Building, 5th Ave. and 23d St.
LONDON
9, Henrietta St., Covent Garden

SAUNDERS'
MEDICAL HAND-ATLASES

IN planning this series of books arrangements were made with representative publishers in the chief medical centers of the world for the publication of translations of the atlases in thirteen different languages, the lithographic plates for all being made in Germany, where work of this kind has been brought to the greatest perfection. The enormous expense of making the plates being shared by the various publishers, the cost to each one was reduced approximately to one-tenth.

Moderate Price

Thus, by reason of their **universal translation** and **reproduction**, affording international distribution, the publishers have been enabled to secure for these atlases the **best artistic and professional talent**, to produce them in the **most elegant style**, and yet to offer them at a **price heretofore unapproached in cheapness**.

Substitute for Clinical Observation

One of the most valuable features of these atlases is that they offer a **ready and satisfactory substitute for clinical observation.** Such observation, of course, is available only to the residents in large medical centers; and even then the requisite variety is seen only after long years of routine hospital work. To those unable to attend important clinics these books will be absolutely indispensable, as presenting in a complete and convenient form the most accurate reproductions of clinical work, interpreted by the most competent of clinical teachers.

Adopted by U. S. Army

As an indication of the great practical value of the atlases and of the immense favor with which they have been received, it should be noted that the **Medical Department of the U. S. Army** has adopted the "Atlas of Operative Surgery" as its standard, and has ordered the book in large quantities for distribution to the various regiments and army posts.

Sobotta and Huber's Human Histology

Atlas and Epitome of Human Histology. By PRIVAT-DOCENT DR. J. SOBOTTA, of Würzburg. Edited, with additions, by G. CARL HUBER, M. D., Junior Professor of Anatomy and Histology, and Director of the Histological Laboratory, University of Michigan, Ann Arbor. With 214 colored figures on 80 plates, 68 text-cuts, and 248 pages of text. Cloth, $4.50 net.

INCLUDING MICROSCOPIC ANATOMY

This work combines an abundance of well-chosen and most accurate illustrations with a concise text, and in such a manner as to make it both atlas and text-book. The great majority of the illustrations were made from sections prepared from human tissues, and always from fresh and in every respect normal specimens. The colored lithographic plates have been produced with the aid of over thirty colors, and particular care was taken to avoid distortion and assure exactness of magnification. The text is as brief as possible ; clearness, however, not being sacrificed to brevity. The editor of the English translation has annotated and altered very freely certain portions of the sections on the adenoid tissues, blood and the blood-forming organs, muscular tissues, special sense organs, and peripheral nerve distributions, in order to make these parts of the work conform to the latest advances in the study of these tissues.

OPINIONS OF THE MEDICAL PRESS

Boston Medical and Surgical Journal
" In color and proportion they are characterised by gratifying accuracy and lithographic beauty. . . . May be highly recommended to those who are without access to histological collections."

Bulletin Johns Hopkins Hospital
" A ready means of getting a good idea of the appearance of normal human tissues, hardened, sectioned, and stained. . . . The additions which the editor of the translation has made are of such value that one wishes he had used his hand more freely."

Unsurpassed for accuracy, pictorial beauty, completeness, cheapness

Grünwald and Newcomb's
Mouth, Pharynx, Nose

Atlas and Epitome of Diseases of the Mouth, Pharynx, and Nose. By Dr. L. Grünwald, of Munich. *From the Second Revised and Enlarged German Edition.* Edited, with additions, by James E. Newcomb, M. D., Instructor in Laryngology, Cornell University Medical School; Attending Laryngologist to the Roosevelt Hospital, Out-Patient Department. With 102 illustrations on 42 colored lithographic plates, 41 text-cuts, and 219 pages of text. Cloth, $3.00 net.

INCLUDING ANATOMY AND PHYSIOLOGY

In designing this atlas the needs of both student and practitioner were kept constantly in mind, and as far as possible typical cases of the various diseases were selected. The illustrations are described in the text in exactly the same way as a practised examiner would demonstrate the objective findings to his class, the book thus serving as a substitute for actual clinical work. The illustrations themselves are numerous and exceedingly well executed, portraying the conditions so strikingly that their study is almost equal to examination of the actual specimens. The editor has incorporated his own valuable experience, including notes on the use of the active principle of the suprarenal bodies.

OPINIONS OF THE MEDICAL PRESS

American Medicine
" Its conciseness without sacrifice of clearness and thoroughness, as well as the excellence of text and illustration are commendable."

Journal of Ophthalmology, Otology, and Laryngology
" A collection of the most naturally colored lithographic plates that has been published in any book in the English language. . . . Very valuable alike to the student, the practitioner, and the specialist."

Each volume contains from 50 to 100 colored plates

Helferich and Bloodgood's Fractures and Dislocations

Atlas and Epitome of Traumatic Fractures and Dislocations. By Professor Dr. H. Helferich, Professor of Surgery at the Royal University, Greifswald, Prussia. Edited, with additions, by Joseph C. Bloodgood, M. D., Associate in Surgery, Johns Hopkins University, Baltimore. *From the Fifth Revised and Enlarged German Edition.* With 216 colored illustrations on 64 lithographic plates, 190 text-cuts, and 353 pages of text. Cloth, $3.00 net.

SHOWING DEFORMITY, X-RAY SHADOW, AND TREATMENT

This department of medicine being one in which, from lack of practical knowledge, much harm can be done, and in which in recent years great importance has obtained, a book, accurately portraying the anatomic relations of the fractured parts, together with the diagnosis and treatment of the condition, becomes an absolute necessity. This present work fully meets all requirements. As complete a view as possible of each case has been presented, thus equipping the physician for the manifold appearances that he will meet with in practice. The illustrations show the visible external deformity, the X-ray shadow, the anatomic preparation, and the method of treatment.

OPINIONS OF THE MEDICAL PRESS

Medical News, New York

"This compact and exceedingly attractive little volume will be most welcome to all who are interested in the practical application of anatomy. The author and editor have made a most successful effort to arrange the illustrations that the interpretation of what they are intended to present is exceedingly easy."

Brooklyn Medical Journal

"There are few books published that better answer the requirements for illustration than this work of Professor Helferich. . . . Such a collection of illustrations must be the result of much labor and thought."

They are Satisfactory Substitutes for Clinical Observation

Sultan and Coley's Abdominal Hernias

Atlas and Epitome of Abdominal Hernias. By PRIVAT-DOCENT DR. GEORG SULTAN, of Göttingen. Edited, with additions, by WILLIAM B. COLEY, M. D., Clinical Lecturer on Surgery, Columbia University (College of Physicians and Surgeons), New York. With 119 illustrations, 36 of them in colors, and 277 pages of text. Cloth, $3.00 net.

DEALING WITH THE SURGICAL ASPECT

This new atlas covers one of the most important subjects in domain of medical teaching, since these hernias are not only exceedingly common, but the frequent occurrence of strangulation demands extraordinarily quick and energetic surgical intervention. During the last decade the operative side of this subject has been steadily growing in importance, until now it is absolutely essential to have a book treating of its surgical aspect. This present atlas does this to an admirable degree. The illustrations are not only very numerous, but they excel, in the accuracy of the portrayal of the conditions represented, those of any other work upon abdominal hernias with which we are familiar. The work will be found a worthy exponent of our present knowledge of the subject of which it treats.

PERSONAL AND PRESS OPINIONS

Robert H. M. Dawbarn, M. D.,

Professor of Surgery and Surgical Anatomy, New York Polyclinic.

" I have spent several interested hours over it to-day, and shall willingly recommend it to my classes at the Polyclinic College and elsewhere."

Boston Medical and Surgical Journal

" For the general practitioner and the surgeon it will be a very useful book for reference. The book's value is increased by the editorial notes of Dr. Coley."

They have already appeared in thirteen different languages

Brühl, Politzer, and MacCuen Smith's Otology

Atlas and Epitome of Otology. By GUSTAV BRÜHL, M. D., of Berlin, with the collaboration of Professor DR. A. POLITZER, of Vienna. Edited, with additions, by S. MACCUEN SMITH, M. D., Clinical Professor of Otology, Jefferson Medical College, Philadelphia. With 244 colored figures on 39 lithographic plates, 99 text-illustrations, and 292 pages of text. Cloth, $3.00 net.

INCLUDING ANATOMY AND PHYSIOLOGY

This excellent volume is the first attempt to supply in English an illustrated clinical handbook to act as a worthy substitute for personal instruction in a specialized clinic. This work is both didactic and clinical in its teaching, the latter aspect being especially adapted to the student's wants. A special feature is the very complete exposition of the minute anatomy of the ear, a working knowledge of which is so essential to an intelligent conception of the science of otology. The illustrations are beautifully executed in colors, and illuminate the text in a singularly lucid manner, portraying pathologic changes with such striking exactness that the student should receive a deeper and more lasting impression than the most elaborate description could produce. Further, the association of Professor Politzer in the preparation of the work, and the use of so many valuable specimens from his notably rich collection especially enhance the value of the work. The text contains everything of importance in the elementary study of otology.

PERSONAL AND PRESS OPINIONS

Clarence J. Blake, M. D.,
Professor of Otology, Harvard University Medical School, Boston.
"The most complete work of its kind as yet published, and one commending itself to both the student and teacher in the character and scope of its illustrations."

Boston Medical and Surgical Journal
"Contains what is probably the best collection of colored plates of the ear, both of normal and pathological conditions, of any hand-book published in the English language. In addition to this the text is presented in an unusually clear and direct manner."

They are offered at a price heretofore unapproached in cheapness

Lehmann, Neumann, and Weaver's Bacteriology

Atlas and Epitome of Bacteriology: INCLUDING A TEXT-BOOK OF SPECIAL BACTERIOLOGIC DIAGNOSIS. By PROF. DR. K. B. LEHMANN and DR. R. O. NEUMANN, of Würzburg. *From the Second Revised and Enlarged German Edition.* Edited, with additions, by G. H. WEAVER, M. D., Assistant Professor of Pathology and Bacteriology, Rush Medical College, Chicago. In two parts. Part I.—632 colored figures on 69 lithographic plates. Part II.—511 pages of text, illustrated. Per part: Cloth, $2.50 net.

INCLUDING SPECIAL BACTERIOLOGIC DIAGNOSIS

This work furnishes a survey of the properties of bacteria, together the causes of disease, disposition, and immunity, reference being constantly made to an appendix of bacteriologic technic. The special part gives a complete description of the important varieties, the less important ones being mentioned when worthy of notice. The lithographic plates, as in all this series, are accurate representations of the conditions as actually seen, and this collection, if anything, is more handsome than any of its As an aid in original investigation the work is invaluable.

OPINIONS OF THE MEDICAL PRESS

American Journal of the Medical Sciences

" Practically all the important organisms are represented, and in such a variety of forms and cultures that any other atlas would rarely be needed in the ordinary hospital laboratory."

The Lancet, London

" We have found the work a more trustworthy guide for the recognition of unfamiliar species than any with which we are acquainted."

There have been 82,000 copies imported since publication

Zuckerkandl and DaCosta's Operative Surgery

Second Edition, Revised and Greatly Enlarged

Atlas and Epitome of Operative Surgery. By Dr. O. Zuckerkandl, of Vienna. Edited, with additions, by J. Chalmers DaCosta, M. D., Professor of the Principles of Surgery and Clinical Surgery, Jefferson Medical College, Philadelphia. With 40 colored plates, 278 text-cuts, and 410 pages of text. Cloth, $3.50 net.

ADOPTED BY THE U. S. ARMY

In this new edition the work has been brought precisely down to date. The revision has not been casual, but thorough and exhaustive, the entire text having been subjected to a careful scrutiny, and many improvements and additions made. A number of chapters have been practically rewritten, and of the newer operations, all those of special value have been described. The number of illustrations has also been materially increased. Sixteen valuable lithographic plates in colors and sixty-one text-figures have been added, thus greatly enhancing the value of the work. There is no doubt that the volume in its new edition will still maintain its leading position as a substitute for clinical instruction.

OPINIONS OF THE MEDICAL PRESS

Philadelphia Medical Journal

"The names of Zuckerkandl and DaCosta, the fact that the book has been translated into 13 different languages, together with the knowledge that it is used in the United States Army and Navy, would be sufficient recommendation for most of us."

Munchener Medicinische Wochenschrift

"We know of no other work that combines such a wealth of beautiful illustrations with clearness and conciseness of language, that is so entirely abreast of the latest achievements, and so useful both for the beginner and for one who wishes to increase his knowledge of operative surgery."

Each volume is edited, with additions, by a leading specialist

Dürck and Hektoen's Special Pathologic Histology

Atlas and Epitome of Special Pathologic Histology.
By Dr. H. Dürck, of Munich. Edited, with additions, by
Ludwig Hektoen, M. D., Professor of Pathology, Rush Medical College, Chicago. In Two Parts. Part I.—Circulatory,
Respiratory, and Gastro-intestinal Tracts. 120 colored figures
on 62 plates, and 158 pages of text. Part II.—Liver, Urinary
and Sexual Organs, Nervous System, Skin, Muscles, and Bones.
123 colored figures on 60 plates, and 192 pages of text. Per
part : Cloth, $3.00 net.

A RARE COLLECTION OF BEAUTIFUL PLATES

The colored lithographs of this volume are beautifully reproduced, and
are extremely accurate representations of the microscopic changes produced
by disease. The great value of these plates is that they represent in the
exact colors the effect of the stains, which is of such great importance for
the differentiation of tissue. The text portion of the book is admirable, and,
while brief, it is entirely satisfactory in that the leading facts are stated, and
so stated that the reader feels he has grasped the subject extensively. The
work is modern and scientific, and altogether forms a concise and systematic
view of pathologic knowledge.

PERSONAL OPINIONS

William H. Welch, M. D.,
Professor of Pathology, Johns Hopkins University, Baltimore.
" I consider Dürck's ' Atlas of Special Pathologic Histology,' edited by Hektoen, a very
useful book for students and others. The plates are admirable."

Frank B. Mallory, M. D.,
Assistant Professor of Pathology, Harvard University Medical School, Boston.
" The information is presented in a very compact form : it is carefully arranged, briefly
and clearly stated, and almost always represents our latest knowledge of the subject."

They represent the best artistic and professional talent

Haab and deSchweinitz's Ophthalmoscopy

Atlas and Epitome of Ophthalmoscopy and Ophthalmoscopic Diagnosis. By Dr. O. Haab, of Zürich. *From the Third Revised and Enlarged German Edition.* Edited, with additions, by G. E. deSchweinitz, M. D., Professor of Ophthalmology, University of Pennsylvania. With 152 colored lithographic illustrations; 85 pages of text. Cloth, $3.00 net.

Not only is the student made acquainted with carefully prepared ophthalmoscopic drawings done into well-executed lithographs of the most important fundus changes, but, in many instances, plates of the microscopic lesions are added. It furnishes a manual of the greatest possible service.

The Lancet, London

" We recommend it as a work that should be in the ophthalmic wards or in the library of every hospital into which ophthalmic cases are received."

Haab and deSchweinitz's External Diseases of Eye

Atlas and Epitome of External Diseases of the Eye. By Dr. O. Haab, of Zürich. Edited, with additions, by G. E. deSchweinitz, M. D., Professor of Ophthalmology, University of Pennsylvania. With 76 colored illustrations on 40 lithographic plates and 228 pages of text. Cloth, $3.00 net.

This new work of the distinguished Zürich ophthalmologist is destined to become a valuable handbook in the library of every practising physician. The conditions attending diseases of the external eye have probably never been more clearly and comprehensively expounded than in the forelying work, in which the pictorial most happily supplements the verbal description.

The Medical Record, New York

" The work is excellently suited to the student of ophthalmology and to the practising physician. It cannot fail to attain a well-deserved popularity."

They are convenient in size and uniformly bound

Schäffer *and* Edgar's Labor *and* Operative Obstetrics

Atlas and Epitome of Labor and Operative Obstetrics.
By Dr. O. Schäffer, of Heidelberg. *From the Fifth Revised and Enlarged German Edition.* Edited, with additions, by J. Clifton Edgar, M. D., Professor of Obstetrics and Clinical Midwifery, Cornell University Medical School. 14 lithographic plates in colors; 139 other cuts; 111 pages of text. $2.00 net.

The book presents the act of parturition and the various obstetric operations in a series of easily understood illustrations. These are accompanied by a text that treats the subject from a practical standpoint.

Dublin Journal of Medical Science, Dublin

"One fault Professor Schäffer's Atlases possess. Their name, and the extent and number of the illustrations, are apt to lead one to suppose that they are merely ' atlases,' whereas the truth really is they are also concise and modern epitomes of obstetrics."

Schäffer & Edgar's Obstetric Diagnosis and Treatment

Atlas and Epitome of Obstetric Diagnosis and Treatment. By Dr. O. Schäffer, of Heidelberg. *From the Second Revised German Edition.* Edited, with additions, by J. Clifton Edgar, M. D., Professor of Obstetrics and Clinical Midwifery, Cornell University Medical School. 122 colored figures on 56 plates; 38 other cuts; 315 pages of text. $3.00 net.

This book treats particularly of obstetric operations, and, besides the wealth of beautiful lithographic illustrations, contains an extensive text of great value. This text deals with the practical, clinical side of the subject.

New York Medical Journal

" The illustrations are admirably executed, as they are in all of these atlases, and the text can safely be commended, not only as elucidatory of the plates, but as expounding the scientific midwifery of to-day."

These are the famous " Lehmann medicinische Handatlanten "

Mracek and Stelwagon's Skin

Atlas and Epitome of Diseases of the Skin. By Prof. Dr. Franz Mracek, of Vienna. Edited, with additions, by Henry W. Stelwagon, M. D., Clinical Professor of Dermatology, Jefferson Medical College, Philadelphia. With 63 colored plates, 39 half-tone illustrations, and 200 pages of text. Cloth, $3.50 net.

This volume, the outcome of years of scientific and artistic work, contains, together with colored plates of unusual beauty, numerous illustrations in black, and a text comprehending the entire field of dermatology. The illustrations are all original and prepared from actual cases in Mracek's clinic.

American Journal of the Medical Sciences

" The advantages which we see in this book and which recommend it to our minds are : First, its handiness; secondly, the plates, which are excellent as regards drawing, color, and the diagnostic points which they bring out. We most heartily recommend it."

Mracek and Bang's Syphilis *and* Venereal Diseases

Atlas and Epitome of Syphilis and the Venereal Diseases. By Prof. Dr. Franz Mracek, of Vienna. Edited, with additions, by L. Bolton Bangs, M. D., late Prof. of Genito-Urinary Surgery, University and Bellevue Hospital Medical College, New York. With 71 colored plates and 122 pages of text. Cloth, $3.50 net.

According to the unanimous opinion of numerous authorities, to whom the original illustrations of this book were presented, they surpass in beauty anything of the kind that has been produced in this field, not only in Germany, but throughout the literature of the world.

Robert L. Dickinson, M. D.,

Art Editor of " The American Text-Book of Obstetrics."

" The book that appeals instantly to me for the strikingly successful, valuable, and graphic character of its illustrations is the ' Atlas of Syphilis and the Venereal Diseases.' I know of nothing in this country that can compare with it."

The lithographs, all made in Germany, are unrivalled

Jakob and Fisher's Nervous System & its Diseases

Atlas and Epitome of the Nervous System and its Diseases. By PROFESSOR DR. CHR. JAKOB, of Erlangen. *From the Second Revised German Edition.* Edited, with additions, by EDWARD D. FISHER, M. D., Professor of Diseases of the Nervous System, University and Bellevue Hospital Medical College, New York. With 83 plates and copious text. · Cloth, $3.50 net.

The matter is divided into Anatomy, Pathology, and Description of Diseases of the Nervous System. The plates illustrate these divisions most completely; especially is this so in regard to pathology. The exact site and character of the lesion are portrayed in such a way that they cannot fail to impress themselves on the memory of the reader.

Philadelphia Medical Journal

" We know of no one work of anything like equal size which covers this important and complicated field with the clearness and scientific fidelity of this hand-atlas."

Shaffer and Norris' Gynecology

Atlas and Epitome of Gynecology. By DR. O. SHAFFER, of Heidelberg. *From the Second Revised and Enlarged German Edition.* Edited, with additions, by RICHARD C. NORRIS, A. M., M. D., Gynecologist to Methodist-Episcopal and Philadelphia Hospitals. With 207 colored figures on 90 plates, 65 text-cuts, and 308 pages of text. Cloth, $3.50 net.

The value of this atlas will be found not only in the concise explanatory text, but especially in the illustrations. The large number of colored plates, reproducing the appearance of fresh specimens, will give the student a knowledge of the changes induced by disease that cannot be obtained from mere description.

Bulletin of Johns Hopkins Hospital, Baltimore

" The book contains much valuable material. Rarely have we seen such a valuable collection of gynecological plates."

These books are next best to actual clinical work

Hofmann and Peterson's Legal Medicine

Atlas of Legal Medicine. By DR. E. VON HOFMANN, of Vienna. Edited by FREDERICK PETERSON, M. D., Chief of Clinic, Nervous Department, College of Physicians and Surgeons, New York. With 120 colored figures on 56 plates and 193 half-tone illustrations. Cloth, $3.50 net.

By reason of the wealth of illustrations and the fidelity of the colored plates, the book supplements all the text-books on the subject. Moreover, it furnishes to every physician, student, and lawyer a veritable treasure-house of information.

The Practitioner, London

" The illustrations appear to be the best that have ever been published in connection with this department of medicine, and they cannot fail to be useful alike to the medical jurist and to the student of forensic medicine."

Golebiewski and Bailey's Accident Diseases

Atlas and Epitome of Diseases Caused by Accidents. By DR. ED. GOLEBIEWSKI, of Berlin. Edited, with additions, by PEARCE BAILEY, M. D., Attending Physician to the Almshouse and Incurable Hospitals, New York. With 71 colored illustrations on 40 plates, 143 text-illustrations, and 549 pages of text. Cloth, $4.00 net.

This work contains a full and scientific treatment of the subject of accident injury; the functional disability caused thereby; the medicolegal questions involved, and the amount of indemnity justified in given cases.

Medical Examiner and Practitioner

" It is a useful addition to life-insurance libraries, for lawyers, physicians, and for every one who is brought in contact with the treatment or consideration of accidents or diseases growing out of them, or legal complications flowing from them."

The " Atlas of Operative Surgery " has been adopted by U. S. Army

Jakob and Eshner's Internal Medicine & Diagnosis

Atlas and Epitome of Internal Medicine and Clinical Diagnosis. By DR. CHR. JAKOB, of Erlangen. Edited, with additions, by AUGUSTUS A. ESHNER, M. D., Professor of Clinical Medicine in the Philadelphia Polyclinic. With 182 colored figures on 68 plates, 64 illustrations in black and white, and 259 pages of text. Cloth, $3.00 net.

In addition to an admirable atlas of clinical microscopy, this volume describes the physical signs of all internal diseases in an instructive manner by means of fifty colored schematic diagrams. As a means of instruction its value is very great; as a reference handbook it is admirable.

British Medical Journal
" Dr. Jakob's work deserves nothing but praise. The information is accurate and up to present-day requirements."

Grünwald and Grayson's Diseases of the Larynx

Atlas and Epitome of Diseases of the Larynx. By DR. L. GRÜNWALD, of Munich. Edited, with additions, by CHARLES P. GRAYSON, M. D., Physician-in-Charge, Throat and Nose Department, Hospital of the University of Pennsylvania. With 107 colored figures on 44 plates, 25 text-illustrations, and 103 pages of text. Cloth, $2.50 net.

This atlas exemplifies a happy blending of the didactic and clinical, such as is not to be found in any other volume upon this subject. The author has given special attention to the clinical portion of the work, the sections on diagnosis and treatment being particularly full.

The Medical Record, New York
" This is a good work of reference, being both practical and concise. . . . It is a valuable addition to existing laryngeal text-books."

For " Special Offer " regarding these atlases see page 1

Lightning Source UK Ltd.
Milton Keynes UK
UKHW020833221118
332788UK00009B/451/P